NEUROSCIENCE RESEARCH PROGRESS

NEURO-IMMUNE INTERACTIONS IN THE ADULT CENTRAL NERVOUS SYSTEM

which will benefit to a wide variety of readers, from undergraduate students to postdoctoral fellows or scientific colleagues from many disciplines.

On behalf of the authors and my-self, I hope that readers find in this book a very useful compendium for their academic and research activities. I want to expresses his gratitude to the staff of *Nova Science Publishers* involved in this book production. I am particularly grateful to my dear mentors: Arturo Alvarez-Buylla at the *University of California at San Francisco*, Jose M Garcia-Verdugo at the *University of Valencia* and Dr. César Ramos-Remus at the *Instituto Mexicano del Seguro Social*, as outstanding sources of insights, personal support and academic guidance. Finally, I would like to express a great appreciation and gratitude to all my colleagues over the years. They are too many to list here, but I want them to know my gratitude. Recent collaborators include Rocio E. Gonzalez-Castañeda, Sonia Luquin, Alfredo Quiñones-Hinojosa, Alma Y. Galvez, Norma Moy, Jorge Guzman and Jorge Collas. Present students include Fernando Gutierrez-Fernandez, Veronica Lopez-Virgen, Tania Campos-Ordoñez, Jimena Rocha, Fabian Adirsch, David Zarate, Salvador Magallon, Maria F. Pinto and many others. I thank you for your hard work, personal support, scientific contributions, and invaluable friendship.

In: Neuro-Immune Interactions …
Editor: Oscar González-Pérez
ISBN: 978-1-62948-646-8

Chapter 1

INFLUENTIAL EFFECTS OF NEURONAL REGULATION OF IMMUNE CELLS ON BRAIN DISEASES

Li Tian[1,*]
Neuroscience Center, University of Helsinki, Helsinki, Finland

ABSTRACT

A homeostatic maintenance of neuroimmune interaction during development and adulthood is critical to prevent the onset or progression of psychiatric diseases. Within the CNS, while studies on glial cells, especially microglia, have highlighted the importance of this cell type in innate immune responses of the CNS, the immune regulatory functions of other cell types, especially neurons are largely unknown. How the neuroimmune crosstalk is homeostatically maintained in neurodevelopment and adult plasticity is even more elusive. Inspiringly, accumulating evidences suggest that neurons may also actively participate in immune responses by controlling glial cells and infiltrated immune cells.

The aim of this review is to address the immune function of both glial cells and neurons, and the roles they play in regulating inflammatory processes and maintaining homeostasis of the CNS. The potential clinical application of this knowledge warrants a deeper understanding of the mutual interactions between neurons and other types of cells during

* Correspondence: li.tian@helsinki.fi, fax: +358-9-19157620, tel. +358-9-19157613.

neurological and immunological processes within the CNS, which will help for the progress on diagnosis, prevention and intervention of various neurological diseases. I will especially emphasize and provide relevant evidences on how neurons mechanistically control the activation of microglia and infiltrated immune cells.

Keywords: Microglia, neuron, immune genes, neuroinflammation, neurological diseases

ABBREVIATIONS

A-β	amyloid β
AD	Alzheimer's disease
APC	antigen presenting cell
ATP	adenosine tri-phosphate
BDNF	brain-derived neurotrophic factor
CD	cluster of differentiation;
CR	complement receptor
CNS	central nervous system
EAE	experimental autoimmune encephalomyelitis
FasL	Fas ligand
GABA	γ-amino butyric acid
ICAM	intercellular adhesion molecule
IFN	interferon
IL	interleukin
LFA-1	leukocyte function-associated antigen-1
IgSF	immunoglobulin superfamily
LPS	lipopolysaccharide
MHC	major histocompatibility complex
MS	multiple sclerosis
NGF	nerve growth factor
NO	nitric oxide
PRR	pattern recognition receptors
SIRP	α signal regulatory protein-α
TGF-β	transforming growth factor β;
Th	T helper
TNF	tumor necrosis factor
Treg	regulatory T cells

TREM	triggering receptor expressed on myeloid cells
VIP	vasoactive intestinal peptide

INTRODUCTION

Our understanding on the reciprocal relationship between the nervous and immune systems has developed rapidly within the past decade. Inflammatory response has been associated with pathological processes in a wide range of brain disorders, including not only the conventional inflammatory conditions in autoimmune diseases, traumatic brain injuries, stroke and neurodegenerative diseases [1, 2], but more importantly also neurodevelopmental defects in schizophrenia, epilepsy and autism [3-5]. However, immune responses are specialized within the brain and differ considerably from those in the periphery. Such differences endow the central nervous system (CNS) with an immune-privileged status, and provide challenges for therapeutic interventions to various CNS diseases [6-8]. Hence, a thorough insight into the immunological processes within the CNS and their involvement in neurodevelopment and neuropathology is pivotal for current researchers. This chapter aims at providing readers the updated knowledge of the immune regulatory functions of the CNS residential cells: glia and neurons (Table 1). Since immune functions of glia are much better known than those of neurons [4, 5, 9], we will emphasize more on the latter ones in this review.

ROLE OF MICROGLIA AS INNATE IMMUNE MODULATOR IN THE BRAIN DEVELOPMENT

Although the CNS is relatively secluded from the peripheral immune system, it has its own residential immune network, in which glial cells (mainly microglia and astrocytes) not only serve supportive and nutritive roles for neurons, but also defend the CNS from stress and pathogenic insults by transiently up-regulating inflammatory processes [9]. These processes are usually kept in check by other endogenous anti-inflammatory and neuroprotective responses that return the CNS back into homeostasis. However, excessive or prolonged glial activation results in a more severe and chronic neuronal damage that eventually propagates neuroinflammation and neurodegeneration, suggesting the delicacy of tipping the balance between neuroprotection and neurotoxicity [10].

Microglia comprises 5-20% of all glial cells in various brain regions. As commonly known, they are the major phagocytic cells that provide the first line of defense for the CNS [11].

Table 1. Pro- and anti-inflammatory molecules expressed by glia and neurons

Properties	Promotion of inflammation	Inhibition of inflammation
Microglia		
Soluble factors	TNF, IFN-γ, IL-1β; **[15, 16, 18, 94]** CXCL1,2,12, CCL2,5,10,19; [41] Glutamate; NO, ATP; [15, 16, 18, 94]MMPs; [95] Complements; [16, 20] HMGB1, heat-shock proteins [90-93]	IL-4, IL-10, IFN-β, TGF-β;[15, 16, 18, 94]BDNF, GDNF;[41]TIMPs[95]
Membrane proteins	TLRs, RAGE, LFA-1, MAC-1, CRs, FcRβ; **[15, 16, 18, 90–94, 96]**	CD45, CD91, CD200R, CD172a, [16, 68] CX3CR1, [46] TREM-2, [73]FasL, Fas [86, 87]
Astrocytes		
Soluble factors	TNF, IFN-γ, IL-1β; [10, 27, 30] CXCL1,2,12, CCL2,5,10,19; [27, 41] Glutamate; NO, ATP; MMPs; [10, 27, 30] Complements; [16, 20, 27] HMGB1, heat-shock proteins [90-93]	IL-4, IL-10, IFN-β, TGF-β;[10, 27, 30]Complement inhibitors; [27] BDNF, GDNF; [41, 52, 53]TIMPs [95]
Membrane proteins	TLRs, RAGE, ICAM-1, CRs [91, 92, 96]	FasL[85, 86]
Neurons		
Soluble factors	CXCL10, CCL21; [8, 39, 41] Glutamate, dopamine; [39] NO, ATP; Substance P; [39] MMPs; [95]HMGB1, heat-shock proteins [90-93]	TGF-β;[43, 44] CX3CL1;[45, 46] GABA;[57, 58] VIP; [42, 55] NE,[60, 61]Proteoglycans; [97, 98] NGF, BDNF, NT3, GDNF, CNTF[41, 52, 53]
Membrane proteins	TLRs[96]	CD22,[65] CD47,[66, 67] CD200,[68] ICAM-5,[78, 79] FasL[85, 86]

It was long thought that microglia differentiate from peripheral macrophages that enter the brain shortly after birth. But a recent mouse study found that the majority of resident microglia derive from yolk sac macrophages formed during primitive hematopoiesis at very early embryonic stage (E7.5) [12]. These primitive macrophages migrate to the developing nervous system and reside throughout life. Local progenitors replenish the microglial population and proliferate in response to stimuli during adulthood. In contrast, other CNS macrophages, found in the perivascular space, meninges, and choroid plexus, derive from infiltrated blood monocytes and are replenished by hematopoietic stem cells in bone marrow. The embryonic engagement of microglial ontogenesis provides a timely basis for them to interact with neurons and affect neurogenesis and differentiation during development [11, 13].

Microglia acquires a ramified but nevertheless active morphology normally, with minimal expression of myeloid-monocytic markers such as Fc receptors-cluster of differentiation (CD) 32 and CD64, complement receptors (CR)-3 and -4, (also named as CD11b and CD11c integrins, respectively), major histocompatibility complex (MHC) class I and II and CD45 [14]. But once challenged by inflammation, it becomes rapidly amoeboid and up-regulates a variety of cell surface receptors involved in innate immune responses. These receptors include pattern recognition receptors, such as toll-like receptors and receptor for advanced glycation end products, and phagocytic receptors, such as CR-3, -4 and triggering receptor expressed on myeloid cells (TREM) [15, 16].

In respect to neuroimmune crosstalk, microglia plays the most direct, and perhaps also the most important, role in sensing and modulating neuronal activities. Phagocytosis is an important mechanism for microglia to control neuronal apoptosis. When apoptosis of neurons occurs, for example, at the early developmental stage, or due to neurodegeneration, clearance of apoptotic cell debris in time through phagocytosis is vital for the reminiscent neurons to avoid collateral inflammation-induced damage [17, 18]. Apoptotic cells express cell surface molecular patterns that act as "eat me" signals. These signals are recognized by microglial PRRs, which rapidly initiate clearing processes [16]. On the other hand, insufficient phagocytic clearance of cell debris following neuronal injury is an important pathogenic factor in propagation of neurodegeneration, as illustrated by numerous studies on Alzheimer's disease (AD) [18].

Besides controlling neuronal apoptosis, microglia secrete a wide variety of cytokines, complements and growth factors that have been implicated in regulating synaptic formation and plasticity [17]. With the help of the complement system, unwanted synapses are efficiently removed by phagocytosis under both developmental and pathological conditions [19].

Mice deficient in complement C1q or C3 exhibited sustained defects in elimination of the CNS synapses [20]. More importantly, the orthodox view that microglial activity is only relevant for the pathological processes of neuronal pruning has been overturned by the recent evidences showing that they are highly sensitive for the neighboring neuronal activities and control dendritic spine density under physiological conditions [21, 22]. Furthermore, a recent elegant work by Derecki et al. demonstrated that microglia from bone marrow of wild type mice attenuated Rett syndrome, an X-linked autism spectrum disorder [23]. Undoubtedly, emerging evidences with the help of modern imaging and analytical technologies will shed light into the physiological functions of microglia in the coming years.

Another important function of microglia is the presentation of foreign antigens to T lymphocytes. In the normal CNS, antigen presenting cells (APC) are mainly confined to dendritic cells and macrophages located in the meninges, choroid plexuses and perivascular spaces [24]. MHC class I and II molecules are expressed at low levels by microglia, as they are actively down-regulated by the immune-quiescent microenvironment of the CNS. However, upon activation, these molecules are up-regulated together with the costimulatory receptors CD40, CD80 (B7-1), CD86 (B7-2) and leukocyte function-associated antigen-1 (LFA-1, CD11a/CD18 integrin), which subsequently induces optimal APC functions and T-cell activation [15, 24].

Innate Immune Functions of Astrocytes

Astrocytes have been traditionally viewed as supportive cells for neurons, which are responsible for the CNS homeostasis and neuronal functions [25] (Fig 1A). Their functions as innate immune cells are somehow less appreciated as compared to microglia. Nevertheless, astrocytes have been known to form the glia limitans around blood vessels, thereby restricting the entry of immune cells through the blood-brain barrier into the CNS parenchyma [26]. Emerging evidences have highlighted the importance of this cell population in the regulation of local innate and adaptive immune responses [27].

Astrocytes express a variety of PRRs involved in innate immunity, including toll-like receptors, scavenger receptors, mannose receptors and CRs [27] (Table 1 & 2). Following PRR engagement, astrocytes secrete cytokines, chemokines and neurotrophins that target neighboring glial cells and neurons [10, 27]. Released cytokines also promote the leakage of BBB, resulting in the recruitment of immune cells from the blood circulation into the CNS parenchyma. These altogether amplify both the initial innate immune responses and the upcoming adaptive immune responses, which can result in the elimination of infectious or injurious insults and restoration of tissue integrity or scar formation [28].

Astrocytes are active players in the AD and multiple sclerosis (MS) [29, 30]. Under pathological conditions, astrocytes undergo a series of structural and functional changes collectively referred to as astrogliosis. Amyloid β-peptide (A-β) plays an important role in astrocyte stimulation [31]. Accumulation of astrocytes around the senile plaques and neurofibrillary tangles is one of the hallmarks of the AD [29]. Upon A-β stimulation, astrocytes secrete various chemokines that recruit microglia and monocyte/macrophages to the plaques with the concomitant release of neurotoxins and pro-inflammatory cytokines that contribute in concert to neurodegeneration [29]. Astrocytes are also involved in the MS disease through release of pro-inflammatory cytokines, matrix metalloproteinases and free radicals that result in recruitment of autoimmune cells, oligodendrocyte destruction and demyelination [30].

Another interesting, yet controversial, property of astrocytes is their antigen-presenting ability. In vitro studies have shown that astrocytes express low levels of MHC and costimulatory molecules upon stimulation by cytokines, and are capable of processing and presenting myelin protein epitopes to T cells, inferring that they can also be APCs [32, 33]. However, given the more efficient antigen presentation capabilities of microglia and other infiltrating APCs in the CNS, the in vivo significance of this function of astrocytes is unclear [9, 24, 30].

Despite of these controversies, the ability of astrocytes to regulate the antigen-presenting activities of other APCs and T-cell activation has been clearly established. The fact that the expression levels of MHC and costimulatory molecules are low even after stimulation in vitro suggests that astrocytes may be prone to induce T helper (Th) 2 rather than Th1 responses. Indeed, earlier studies showed that while microglial cells seem to be efficient in activating both Th1 and Th2 cells, astrocytes stimulate only Th2 cells [34]. Microglia and astrocytes also produce chemokines that differentially affect the recruitment of Th1 and Th2 cells [35].

Additionally, astrocytes have been shown to induce anergy of Th cells via cytotoxic T-lymphocyte antigen 4 (CTLA-4, CD152) [36] or promote recruitment and proliferation of regulatory T cells (Treg) via the anti-inflammatory cytokine transforming growth factor β (TGF-β) [37] and chemokine CXCL12 (stromal cell-derived factor-1) [38]. Astrocytes can also secrete other anti-inflammatory cytokines or soluble factors, including interleukin (IL)-10, interferon (IFN)-β and neurotrophins, which are able to suppress T cell and microglial activation [10, 27, 30]. So it seems that a complex network of neurons, astrocytes, microglia and T cells is involved in determining the balance of pro- versus anti-inflammatory signals, which in turn affect the outcome of immune responses within the CNS.

Collectively, the above information indicates that both microglia and astrocytes play an active and dual role in the CNS inflammatory diseases. They not only have the ability to enhance immune responses and promote neurodegeneration, but can also be protective and limit the CNS inflammation.

Neuronal Regulation of Microglial Activation

One can envisage that the regulation of such immune activity is crucial as too little or too much can both lead to impaired neurogenesis and cognitive functions of the CNS. Since neurons in the brain are very sensitive to changes in their surrounding milieu, and are poor to regenerate once damaged, a number of mechanisms exit to limit the immune-mediated neurotoxicity and the collateral tissue damage, which were collectively denoted as immune privilege [6, 7]. While a plethora of data has highlighted the immune functions of microglia and astrocytes, the roles that neurons play in this arena are under-toned [8, 39]. Neurons have primarily been regarded as victims of immune attack, and their participation in the CNS immune responses as passive. Here, we recount the current advances in this research field and summarize the mechanisms on neuronal regulation of innate and adaptive immunities. We believe that the CNS actively interacts with the immune system and provides several specific mechanisms to regulate the central immune responses, which involves not only microglia and astrocytes, but also neurons themselves [8, 39].

Neurons may inactivate infiltrated immune cells and microglia by both contact-dependent and -independent mechanisms [8]. There are a number of neuronal soluble factors that potentially attenuate microglial cell activation. These include anti-inflammatory cytokines [40], chemokines [41], neuropeptides [42], neurotrophins [41] and neurotransmitters [39].

TGF-β is the major anti-inflammatory cytokine needed for an organism to nurture Treg cells and keep autoimmune T cells at bay under the steady state. In the CNS, it is constitutively expressed in neurons [40, 43]. Its importance in down-regulating microglial and autoimmune T cell responses is substantiated by increased microglial activity and neuronal loss in the brains of TGF-β-deficient mice [44]. Additionally, fractalkine (CX3CL1, neurotactin) is the predominant chemokine expressed and released by neurons in the CNS, whereas its receptor CX3CR1 is primarily expressed in microglia. Fractalkine and its receptor play an important role in mediating interaction between neurons and microglia [45], which, on the one hand, controls inflammatory neurotoxicity in the brain as CX3CR1-deficient mice showed a massive activation of microglial cells upon repeated lipopolysaccharide (LPS) injection [46], and on the other hand, regulates the neuronal plasticity as the dendritic spines were increased in CX3CR1-deficient mice due to the inefficient synaptic pruning [22]. Furthermore, stressed neurons also secret semaphorin-3A and other substances to induce the apoptosis of activated microglia [47-49].

Neurotrophins are another group of soluble factors used by neurons to control immune cell functions. They play critical roles in neuronal survival, migration and differentiation, and are potential drugs for the treatment of neurodegenerative diseases [50]. One aspect of their multiple effects on neurons is dampening inflammation-induced damage in the CNS. Among them, nerve growth factor (NGF) and brain-derived neurotrophic factor (BDNF) were investigated. NGF influences B-cell and T-cell functions and regulates macrophage migration into inflamed lesions outside of the nervous system [51]. Within the CNS, NGF was previously shown to inhibit MHC class II expression in microglia [52]. And BDNF was demonstrated to downregulate the costimulatory molecules B7 and CD40 expression in microglia [53].

Additionally, neurons are equipped with various immunosuppressive neuropeptides, such as vasoactive intestinal peptide (VIP), and adenosine tri-phosphate (ATP). VIP is a widely distributed anti-inflammatory neuropeptide by inhibition of proinflammatory mediators, such as IL-6, tumor necrosis factor (TNFα), IL-12 and nitric oxide (NO) [54], which has been shown to protect against beta-amyloid-induced neurodegeneration by inhibiting microglial activation [55]. For ATP and its metabolite adenosine, although their neuroprotective effects have been explained mainly by actions on neurons, modulation of microglial functions is likely to be as important as they can affect many microglial signaling pathways [56].

Concerning the major neurotransmitters, their immune regulatory roles in the brain are somewhat mixed. While glutamate is mostly involved in promoting microglial activation and neuroinflammation [56], γ-amino butyric acid (GABA) and acetylcholine attenuate pro-inflammatory responses. GABA, a main inhibitory neurotransmitter in the brain, has been shown to attenuate LPS-induced IL-6 and IL-10 production in microglia [57], and affect the entry of pathogenic T lymphocytes into the brain and T cell proliferation [58]Furthermore, acetylcholine have been shown to attenuate pro-inflammatory response of microglial cultures [59]. For catechol amines, they have been reported to induce both microglial activation and suppression. Norepinephrine is a catecholamine that dampens cellular immunity systemically and suppresses neuroinflammation in the brain [60]. LPS-induced TNFα production in hippocampus is inversely correlated with the release of NE in an animal model of depression [61]. However, it may also promote local inflammation by activating α- or β-adrenergic receptors both centrally and peripherally [59, 62, 63].

Several neuronal membrane glycoproteins, such as CD22 [64, 65], CD47 [66, 67], CD200 [68-70] and neural cell adhesion molecule [71, 72] have been shown to prevent microglial activation through interaction with their respective counter-receptors. Moreover, the receptor TREM-2 on microglia was shown to mediate the phagocytosis of apoptotic neurons while decreasing microglial pro-inflammatory responses, although its neuronal ligand has not been identified yet [73, 74].

The immunoglobulin superfamily (IgSF) member CD200 (OX2) is broadly expressed in neurons, endothelial and immune cells, while its receptor, CD200R, which is also an IgSF molecule, is expressed predominantly by cells of the myeloid lineage, including microglia [68] and T cells [75]. Knocking out CD200 in mice results in spontaneous microglial activation [68]. Similarly, antibody-mediated blocking of CD200R also leads to an aggravated clinical course of experimental autoimmune encephalomyelitis (EAE), accompanied by increased infiltration of T cells and macrophages [68]. Blocking CD200R on macrophages *in vitro* leads to enhanced IFN-γ-induced release of IL-6 and neuronal cell death in co-cultures with hippocampal neurons expressing CD200 [69].

Another IgSF and sialic acid-binding molecule, CD22, has been implicated in attenuation of the CNS immune responses as well. CD22 is expressed in cultured cortical neurons, and might mediate the binding of neurons to microglia through CD45 [65]. Ligation of microglial CD45 by CD22 has been shown to prevent the LPS-induced microglial production of the pro-inflammatory cytokine TNF [64, 65].

Additionally, the integrin-associated protein CD47 may also be important in down-regulating immune responses in the CNS. CD47 has been identified as a cellular ligand for the signal regulatory protein-α (SIRPα, CD172a), which is also an IgSF member. Studies on SIRPα deficient mice reveal that SIRPα is a negative regulator of macrophage phagocytosis [66], and ligation of monocyte SIRPα by CD47 downregulates their TNF production [67].

Furthermore, when mixed with glial cells *in vitro*, neurons inhibit the LPS-stimulated production of NO and TNF by glial cells. This effect is partially mediated through the IgSF adhesion molecule neural cell adhesion molecule (NCAM) [71, 72]. Chronic stimulation and interaction with apoptotic neurons induce microglial cells to release neuroprotective agents while inhibiting the production of NO and pro-inflammatory cytokines [1]. Furthermore, the receptor TREM-2 on microglia was shown to mediate the phagocytosis of apoptotic neurons while decreasing microglial pro-inflammatory responses, although its neuronal ligand has not been identified yet [73, 74].

NEURONAL REGULATION OF INFILTRATED IMMUNE CELLS IN THE CNS

Given that peripheral immune cells do not normally penetrate into the brain parenchyma, but instead stay in the perivascular space and on meninges, one might predict that soluble factors in the brain thus provide an important means for neurons to control their activities. However, experimental evidences demonstrating the molecular mechanisms of such regulation are currently still scant. As mentioned earlier, TGF-β is the major anti-inflammatory cytokine in the brain, which nurtures Treg and keeps autoimmune T cells at bay under the steady state [76]. Additionally, GABA has been shown to affect the entry of pathogenic T lymphocytes into the brain and T cell proliferation [58].

We have previously shown that the neuronal intercellular adhesion molecule-5 (ICAM-5), an integrin ligand that regulates dendritic filopodia elongation and spine plasticity [77, 78], down-regulates T-cell activation through interfering with the costimulatory function of integrin LFA-1 [79]. In addition, semaphorins and their receptors plexins, in concert with neuropilin, have also been shown to attenuate T-cell activation and mitigate experimental autoimmune encephalomyelitis (EAE) [49, 80-83]. Alternatively, neurons have been shown to convert T cells into Treg cells irrespective of their antigen specificity, which in turn suppresses EAE [76, 84]. And as suggested in the previous section, T-cell derived CD200R may also be important in dampening autoimmune responses in EAE [68].

Furthermore, neurons, microglia and astrocytes have been shown to up-regulate Fas ligand (FasL, CD95L) under inflammatory conditions, which can induce apoptosis of activated T or microglial cells through the FasL-Fas pathway [85, 86]. Administration of anti-FasL antibody to Lewis rat with EAE in the clinically recovery phase has been shown to reduce T cell apoptosis, increase accumulation of T cells and macrophages at the site of inflammation, and delay spontaneous recovery of the animals [87]. Both T and microglial cells are more sensitive to Fas-dependent cell apoptosis than neurons and astrocytes [88, 89], indicating the robustness of the later two cell types in limiting inflammatory insults through this pathway (Table 2).

It should be noted that the ability of neurons to limit immune responses in the CNS is largely dependent on their own integrity. At the early stage of pathological conditions, self-limiting machineries, such as apoptotic destruction of activated T cells, microglial cells and injured neurons, may initially be able to keep the balance of protection versus damage [16]. Once this is compromised, the inflammatory processes will be accelerated by neurons which turn on the expression of multiple pro-inflammatory cytokines and neurotoxic proteins such as A-β peptide, heat-shock proteins and high mobility group box 1 (HMGB1, amphoterin) [90, 91]. These endogenous "dangerous signals", also termed as damage-associated molecular pattern (DAMP) molecules, then agitate the already activated glial cells, and hence probably lead to their over-activation, which eventually exacerbates neuronal damages [92, 93].

CONCLUSION

Neurons, glia and immune cells form a coordinated network to maintain the homeostasis and restrict neuroinflammation in the CNS. This integrative network is not only involved in the pathogenesis of neuroinflammation, but more importantly, may also play a major role in the normal brain functions. The particular impact of glial and immune cells on the physiological versus pathological process in the CNS is dependent on a number of factors that influence their state of activation. Here, we have summarized that neurons, the major effector cells for cognitive and motor function of an organism, provide environmental milieu that regulate microglial and immune cell activation. Since inflammation is a double-edged sword for the CNS, improved knowledge on both beneficial and detrimental factors provided by neurons for the progress of inflammation should help develop better ways to treat various neurological diseases.

Acknowledgments

This chapter was supported by the Academy of Finland and the Magnus Ehrnrooth Foundation. The author declares no conflict of interests.

References

[1] A. Klegeris, E.G. McGeer, and P.L. McGeer, Therapeutic approaches to inflammation in neurodegenerative disease, *Curr. Opin. Neurol.* 20, 351 (2007).

[2] L. Steinman, A molecular trio in relapse and remission in multiple sclerosis, *Nat. Rev. Immunol.* 9, 440 (2009).

[3] A. Vezzani and T. Granata, Brain inflammation in epilepsy: experimental and clinical evidence, *Epilepsia.*46, 1724 (2005).

[4] N. Muller, Inflammation and the glutamate system in schizophrenia: implications for therapeutic targets and drug development, *Expert Opin. Ther.Targets.* 12, 1497 (2008).

[5] U. Meyer, J. Feldon, and O. Dammann, Schizophrenia and Autism: Both Shared and Disorder-Specific Pathogenesis Via Perinatal Inflammation?, *Pediatr Res.* 69(5 Pt 2), 26R (2011).

[6] M.J. Carson, J.M. Doose, B. Melchior, C.D. Schmid, and C.C. Ploix, CNS immune privilege: hiding in plain sight, *Immunol. Rev.* 213, 48 (2006).

[7] I. Galea, I. Bechmann, and V.H. Perry, What is immune privilege (not)?, *Trends Immunol.*28,12 (2007).

[8] L. Tian, H. Rauvala, and C.G. Gahmberg, Neuronal regulation of immune responses in the central nervous system, *Trends Immunol.* 30,91 (2009).

[9] S.L. Bailey, P.A. Carpentier, E.J. McMahon, W.S. Begolka, and S.D. Miller, Innate and adaptive immune responses of the central nervous system, *Crit. Rev. Immunol.* 26,149 (2006).

[10] R. Hohlfeld, M. Kerschensteiner, and E. Meinl, Dual role of inflammation in CNS disease, *Neurology.* 68, S91 (2007).

[11] A. Aguzzi, B.A. Barres, and M.L. Bennett, Microglia: scapegoat, saboteur, or something else?, *Science.* 339,156 (2013).

[12] F. Ginhoux, M. Greter, M. Leboeuf, S. Nandi, P. See, S. Gokhan, M.F. Mehler, S.J. Conway, L.G. Ng, E.R. Stanley, I.M. Samokhvalov, and M. Merad, Fate mapping analysis reveals that adult microglia derive from primitive macrophages, *Science.* 330,841 (2010).

[13] P.A. Carpentier and T.D. Palmer, Immune influence on adult neural stem cell regulation and function, *Neuron.* 64, 79 (2009).

[14] G.J. Guillemin and B.J. Brew, Microglia, macrophages, perivascular macrophages, and pericytes: a review of function and identification, *J. Leukoc. Biol.* 75, 388 (2004).

[15] B.R. Tambuyzer, P. Ponsaerts, and E.J. Nouwen, Microglia: gatekeepers of central nervous system immunology, *J. Leukoc. Biol.* 85, 352 (2009).

[16] M.R. Griffiths, P. Gasque, and J.W. Neal, The multiple roles of the innate immune system in the regulation of apoptosis and inflammation in the brain, *J. Neuropathol. Exp. Neurol.* 68,217 (2009).

[17] A. Bessis, C. Bechade, D. Bernard, and A. Roumier, Microglial control of neuronal death and synaptic properties, *Glia.*55, 233 (2007).

[18] I. Napoli and H. Neumann, Microglial clearance function in health and disease, *Neuroscience.* 158, 1030 (2009).

[19] V.H. Perry and V. O'Connor, C1q: the perfect complement for a synaptic feast?, *Nat. Rev. Neurosci.* 9,807 (2008).

[20] B. Stevens, N.J. Allen, L.E. Vazquez, G.R. Howell, K.S. Christopherson, N. Nouri, K.D. Micheva, A.K. Mehalow, A.D. Huberman, B. Stafford, A. Sher, A.M. Litke, J.D. Lambris, S.J. Smith, S.W. John, and B.A. Barres, The classical complement cascade mediates CNS synapse elimination, *Cell.* 131,1164 (2007).

[21] M.E. Tremblay, R.L. Lowery, and A.K. Majewska, Microglial interactions with synapses are modulated by visual experience, *PLoS Biol.* 8, e1000527(2010).

[22] R.C. Paolicelli, G. Bolasco, F. Pagani, L. Maggi, M. Scianni, P. Panzanelli, M. Giustetto, T.A. Ferreira, E. Guiducci, L. Dumas, D. Ragozzino, and C.T. Gross, Synaptic pruning by microglia is necessary for normal brain development, *Science.* 333,1456 (2011).

[23] N.C. Derecki, J.C. Cronk, Z. Lu, E. Xu, S.B.G. Abbott, P.G. Guyenet, and J. Kipnis, Wild-type microglia arrest pathology in a mouse model of Rett syndrome, *Nature.* 484, 105 (2012).

[24] B. Becher, I. Bechmann, and M. Greter, Antigen presentation in autoimmunity and CNS inflammation: how T lymphocytes recognize the brain, *J. Mol. Med.* 84,532 (2006).
[25] P.G. Haydon and G. Carmignoto, Astrocyte control of synaptic transmission and neurovascular coupling, *Physiol. Rev.* 86, 1009 (2006).
[26] I. Bechmann, I. Galea, and V.H. Perry, What is the blood-brain barrier (not)?, *Trends Immunol.* 28,5 (2007).
[27] C. Farina, F. Aloisi, and E. Meinl, Astrocytes are active players in cerebral innate immunity, *Trends Immunol.* 28, 138 (2007).
[28] B. Engelhardt, Immune cell entry into the central nervous system: involvement of adhesion molecules and chemokines, *J. Neurol. Sci.* 274, 23 (2008).
[29] C. Schwab and P.L. McGeer, Inflammatory aspects of Alzheimer disease and other neurodegenerative disorders, *J. Alzheimers Dis.* 13, 359 (2008).
[30] A. Nair, T.J. Frederick, and S.D. Miller, Astrocytes in multiple sclerosis: a product of their environment, *Cell Mol. Life Sci.* 65, 2702 (2008).
[31] T. Wyss-Coray, J.D. Loike, T.C. Brionne, E. Lu, R. Anankov, F. Yan, S.C. Silverstein, and J. Husemann, Adult mouse astrocytes degrade amyloid-beta in vitro and in situ, *Nat. Med.* 9, 453 (2003).
[32] L. Tan, K.B. Gordon, J.P. Mueller, L.A. Matis, and S.D. Miller, Presentation of proteolipid protein epitopes and B7-1-dependent activation of encephalitogenic T cells by IFN-gamma-activated SJL/J astrocytes, *J. Immunol.* 160, 4271 (1998).
[33] J.M. Soos, J. Morrow, T.A. Ashley, B.E. Szente, E.K. Bikoff, and S.S. Zamvil, Astrocytes express elements of the class II endocytic pathway and process central nervous system autoantigen for presentation to encephalitogenic T cells, *J. Immunol.* 161, 5959 (1998).
[34] F. Aloisi, F. Ria, G. Penna, and L. Adorini, Microglia are more efficient than astrocytes in antigen processing and in Th1 but not Th2 cell activation, *J. Immunol.* 160, 4671 (1998).
[35] W.J. Karpus and K.J. Kennedy, MIP-1alpha and MCP-1 differentially regulate acute and relapsing autoimmune encephalomyelitis as well as Th1/Th2 lymphocyte differentiation, *J. Leukoc. Biol.* 62,681 (1997).
[36] U. Gimsa, A. ORen, P. Pandiyan, D. Teichmann, I. Bechmann, R. Nitsch, and M.C. Brunner-Weinzierl, Astrocytes protect the CNS: antigen-specific T helper cell responses are inhibited by astrocyte-induced upregulation of CTLA-4 (CD152), *J. Mol. Med.* 82, 364 (2004).

[37] V. Trajkovic, O. Vuckovic, S. Stosic-Grujicic, D. Miljkovic, D. Popadic, M. Markovic, V. Bumbasirevic, A. Backovic, I. Cvetkovic, L. Harhaji, Z. Ramic, and M. MostaricaStojkovic, Astrocyte-induced regulatory T cells mitigate CNS autoimmunity, *Glia.*47, 168 (2004).

[38] M. Meiron, Y. Zohar, R. Anunu, G. Wildbaum, and N. Karin, CXCL12 (SDF-1alpha) suppresses ongoing experimental autoimmune encephalomyelitis by selecting antigen-specific regulatory T cells, *J. Exp. Med.* 205,2643 (2008).

[39] K. Biber, H. Neumann, K. Inoue, and H.W. Boddeke, Neuronal 'On' and 'Off' signals control microglia, *Trends Neurosci.* 30,596 (2007).

[40] S.M. Wahl, J. Wen, and N. Moutsopoulos, TGF-beta: a mobile purveyor of immune privilege, *Immunol. Rev.* 213,213 (2006).

[41] M. Kerschensteiner, E. Meinl, and R. Hohlfeld, Neuro-immune crosstalk in CNS diseases, *Neuroscience.* 158, 1122 (2009).

[42] E. Reinke and Z. Fabry, Breaking or making immunological privilege in the central nervous system: the regulation of immunity by neuropeptides, *Immunol. Lett.* 104, 102 (2006).

[43] D. Boche, C. Cunningham, F. Docagne, H. Scott, and V.H. Perry, TGFbeta1 regulates the inflammatory response during chronic neurodegeneration, *Neurobiol. Dis.* 22,638 (2006).

[44] T.C. Brionne, I. Tesseur, E. Masliah, and T. Wyss-Coray, Loss of TGF-beta 1 leads to increased neuronal cell death and microgliosis in mouse brain, *Neuron.* 40, 1133 (2003).

[45] J.K. Harrison, Y. Jiang, S. Chen, Y. Xia, D. Maciejewski, R.K. McNamara, W.J. Streit, M.N. Salafranca, S. Adhikari, D.A. Thompson, P. Botti, K.B. Bacon, and L. Feng, Role for neuronally derived fractalkine in mediating interactions between neurons and CX3CR1-expressing microglia, *Proc. Natl. Acad. Sci. U. S. A.* 95, 10896 (1998).

[46] A.E. Cardona, E.P. Pioro, M.E. Sasse, V. Kostenko, S.M. Cardona, I.M. Dijkstra, D. Huang, G. Kidd, S. Dombrowski, R. Dutta, J.C. Lee, D.N. Cook, S. Jung, S.A. Lira, D.R. Littman, and R.M. Ransohoff, Control of microglial neurotoxicity by the fractalkine receptor, *Nat. Neurosci.* 9,917 (2006).

[47] H.H. Majed, S. Chandran, S.P. Niclou, R.S. Nicholas, A. Wilkins, M.G. Wing, K.E. Rhodes, M.G. Spillantini, and A. Compston, A novel role for Sema3A in neuroprotection from injury mediated by activated microglia, *J. Neurosci.* 26, 1730 (2006).

[48] E. Polazzi and A. Contestabile, Overactivation of LPS-stimulated microglial cells by co-cultured neurons or neuron-conditioned medium, *J. Neuroimmunol.* 172, 104 (2006).
[49] N. Takegahara and A. Kumanogoh, Involvement of semaphorins and their receptors in neurological diseases, *Clinical and Experimental Neuroimmunology.* 1,33 (2010).
[50] M.M. Bespalov and M. Saarma, GDNF family receptor complexes are emerging drug targets, *Trends Pharmacol. Sci.* 28, 68 (2007).
[51] R. Linker, R. Gold, and F. Luhder, Function of neurotrophic factors beyond the nervous system: inflammation and autoimmune demyelination, *Crit. Rev. Immunol.*29,43 (2009).
[52] H. Neumann, T. Misgeld, K. Matsumuro, and H. Wekerle, Neurotrophins inhibit major histocompatibility class II inducibility of microglia: involvement of the p75 neurotrophin receptor, *Proc. Natl. Acad. Sci. U. S. A.* 95, 5779 (1998).
[53] R. Wei and G.M. Jonakait, Neurotrophins and the anti-inflammatory agents interleukin-4 (IL-4), IL-10, IL-11 and transforming growth factor-beta1 (TGF-beta1) down-regulate T cell costimulatory molecules B7 and CD40 on cultured rat microglia, *J. Neuroimmunol.* 95,8 (1999).
[54] J.A. Waschek, VIP and PACAP: neuropeptide modulators of CNS inflammation, injury, and repair, *Br. J. Pharmacol.*169, 512 (2013).
[55] M. Delgado, N. Varela, and E. Gonzalez-Rey, Vasoactive intestinal peptide protects against beta-amyloid-induced neurodegeneration by inhibiting microglia activation at multiple levels, *Glia.* 56, 1091 (2008).
[56] M. Domercq, N. Vazquez-Villoldo, and C. Matute, Neurotransmitter signaling in the pathophysiology of microglia, *Front. Cell.Neurosci.* 7, 49(2013).
[57] S.A. Kuhn, F.K. van Landeghem, R. Zacharias, K. Farber, A. Rappert, S. Pavlovic, A. Hoffmann, C. Nolte, and H. Kettenmann, Microglia express GABA(B) receptors to modulate interleukin release, *Mol. Cell. Neurosci.* 25, 312 (2004).
[58] H. Bjurstom, J. Wang, I. Ericsson, M. Bengtsson, Y. Liu, S. Kumar-Mendu, S. Issazadeh-Navikas, and B. Birnir, GABA, a natural immunomodulator of T lymphocytes, *J. Neuroimmunol.* 205, 44 (2008).
[59] D. Carnevale, R. De Simone, and L. Minghetti, Microglia-neuron interaction in inflammatory and degenerative diseases: role of cholinergic and noradrenergic systems, *CNS Neurol. Disord. Drug Targets.* 6, 388 (2007).

[60] M.T. Heneka and M.K. O'Banion, Inflammatory processes in Alzheimer's disease, *J. Neuroimmunol.* 184, 69(2007).

[61] J. Szelenyi and E.S. Vizi, The catecholamine cytokine balance: interaction between the brain and the immune system, *Ann. N. Y. Acad. Sci.* 1113, 311 (2007).

[62] E.S. Wohleb, M.L. Hanke, A.W. Corona, N.D. Powell, L.M. Stiner, M.T. Bailey, R.J. Nelson, J.P. Godbout, and J.F. Sheridan, beta-Adrenergic receptor antagonism prevents anxiety-like behavior and microglial reactivity induced by repeated social defeat, *J. Neurosci.* 31, 6277 (2011).

[63] G. Pongratz and R.H. Straub, Role of peripheral nerve fibres in acute and chronic inflammation in arthritis, *Nat. Rev. Rheumatol.* 9, 117 (2013).

[64] J. Tan, T. Town, T. Mori, Y. Wu, M. Saxe, F. Crawford, and M. Mullan, CD45 opposes beta-amyloid peptide-induced microglial activation via inhibition of p44/42 mitogen-activated protein kinase, *J. Neurosci.* 20, 7587 (2000).

[65] R.T. Mott, G. Ait-Ghezala, T. Town, T. Mori, M. Vendrame, J. Zeng, J. Ehrhart, M. Mullan, and J. Tan, Neuronal expression of CD22: novel mechanism for inhibiting microglial proinflammatory cytokine production, *Glia.* 46, 369 (2004).

[66] P.A. Oldenborg, H.D. Gresham, and F.P. Lindberg, CD47-signal regulatory protein alpha (SIRPalpha) regulates Fcgamma and complement receptor-mediated phagocytosis, *J. Exp. Med.* 193,855 (2001).

[67] R.E. Smith, V. Patel, S.D. Seatter, M.R. Deehan, M.H. Brown, G.P. Brooke, H.S. Goodridge, C.J. Howard, K.P. Rigley, W. Harnett, and M.M. Harnett, A novel MyD-1 (SIRP-1alpha) signaling pathway that inhibits LPS-induced TNFalpha production by monocytes, *Blood.* 102, 2532 (2003).

[68] R.M. Hoek, S.R. Ruuls, C.A. Murphy, G.J. Wright, R. Goddard, S.M. Zurawski, B. Blom, M.E. Homola, W.J. Streit, M.H. Brown, A.N. Barclay, and J.D. Sedgwick, Down-regulation of the macrophage lineage through interaction with OX2 (CD200), *Science.* 290, 1768 (2000).

[69] S.G. Meuth, O.J. Simon, A. Grimm, N. Melzer, A.M. Herrmann, P. Spitzer, P. Landgraf, and H. Wiendl, CNS inflammation and neuronal degeneration is aggravated by impaired CD200-CD200R-mediated macrophage silencing, *J. Neuroimmunol.* 194, 62 (2008).

[70] D.A. Costello, A. Lyons, S. Denieffe, T.C. Browne, F.F. Cox, and M.A. Lynch, Long term potentiation is impaired in membrane glycoprotein CD200-deficient mice: a role for Toll-like receptor activation, *J. Biol. Chem.* 286, 34722 (2011).

[71] M.K. McMillian, L. Thai, J.S. Hong, J.P. O'Callaghan, and K.R. Pennypacker, Brain injury in a dish: a model for reactive gliosis, *Trends Neurosci.* 17, 138 (1994).

[72] R.C. Chang, P. Hudson, B. Wilson, L. Haddon, and J.S. Hong, Influence of neurons on lipopolysaccharide-stimulated production of nitric oxide and tumor necrosis factor-alpha by cultured glia, *Brain Res.* 853, 236 (2000).

[73] K. Takahashi, C.D. Rochford, and H. Neumann, Clearance of apoptotic neurons without inflammation by microglial triggering receptor expressed on myeloid cells-2, *J. Exp. Med.* 201 647 (2005).

[74] H. Neumann and K. Takahashi, Essential role of the microglial triggering receptor expressed on myeloid cells-2 (TREM2) for central nervous tissue immune homeostasis, *J. Neuroimmunol.* 184,92 (2007).

[75] K. Minas and J. Liversidge, Is the CD200/CD200 receptor interaction more than just a myeloid cell inhibitory signal?, *Crit. Rev. Immunol.* 26, 213 (2006).

[76] Y. Liu, I. Teige, B. Birnir, and S. Issazadeh-Navikas, Neuron-mediated generation of regulatory T cells from encephalitogenic T cells suppresses EAE, *Nat. Med.* 12,518 (2006).

[77] L. Tian, M. Stefanidakis, L. Ning, P. Van Lint, H. Nyman-Huttunen, C. Libert, S. Itohara, M. Mishina, H. Rauvala, and C.G. Gahmberg, Activation of NMDA receptors promotes dendritic spine development through MMP-mediated ICAM-5 cleavage, *J. Cell Biol.* 178, 687 (2007).

[78] C.G. Gahmberg, L. Tian, L. Ning, and H. Nyman-Huttunen, ICAM-5-A novel two-facetted adhesion molecule in the mammalian brain, *Immunol. Lett.* 117, 131 (2008).

[79] L. Tian, J. Lappalainen, M. Autero, S. Hanninen, H. Rauvala, and C.G. Gahmberg, Shedded neuronal ICAM-5 suppresses T-cell activation, *Blood.* 111, 3615 (2008).

[80] Y. Lepelletier, I.C. Moura, R. Hadj-Slimane, A. Renand, S. Fiorentino, C. Baude, A. Shirvan, A. Barzilai, and O. Hermine, Immunosuppressive role of semaphorin-3A on T cell proliferation is mediated by inhibition of actin cytoskeleton reorganization, *Eur. J. Immunol.* 36, 1782 (2006).

[81] A. Catalano, P. Caprari, S. Moretti, M. Faronato, L. Tamagnone, and A. Procopio, Semaphorin-3A is expressed by tumor cells and alters T-cell signal transduction and function, *Blood.* 107,3321 (2006).

[82] A.K. Czopik, M.S. Bynoe, N. Palm, C.S. Raine, and R. Medzhitov, Semaphorin 7A is a negative regulator of T cell responses, *Immunity.* 24,591 (2006).

[83] M. Yamamoto, K. Suzuki, T. Okuno, T. Ogata, N. Takegahara, H. Takamatsu, M. Mizui, M. Taniguchi, A. Chedotal, F. Suto, H. Fujisawa, A. Kumanogoh, and H. Kikutani, Plexin-A4 negatively regulates T lymphocyte responses, *Int. Immunol.* 20,413 (2008).

[84] M.S. Bynoe, P. Bonorino, and C. Viret, Control of experimental autoimmune encephalomyelitis by CD4+ suppressor T cells: peripheral versus in situ immunoregulation, *J. Neuroimmunol.* 191,61 (2007).

[85] D.W. Ethell and L.A. Buhler, Fas ligand-mediated apoptosis in degenerative disorders of the brain, *J. Clin.Immunol.* 23, 439 (2003).

[86] C. Choi and E.N. Benveniste, Fas ligand/Fas system in the brain: regulator of immune and apoptotic responses, *Brain Res. Brain Res. Rev.* 44, 65 (2004).

[87] G. Wildbaum, J. Westermann, G. Maor, and N. Karin, A targeted DNA vaccine encoding fas ligand defines its dual role in the regulation of experimental autoimmune encephalomyelitis, *J. Clin. Invest.* 106, 671 (2000).

[88] C.P. Beier, J. Wischhusen, M. Gleichmann, E. Gerhardt, A. Pekanovic, A. Krueger, V. Taylor, U. Suter, P.H. Krammer, M. Endres, M. Weller, and J.B. Schulz, FasL (CD95L/APO-1L) resistance of neurons mediated by phosphatidylinositol 3-kinase-Akt/protein kinase B-dependent expression of lifeguard/neuronal membrane protein 35, *J. Neurosci.* 25, 6765 (2005).

[89] J.H. Song, A. Bellail, M.C. Tse, V.W. Yong, and C. Hao, Human astrocytes are resistant to Fas ligand and tumor necrosis factor-related apoptosis-inducing ligand-induced apoptosis, *J. Neurosci.* 26, 3299 (2006).

[90] U. Andersson and H. Rauvala, Introduction: HMGB1 in inflammation and innate immunity, *J. Intern. Med.* 270, 296 (2011).

[91] K.J. Tracey, Reflex control of immunity, *Nat. Rev. Immunol.* 9, 418 (2009).

[92] S. Muhammad, W. Barakat, S. Stoyanov, S. Murikinati, H. Yang, K.J. Tracey, M. Bendszus, G. Rossetti, P.P. Nawroth, A. Bierhaus, and M.

Schwaninger, The HMGB1 receptor RAGE mediates ischemic brain damage, *J. Neurosci.* 28, 12023 (2008).

[93] H. Gao, H. Zhou, F. Zhang, B.C. Wilson, W. Kam, and J. Hong, HMGB1 acts on microglia Mac1 to mediate chronic neuroinflammation that drives progressive neurodegeneration, *J. Neurosci.* 31, 1081 (2011).

[94] S. Rivest, Regulation of innate immune responses in the brain, *Nat. Rev. Immunol.* 9, 429 (2009).

[95] E. Candelario-Jalil, Y. Yang, G.A. Rosenberg, Diverse roles of matrix metalloproteinases and tissue inhibitors of metalloproteinases in neuroinflammation and cerebral ischemia, *Neuroscience.* 158, 983 (2009).

[96] E. Okun, K.J. Griffioen, J.D. Lathia, S.C. Tang, M.P. Mattson, T.V. Arumugam, Toll-like receptors in neurodegeneration, *Brain Res. Rev.* 59, 278 (2009).

[97] U. Rauch, Extracellular matrix components associated with remodeling processes in brain, *Cell Mol. Life Sci.* 61,2031 (2004).

[98] Q. Ma, U. Cornelli, I. Hanin, W.P. Jeske, R.J. Linhardt, J.M. Walenga, J. Fareed, J.M. Lee, Heparin oligosaccharides as potential therapeutic agents in senile dementia, *Curr. Pharm. Des.*13, 1607 (2007).

In: Neuro-Immune Interactions …
Editor: Oscar González-Pérez
ISBN: 978-1-62948-646-8

Chapter 2

SYSTEMIC INFLAMMATORY REACTION AND PATHOPHYSIOLOGICAL ALTERATION IN THE BRAIN

Grzegorz A. Czapski [*] ***and Joanna B. Strosznajder***
Mossakowski Medical Research Centre Polish Academy of Sciences,
Warsaw, Poland

ABSTRACT

Inflammation-related signaling plays an essential role in the physiology and pathology of the central nervous system (CNS). However, the precise mechanisms underlying interactions between systemic inflammatory reaction (SIR) and molecular, functional and morphological alterations in the brain are not fully understood. For a long period of time the brain was assumed to be an immunologically privileged organ due to anatomical and physiological barriers. During the last decade several novel findings have elucidated the nature of neuroinflammation and interactions between the immune system and brain physiology and pathology.

In this chapter we demonstrate the sequence of molecular events that take place in the brain following activation of SIR. Rapid changes in the expression of several pro-inflammatory genes (iNOS, cPLA2, COX-2,

[*] Corresponding author: Grzegorz A. Czapski, Ph.D., Department of Cellular Signaling, Mossakowski Medical Research Centre Polish Academy of Sciences, Pawinskiego 5, 02-106 Warsaw, Poland, Tel/Fax: +48 22 6086613, Email: gczapski@imdik.pan.pl.

5/12-LOX, NOX), oxidative stress, modifications of macromolecules, and activation of pro-apoptotic and autophagic processes were observed. Our results demonstrate activation of poly(ADP-ribose) polymerase-1 (PARP-1), a key enzyme involved in the regulation of gene transcription and cell survival/death in brain aging, as well as ischemia and inflammation.

Our data demonstrated the role of PARP-1 in the release of AIF from the mitochondria, which may induce caspase-independent neuronal apoptotic death. Moreover, SIR leads to upregulation of gene expression for other members of the PARP family in the hippocampus. Molecular and ultrastructural changes in the brain during SIR suggest a close relationship between the immune system and CNS, which could be critical in the progression of neurodegenerative diseases. We propose that modulation of the cPLA2 signaling pathway and PARP-1 ought to be taken into consideration in the neuroprotective strategy.

Introduction

Inflammation-related signaling plays an essential role in the physiology and pathology of the central nervous system (CNS). For a long period of time the brain was assumed to be an immunologically privileged organ due to anatomical and physiological barriers. Recent findings have elucidated the nature of neuroinflammation and the relationship between the immune system and the brain.

It is evident that peripheral activation of the immune system may significantly affect brain function. The pattern of behavioral changes observed during peripheral inflammation, known as "sickness behavior", combines several symptoms, including fever, activation of the hypothalamic-pituitary-adrenal (HPA) axis, reduction of food intake and other behavioral activities as well as withdrawal from the physical and social environment. It is believed that all of these symptoms could be an evolutionary adaptation limiting the spread of an infectious factor in the population [1]. These phenomena are mediated by the action of pro-inflammatory cytokines. It is generally assumed that aging increases the brain's vulnerability to pro-inflammatory signaling from the periphery. Moreover, systemic inflammatory response (SIR) may significantly affect physiological aging and the progression of neurological diseases. However, recently published data have shown that SIR may evoke long-lasting molecular and morphological changes in the CNS in patients with normal cognition also. The most evident alterations in the brain were observed after sepsis. Encephalopathy, which occurs in >50% of septic patients, comprises a variety of alterations, including alteration of the gene expression pattern, mitochondrial dysfunction, deregulation of calcium homeostasis and disturbances in neurotransmission [2,3]. Moreover, severe sepsis evokes substantial and persistent impairments in learning and memory. Recent studies demonstrated that 70% of sepsis survivors had cognitive sequelae at hospital discharge, and 45% one year later [4-6]. Because the population of long-term survivors is increasing in developed countries, the rise in the group of cognitively impaired patients is becoming a common and rapidly growing public health problem [7]. Understanding the molecular mechanisms involved in pathological alterations in the brain which lead to impairment of memory and cognition during SIR is an important challenge for researchers and may indicate novel targets for the neuroprotective strategy.

Experimental studies in the field of SIR-associated pathology were carried out using several animal models of sepsis and SIRS syndrome [8]. Peripheral administration of lipopolysaccharide (LPS) is the most common method of activating innate immunity leading to SIR. This method mimics the conditions of bacterial infection or sepsis. LPS, a component of the cell wall of Gram-negative bacteria, is responsible for ~45% of human sepsis cases [8]. The immune system detects the presence of LPS in the inner environment by specific Toll-like receptors 4 (TLR4) belonging to the family of pattern recognition receptors (PRR) TLRs. Toll-like receptors are transmembrane proteins expressed in many types of cells. The broad expression of TLR4 was confirmed in the cells of the CNS: in the microglia, astrocytes, oligodendrocytes, endothelial cells as well as in the neural stem/progenitor cells and in some populations of neurons [9-12]. Activation of TLR4 by LPS requires its homodimerization and cooperation of many accessory molecules, such as LBP, MD2, CD14 [13]. Upon stimulation, TLR4 signaling leads to enhanced release of several cytokines and other inflammatory mediators. The exact mechanisms responsible for transmission of the pro-inflammatory signals from the periphery to the brain are not completely understood. Pathways of special significance are: 1) stimulation of the primary afferent neurons or vagal afferent fibers by pathogen-associated molecular patterns (PAMPs) or cytokines at the site of infection 2) a cascade of cell-to-cell signal transduction in the CNS, starting from cells exposed to circulating molecules (PAMPs or cytokines), e.g., endothelial cells or phagocytic cells in the circumventricular organs (CVOs) and the choroid plexus [14]. Cerebral endothelial cells play a key role in the transfer of inflammatory signaling through the blood-brain barrier (BBB) to the CNS. The areas enabling easy communication between the peripheral immune system and the CNS are the periventricular organs, blood vessels and meninges [15]. Under physiological conditions the BBB protects the brain against a number of potentially harmful substances circulating in the blood, including LPS. Because very small amounts of circulating LPS (0.025% of an intravenously injected dose) cross the BBB to enter the CNS, it seems unlikely that direct stimulation of TLR4 receptors in brain parenchyma by circulating LPS would be a pathway of noticeable significance [16]. However, recent studies suggested that functioning TLR4s in CNS-resident cells are necessary for the inflammatory reaction to develop within the brain after peripheral administration of LPS. The role of hematogenous TLR4 receptors seems to be of lesser importance [17,18]. Moreover, LPS circulating in the blood may impair the integrity of BBB, thus enabling increased diffusion of neurotoxic substances to the brain. There is also evidence that circulating cytokines can cross the BBB [19]. On the other hand, the question arises whether concentrations of these peripheral cytokines inside the brain can reach levels that are high enough to activate immune processes. Additionally, recent studies clearly demonstrated that the impact of peripheral administration of LPS on inflammatory and neurodegenerative processes within the brain is independent of circulating cytokines IL-1β and IL-6, regardless of their high elevation in the serum [20].

In this chapter we summarize our previously published results concerning molecular alterations in the brain during an experimental model of SIR. In our studies we analyzed gene expression for the cPLA2-mediated signaling pathway and oxidative stress-related alterations leading to DNA damage and PARP-1 activation [21-26]. We focused on the hippocampus that is crucial brain structure involved in memory and cognition, and one that is the most sensitive to several neurodegenerative insults and neuroinflammatory processes [27-30]. All of these events may lead to impairment of the cognitive processes during SIR.

ALTERATIONS OF GENE EXPRESSION IN THE HIPPOCAMPUS DURING SIR

The brain is one of the first organs that is affected during sepsis [31]. Peripheral administration of LPS evokes significant changes in gene expression in the brain, thus demonstrating that a peripheral inflammatory reaction may affect brain functions, including local synthesis of proinflammatory cytokines in certain brain structures [32,33]. It was suggested that the vagal afferent fibers play a prominent role in communication between the immune system and the brain [33,34]. However, the effect of SIR on the brain may be dependent on several other factors and experimental conditions (LPS dose, toxicity, animal strain).

In our studies, i.e., using a mouse model of SIR induced by LPS (1 mg/kg b.w.; i.p.), characteristic symptoms of sickness behavior, including anorexia, adipsia, lethargy and reduced social activity were observed, which had also been described previously by Dantzer et al. [35]. The levels of mRNA for an inducible isoform of nitric oxide synthase (iNOS), tumor necrosis factor alpha (TNFα), toll-like receptor 4 (TLR4), cytosolic phospholipase A2 (cPLA2), cyclooxygenase-2 (COX-2) and lipoxygenases-5 and -12 were significantly increased with differential dynamics (Figure 1). The maximum level of mRNA for iNOS and TNFα was observed as early as 3 h post-injection. The increase in mRNA for cPLA2 was biphasic, with maxima at 6 and 24 h post-injection. The increase in expression of the COX-2 gene reached the highest level at 6 h. The maximum expression of 5-LOX and 12-LOX was observed at 12–24 and 24–48 h post-injection, respectively. The level of mRNA for TLR4 increased gently but constantly up to 48 h. These results demonstrated that in the hippocampus of LPS-treated animals the tightly regulated sequence of activation/deactivation of genes leads to the production of several proteins that are crucial for maintenance of the neuroinflammatory reaction. The release of arachidonic acid (AA) catalyzed by cPLA2 provides a substrate for COX-2 and LOXs for synthesis of several lipid mediators that are necessary for an inflammatory reaction. It was recently presented that LPS-induced expression of the gene for iNOS in the glial cells is dependent on PLA2 activation [36]. Pro-inflammatory gene expression is associated with activation of the microglia in the hippocampus [29]. It is worth noting that enhancing the activity of many of these enzymes may lead to increased production of free radicals and other reactive oxygen and nitrogen species (ROS and RNS, respectively).

Oxidative Stress and Pro-Apoptotic Signaling in the Hippocampus during Sir: The Consequence of a Neuroinflammatory Reaction

Oxidative stress is a component of countless disorders, including sepsis-evoked encephalopathy [37]. The brain is an organ that is especially vulnerable to oxidative damage due to the 1) high oxygen consumption that is necessary for production of high amounts of ATP needed to maintain neuronal intracellular ion homoeostasis, 2) high amounts of polyunsaturated fatty acids, 3) high level of iron, 4) presence of excitotoxic amino acids and 5) relatively low level of antioxidant defense [38]. A rapid increase in expression of iNOS, cPLA2, COX-2, LOXs, and NADPH subunits [24,25] is inevitably followed by enhancement of production of reactive oxygen species (ROS) and by oxidative modifications of macromolecules in the brain (Figure 2). Oxidative/nitrosative stress in the brain after sepsis may be long-lasting phenomena. Alterations of the oxidative parameters in the brain have been observed in rats even 30 and 60 days after sepsis [39].

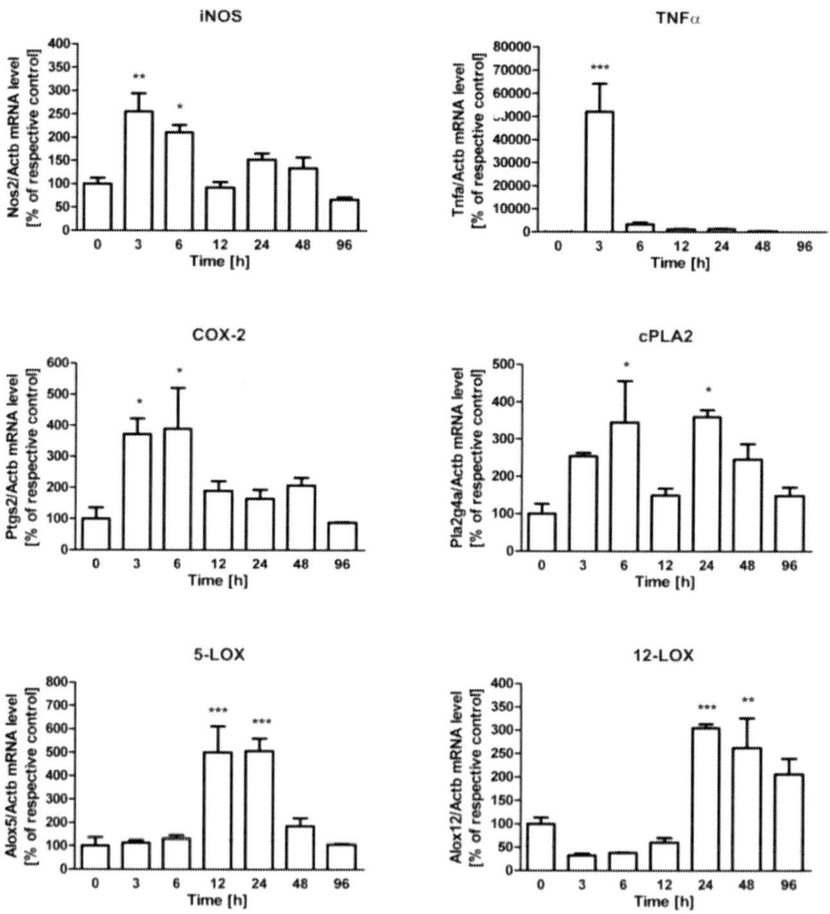

Figure 1. Continued on next page.

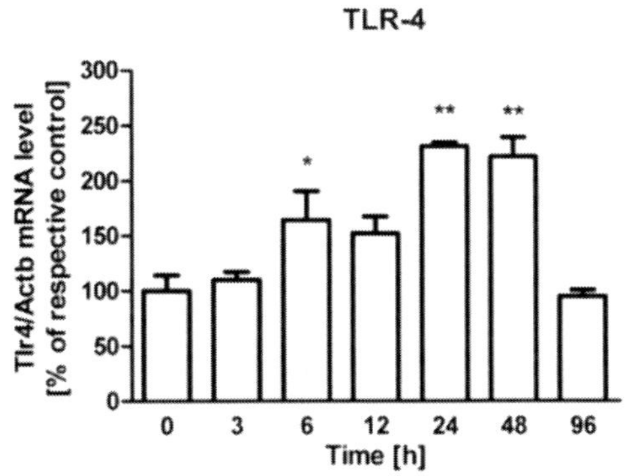

Figure 1. Relative changes in mRNA levels in the hippocampus after LPS treatment. LPS (1 mg/kg b.w.) was injected intraperitoneally and gene expression was analyzed at 0, 3, 6, 12, 24, 48 or 96 h after injection by quantitative RT-PCR. The results were normalised to β-actin gene expression and are presented as the mean ± SEM from three independent experiments. *, **, ***$p<0.05$, 0.01 and 0.001 compared with the respective control. Adapted from Czapski et al., 2010 [24].

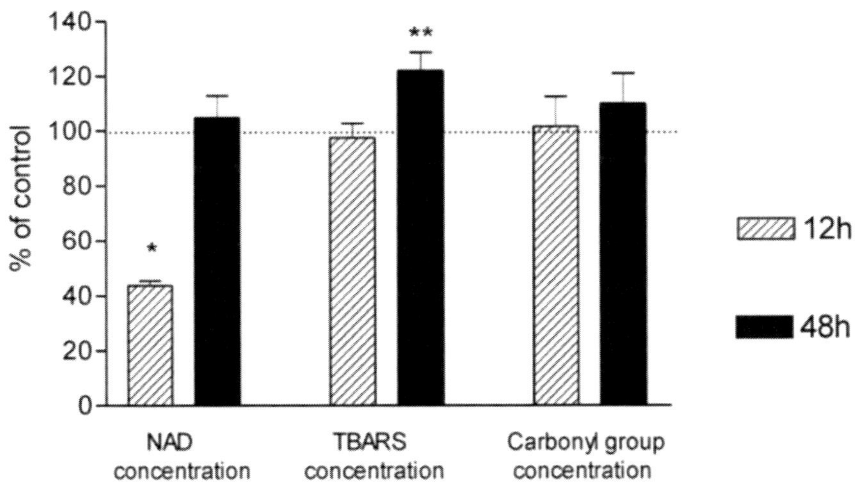

Figure 2.The effect of lipopolysaccharide on oxidative stress in the brain. Twelve and 48 h after LPS administration (1 mg/kg ip), mice were decapitated, and whole brains were analyzed. The effect of LPS on NAD^+ concentration and oxidation of macromolecules was analyzed. * and ** – statistical significance compared to control group $p < 0.05$ and 0.01, respectively. Results are the means ± SEM, n = 4 to 11. Adapted from Czapski et al., 2004 [21].

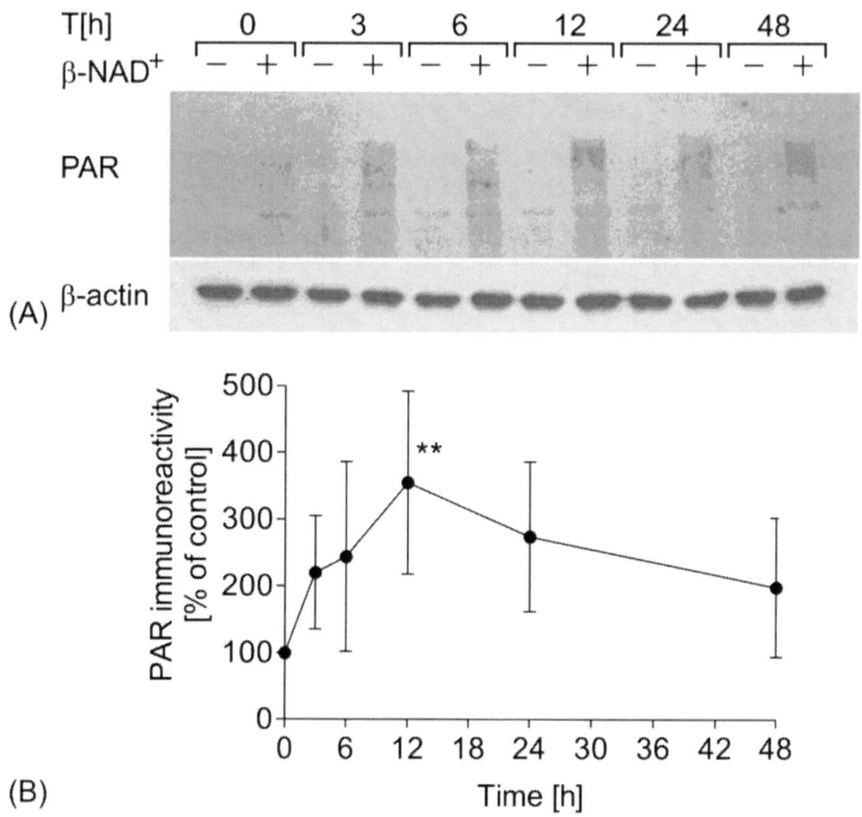

Figure 3. The effect of systemic lipopolysaccharide administration on PARP-1 activation in the brain. After LPS administration (1 mg/kg i.p.) mice were decapitated, and PAR formation in midbrain in vitro was analyzed by Western blotting method, as described above. Representative picture is presented, including loading control. Asterisks (**) indicate statistical significance compared to control group. Results are the means ± S.E.M., n=3. Adapted from Czapski et al., 2006 [22].

Oxidative damage of lipids and proteins may have a significant impact on their function, but the modified molecules may be replaced by continuously synthesized new molecules. A true problem for the cell may be oxidatively modified DNA, however, it can be repaired. Poly(ADP-ribose)polymerase-1 (PARP-1) possesses the crucial function in the DNA repair mechanism. This nuclear enzyme is the most sensitive detector of single- and double-strand breaks in the DNA. Upon activation, PARP-1 synthesizes long, branched polymers of ADP-ribose and attaches them covalently to DNA-related proteins. Because poly(ADP-ribose) has a high negative charge, such modification of histones and other DNA-binding proteins evokes their dissociation from the DNA. In consequence, exposition of the damaged DNA to BER and NER repair complexes occurs. Activation of PARP-1 is crucial for successful DNA repair in low and mild DNA damage. However, massive DNA damage may lead to sustained overactivation of PARP-1 and, in consequence, to depletion of its substrate nicotinamide adenine dinucleotide (NAD^+). The concentration of NAD^+, which is about 400–500 μM in healthy mammalian cells, in response to a powerful genotoxic stimulus, is reduced to 10–20% of the basal level [40]. As shown in Figure 2, peripheral administration of LPS evokes a rapid decrease in the NAD^+ level in the mouse brain, which is accompanied by increased PARP activity (Figure 3). It was proposed that this depletion of cellular NAD^+ may, in consequence, lead to further energy failure and cell death, as two-four molecules of ATP are necessary for resynthesis of one molecule of NAD^+ [41]. PARP-1-dependent NAD^+ depletion was suggested to be an important mechanism of necrotic neuronal cell death [42,43]. However, overactivation of PARP-1 leads to accumulation of poly(ADP-ribose) molecules (PAR), which have recently been recognized, as signaling molecules, as being capable of translocation to the mitochondria and of inducing the release of the mitochondrial protein – apoptosis inducing factor (AIF) [44,45]. These events may lead to mitochondrial failure. AIF is an important protein in the function of complexes I and III of the mitochondrial electron transport chain, e.g., it is responsible for assembly and stabilization of these complexes [46,47]. AIF also exerts antioxidative properties and protects the mitochondria against oxidative/nitrosative stress. However, after translocation into the nucleus, AIF stimulates endonuclease activity and degrades the DNA to fragments ~50 kpb. Through this mechanism AIF is responsible for caspase-independent apoptosis, termed "parthanatos". Recent analysis of the causal relationships between PARP-1 activation, NAD^+ depletion and the release of AIF demonstrated that NAD^+ depletion and glycolytic failure are upstream of mitochondrial AIF release [48]. NAD^+ depletion has been suggested as being necessary and sufficient for poly(ADP-ribose) polymerase-1-mediated AIF release and neuronal death.

Recent studies have demonstrated that SIR induced activation of pro-apoptotic processes in the hippocampus – the most vulnerable brain structure [29,49,50]. The presence of apoptotic, TUNEL-positive cells was noticed in the hippocampus during SIR. An additional examination revealed that about 15% of TUNEL-positive cells resembled neurons and 80% were identified as glial cells.

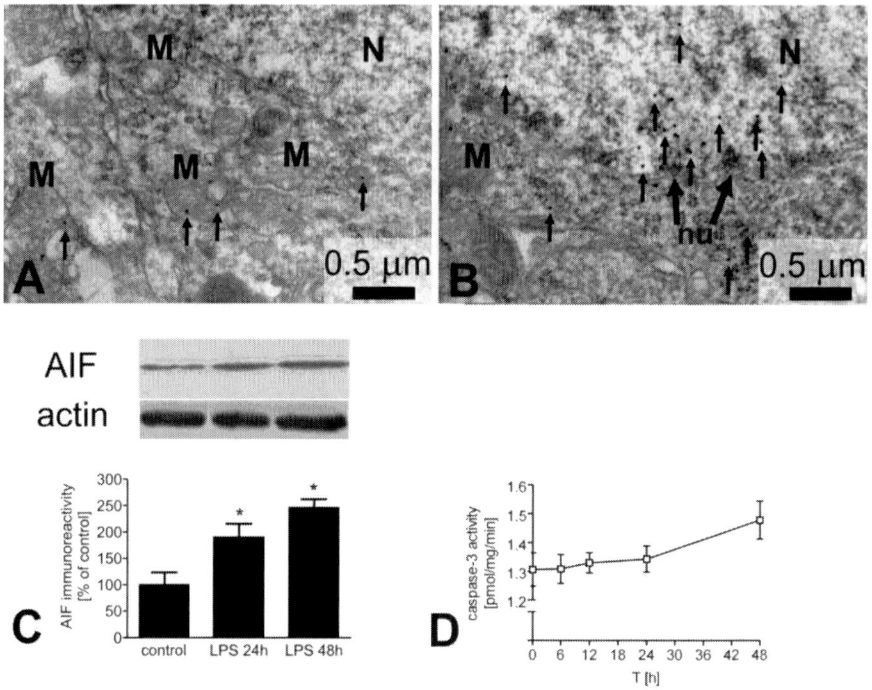

Figure 4. The effect of systemic LPS administration on apoptosis-inducing factor (AIF) translocation and caspase-3 activity in the hippocampus.

Immunocytochemical studies on the hippocampal CA1 sector showed AIF translocation from the mitochondria (M) to the nucleus (N) 48 h after LPS treatment. A—Control conditions. Note the presence of AIF (arrows) only in mitochondria. B—After LPS treatment. Arrows indicate a large number of gold particles representing AIF in the nucleus close to a nuclear pore. C—Immunochemical analysis of the LPS-evoked, time-dependent translocation of AIF from the mitochondria to the nucleus. LPS (1 mg/kg b.w.) was administered intraperitoneally. Twenty-four or 48 h after treatment, a nuclear fraction was prepared from whole hippocampus. Proteins were analyzed by SDS-PAGE and Western blotting (representative picture is shown) followed by densitometry. The data were normalised to corresponding actin bands. The results are presented as the mean±SEM from three to five independent experiments. *$p<0.05$, compared with control (one-way ANOVA with Newman–Keuls post-hoc test). D—Caspase-3 activity in the hippocampus after systemic LPS administration. Six, 12, 24 or 48 h after LPS administration (1 mg/kg b.w.), the hippocampus was isolated and caspase-3 activity was measured. The obtained results are the mean ± SEM from three independent experiments performed in triplicate. Adapted from Czapski et al., 2010 [24].

In parallel, SIR induced upregulation of pro-apoptotic Bax, and downregulation of anti-apoptotic Bcl-2 protein was observed. Moreover, the presence of some cells showing morphological characteristics of necrosis was also noticed [29]. Our analysis using the immunocytochemical and immunochemical method demonstrated activation of the PARP-1/AIF-related apoptotic pathway in the hippocampus during SIR (Figure 4). In control conditions AIF is located mainly in the mitochondria, nevertheless, individual molecules of AIF were also observed in the cytoplasm and the Golgi apparatus. SIR induced the release of AIF from the mitochondria and translocation to the nucleus. A semi-quantitative analysis of the nuclear fraction from the hippocampus demonstrated that the level of AIF in the nuclear fraction was continuously increasing over time. Caspase-3 activity was not increased in the hippocampus in these conditions. We obtained similar results previously in the midbrain after systemic administration of LPS [22,23]. We described the significant role of PARP-1/PAR/AIF-mediated neuronal death in the hippocampus after forebrain ischemia [51,52]. Moreover, Hamby [53] also demonstrated the role of PARP-1 in apoptotic neuronal death after global ischemia. The neuroprotective effect of the PARP inhibitor was connected with anti-inflammatory action.

However, in sepsis some studies did not confirm the presence of evident apoptotic processes, or they demonstrated very weak activation of apoptosis in experimental models of sepsis [54]. All of these data indicate that molecular alterations which are initiated in the hippocampus during SIR, including activation of some pro-apoptotic pathways, do not unavoidably lead to neuronal loss [55]. To explore whether several molecular alterations evoke any changes on the subcellular level, we performed an electron microscopic examination of the hippocampal CA1 region in mice subjected to SIR [24]. Our analysis showed characteristic morphological features of three self-destructive processes, i.e., apoptosis, autophagy and necrosis, in some neurons of the hippocampus (Figures 5–6). We observed in particular in the hippocampal neurons of LPS-treated animals deep invaginations of the nuclear membrane into the nucleoplasm, a shrunken, dark cytoplasm, the presence of numerous, heterogenous lysosomes (dense bodies, multivesicular bodies, lamellar bodies), and swelling of some mitochondria. D'Avila and coworkers used the mouse model of sepsis evoked by cecal ligation and puncture (CLP) for systematic examination of mitochondrial function in brain tissues during sepsis [56].

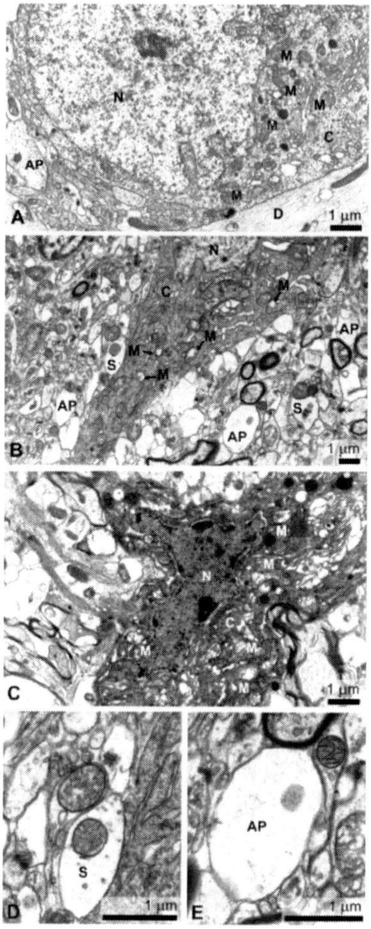

Figure 5. Alterations of ultrastructure of neuronal cells evoked by SIR in CA1 layer of the hippocampus. A—An electron microscopic analysis of ultrastructurally unchanged neuronal cells in control conditions. The correct structure of the mitochondria (M) and the nucleus (N) with evenly distributed chromatin is visible. Cytoplasm (C) is rich in ribosomes and polyribosomes. AP—astrocytic processes, D—dendrites. B, C—Ultrastructure of a neuronal cell in the hippocampus 48 h after LPS (1 mg/kg b.w.) administration. The cytoplasm (C) is shrunken and dark. A deep invagination of the nuclear (N) membrane into the nucleoplasm and the swelling of some mitochondria (M) are seen. Swollen astrocytic processes (AP) and swollen synapses (S) with electron light synaptoplasmand a few synaptic vesicles are visible. D, E—A higher magnification of the selected areas of B showing a swollen synapse (S) and a swollen astrocytic process (AP). The presented pictures are typical of the three animals used in each experimental group. Adapted from Czapski et al., 2010 [24].

Brain mitochondria isolated from whole brains of septic animals presented uncoupling of oxidative phosphorylation, a general reduction in the content of the cytochromes, and a decrease in the activity of cytochrome c oxidase, thus demonstrating that their function may be impaired and that brain tissue bioenergetic efficiency may be reduced during sepsis. These alterations were observed as early as 24 h after induction of SIR.

Another interesting feature of pathologically changed neurons of the hippocampus was degeneration of dendrites, which was manifested by an enlargement of the autophagic vacuoles containing ultrastructurally changed cytoplasmic material or cellular debris (Figure 6). Additionally, many swollen synapses in the pre-synaptic part and swollen astrocytic processes were observed in the neuropil, thus indicating that some degenerative processes within the dendrites were initiated. Similar degenerative processes within the neuropil leading to degeneration of the dendritic trees were observed in an acute model of LPS toxicity, after intraperitoneal [57], intranigral [58] and intracerebroventricular [59] administration. It was suggested that the loss of dendritic processes is mediated by macrophagy and autophagy [60].

An important question is whether all of these SIR-induced apoptotic and autophagic processes in the brain evoke irreversible brain lesions. Mild cases of sepsis-induced encephalopathy are not related with perpetual brain damage. However, the existence of long-term cognitive impairment that is present in patients who suffered from severe sepsis suggests that some permanent changes do occur in the brain [61]. An analysis of autopsic brain samples from patients who died due to sepsis or septic shock demonstrated a high frequency of ischemic or hemorrhagic injuries [62]. Also, apoptotic neurons and multifocal necrotizing lesions have been observed in the brains of patients who died from septic shock [63]. In some studies protein A100β was proposed as a serum marker of cell death during sepsis [64]. This protein is released after damage to the neurons or astroglia. Additionally, an elevated level of A100β in blood serum may indicate blood-brain barrier (BBB) damage, as in normal conditions A100β cannot pass BBB. However, some contradictory data have demonstrated that the A100β level did not correlate with the severity of sepsis-evoked encephalopathy and cannot be used to predict neurological recovery [65].

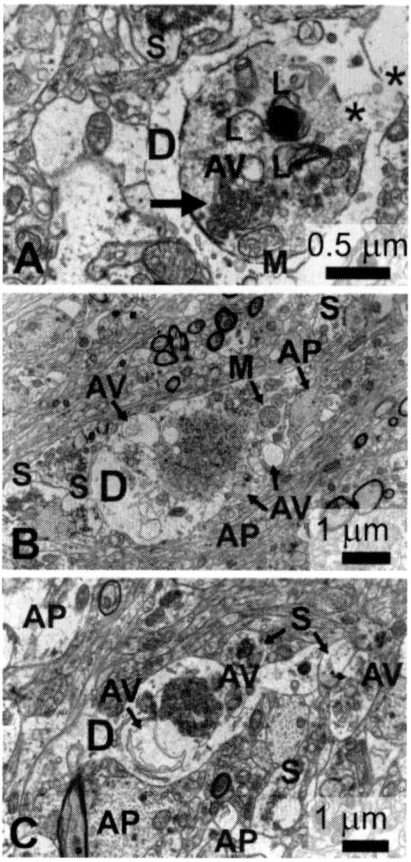

Figure 6. Ultrastructurally changed dendrites in the CA1 layer of the hippocampus after systemic LPS administration. A. Dendrite (D) degeneration is clearly visible: cellular organelles, including abnormal mitochondria (M), heterogeneous lysosomes (L) and unrecognized aggregate of electron-dense material (arrow), enclosed by membrane forms an autophagic vacuole (AV) with characteristic morphological features. Note the loose continuity of membrane autophagic vacuole and dendritic basement membrane (asterisk). B—Degenerating dendrite (D); the accumulation of fibrillar material of different sizes and small vacuoles co-localise with the well-preserved mitochondria (M). New autophagic vacuoles (early stage-vacuoles AV) are present. The swelling of synapses (S) and astrocytic processes (AP) in neuropil are visible. C—Autophagic vacuoles of a different size (AV) containing cellular debris and lysosome lamellar formation can be observed. In the neuropil, many swollen synapses (S) and astrocytic processes (AP) are clearly visible. The presented pictures are typical of the three animals used in each experimental group. Adapted from Czapski et al., 2010 [24].

THE ROLE OF PARP IN THE REGULATION OF TRANSCRIPTION IN THE BRAIN DURING SIR

The family of poly(ADP-ribose) polymerases (PARP, also known as PARS and ADPRT) consists of 18 distinct proteins detected by homology searching and in silico analysis [66,67]. In the brain, PARP-1 is a predominant isoform that is responsible for over 90% of poly(ADP-ribosyl)ation [66,68-71]. The function of PARP is not limited to its involvement in DNA repair mechanisms, NAD^+ depletion and induction of AIF-dependent apoptosis, as was described above. The additional role of PARP-1 is related to its influence on gene transcription, mainly by interaction with several transcription factors (TFs). PARP-1 plays a crucial role in progression of the pro-inflammatory cascade in infectious and non-infectious diseases [72,73]. Transcriptional activity is mainly reduced by poly(ADP-ribosyl)ation, but is increased by direct binding of PARP-1 to the TF. However, PARP-1 may affect the function of transcription factors in several ways. The mechanisms of interactions between PARP-1 and TF were successfully studied based on the example of transcription factor NF-κB due to its leading role in regulating the expression of inflammation-related genes [74-76]. A functional relationship between PARP-1 and NF-κB during systemic inflammation was first reported by Oliver et al. [77]. Then it was suggested that protein-protein interaction is primarily responsible for activation of NF-κB by PARP-1 [78,79]. The authors excluded the importance of poly(ADP-ribosyl)ation and proposed that the enzymatic activity of PARP-1 has no effect on the regulation of NF-κB. In the absence of the substrate (NAD^+), the direct binding of PARP-1 to the transcription factor promotes transcription. However, this issue remains disputable until today because other studies, including studies by our group, have shown that pharmacological inhibition of the enzymatic activity of PARP-1 reduces activation of both NF-κB and the expression of NF-κB-dependent genes (e.g., iNOS) [25,80-83]. Additionally, PARP-1 may directly influence the signaling cascades controlling the activity of TFs. It was shown that PARP-1 may regulate the function of NF-κB by affecting the PI3-kinase/AKT pathway, Gsk-3β and MAP kinase cascades [84-88]. The function of many transcription factors (i.e., p53, YY1, CREB, SP1) may be regulated by direct PARP-1-catalyzed poly (ADP-ribosyl)ation [89-92]. PARP-1 may also directly interact with several TFs, e.g., RelA/p65, NFκB1/p50, Oct-1, TP53, YY1, SP1 (see a review of Hassa and Hottiger, [93]). Also, the binding of large polymers of PAR to a specific binding domain (e.g., in p53) may affect the activity of the TFs due to a high negative charge of PAR [71]. Moreover, poly(ADP-ribose) was proposed to act as a biological glue promoting PARP-TF protein-protein interactions [93]. In addition, PARP-1 may directly bind to a promoter region and work as an activator/repressor of transcription.

In our studies we determined the PARP family's role in the regulation of pro-inflammatory gene expression in the hippocampus of LPS-treated animals [25]. Moreover, we analyzed the expression and activity of PARP in the hippocampus 12 h after intraperitoneal administration of LPS. The transcripts for Parp1-9, Parp11, Parp12, Parp14 and Parp16 were detected in the mouse hippocampus. A quantitative analysis using the RT-PCR method demonstrated that the level of mRNA for Parp1, Parp3, Parp9, Parp12 and Parp14 was increased in LPS-treated animals. Expression of Parp8 and Parp11 was slightly downregulated.

Because the researchers' attention was focused on PARP-1, as the major PARP isoform within the brain, our knowledge about other PARP family members and about the network of interactions between them is poor. However, it seems that interaction between various PARP isoforms may play an important role in the regulation of inflammatory signaling [94]. PARP-3, just as PARP-1 and PARP-2, contributes to DNA repair, but it is involved in a distinct DNA repair pathway; PARP-3 is also a regulator of mitotic progression [95-99]. Additionally, PARP-3 may have a regulatory function, as it activates PARP-1 in the absence of DNA [100]. PARP-9 and PARP-14, belonging to the subfamily of macroPARPs, contain a macro domain which may negatively regulate the activity of PARP-1 on specific promoters [101-103]. These isoforms are upregulated by immune signaling and can be responsible for control of an inflammatory reaction [104-107].

Our data showed that SIR evoked a significant increase in PARP activity in the hippocampus, and that an inhibitor of PARP, 3-aminobenzamide (3AB), efficiently prevented this activation (Figure 7). To examine the possible interaction of PARP family genes with transcription processes, a microarray analysis of the gene expression pattern was performed. The analysis demonstrated an alteration of expression of 262 genes in the hippocampus during SIR (Fold change > 2) [25]. Bioinformatic analysis predicted a list of 228 transcription factors (TFs) that may be potentially responsible for these alterations of gene expression. The top TFs were STAT3, TRIM24, STAT1, NF-κB and CEBPB. Further analysis demonstrated that among these 228 TFs, 41 may interact with PARP family members. In the group of 262 genes affected during SIR, 139 are regulated by 41 PARP-dependent transcription factors. These data demonstrated that PARP may directly or indirectly control the expression of a broad panel of genes during an inflammatory reaction.

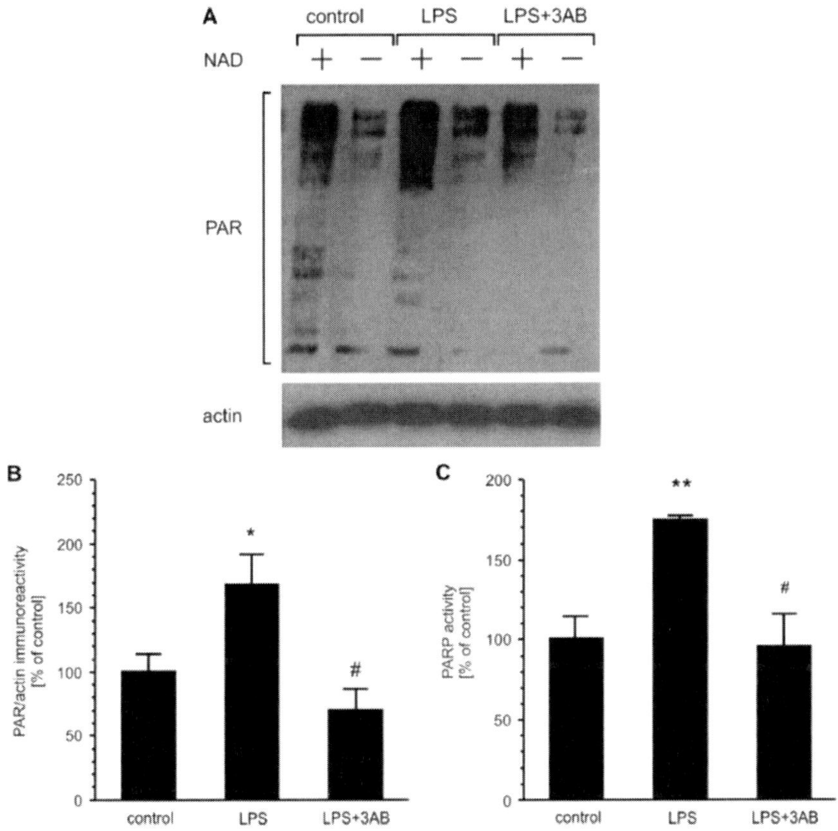

Figure 7. The effect of LPS-evoked systemic inflammation on PARP activity in the hippocampus and the level of PAR. LPS (1 mg/kg b.w.) and 3-aminobenzamide (30 mg/kg b.w.) were injected intraperitoneally, after 12 h the mice were decapitated and the hippocampi were collected. (A) Representative immunoblot of PAR, including loading control. (B) Densitometric analysis of PAR formation in vitro, as analyzed by immunochemical method. Data were normalized to Actin immunoreactivity. (C) PARP activity determined by the radiochemical method. $p < 0.05$, $p < 0.01$ compared with the control group. # $p < 0.05$ compared with the LPS-treated group. n = 5–7. Adapted from Czapski et al., 2013 [25].

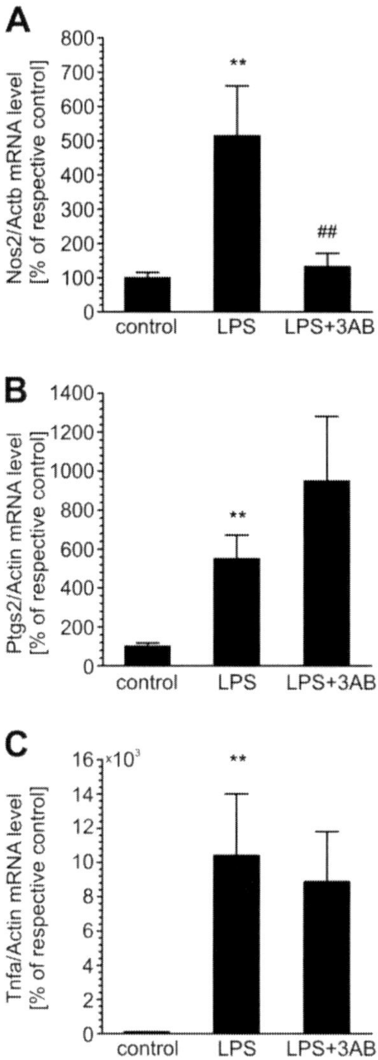

Figure 8. The effect of PARP inhibition on SIR-induced expression of pro-inflammatory genes in the hippocampus.

LPS (1 mg/kg b.w.) and 3-aminobenzamide (30 mg/kg b.w.) were injected intraperitoneally, after 3 h the mice were decapitated and the hippocampi were collected. The level of mRNA for genes coding iNOS (A), COX-2 (B) and TNFa (C) was analyzed by quantitative PCR method. Actb was used as a reference gene. ** $p < 0.01$, compared to the control group, ## $p < 0.01$, compared to the LPS-treated group. n =3. Adapted from Czapski et al., 2013 [25].

To analyze whether inhibition of PARP activity may have a considerable impact on expression of pro-oxidative genes in the hippocampus, the level of mRNA for selected genes was measured in the hippocampi of animals subjected to SIR. As is shown in Figure 8, there is a selective effect of 3AB on expression of the pro-inflammatory genes. The level of mRNA for iNOS was efficiently reduced in 3AB-treated animals, but inhibition of PARP activity had no effect on the expression of TNFα, COX-2 and subunits of NADPH oxidase. This effect of 3AB on expression of the gene for iNOS explains our previous observations which demonstrated the anti-oxidative consequences of inhibition of PARP in LPS-treated animals [22].

The anti-inflammatory effect of the PARP inhibitor was reported previously in several studies [72,108,109]. In human sepsis and in experimental animal models a relevant increase in PARP-catalyzed PAR synthesis in the peripheral organs was observed [110]. In a rodent model of systemic endotoxemia, pretreatment with the PARP inhibitor, PJ34, considerably decreased the levels of pro-inflammatory mediators (i.e., TNF-α, IL-1β, nitrite/nitrate) in the plasma, repressed neutrophil infiltration, NO production and rescued the animals from LPS-induced death [85,111]. In a similar model, PJ34 attenuated LPS-induced renal impairment [112]. The effect of PARP on the inflammatory reaction may vary depending on the genetic background. It was recently shown that PARP-1 controls IL-10 expression in an allele-dependent mode. PARP-1 interacts with the promoter region of the human gene for IL-10, thus acting as a transcription repressor. Single nucleotide polymorphism (-1082G>A) of the IL-10 gene promoter region has a relevant impact on this interaction, which results in remarkably diverse levels of IL-10 transcription [113].

An alternative strategy for modulation of PARP-1 activity may be modulation of the signaling pathways or posttranslational modifications affecting this enzyme [114]. Besides single- and double-strand breaks in the DNA and interaction with PARP-3, also auto-poly(ADP-ribosylation), phosphorylation, acetylation and sumoylation may affect PARP-1 activity [100,115-117]. These modifications may modulate the function of PARP in inflammatory processes, which was demonstrated in several studies *in vitro* and *in vivo*. It was shown that acetylation of PARP-1 at specific lysine residues by the p300/CREB-binding protein is required for the interaction of PARP-1 with p50 and for synergistic coactivation of NF-κB [115]. This phosphorylation is important for the regulation of PARP-1 activity, but the impact of individual phosphorylation sites needs clarification. PARP-1 activity may be phosphorylated by many kinases [118]. Phosphoproteomic analysis revealed that protein kinase C beta (PKCβ), extracellular signal-related kinase-1 (ERK-1), extracellular signal-related kinase-2 (ERK-2), casein kinase II (CK II), cyclin-dependent kinase 5 (CDK5), c-Jun-N-terminal kinase 1 (JNK-1 also known as MAPK8), and calcium/calmodulin-dependent protein kinase type II (CaMK II) are capable of phosphorylation of PARP-1. By using the protein kinase siRNA library targeting 779 human protein kinase and kinase-associated genes, Turner and coworkers found a number of kinases (e.g., CDK5, MAPK12, PLK3, PNKP, STK22c and STK36) whose silencing potently sensitized cells to the PARP-1 inhibitor [119]. However, until today, kinase-dependent regulation of PARP-1 activity in neuroinflammation has been faintly studied. ERK1/2 is capable of PARP-1 phosphorylation on Ser372 and Thr373, and the ERK inhibitor (PD98059) was demonstrated to reduce PARP activity [120;]. Also, JNK1 acts as an upstream regulator of PARP-1, so there is a positive feedback loop between JNK and PARP-1 [121]. Recently published data indicated that CDK5 plays an important role in the regulation of inflammatory processes [122,123]. This may be at least in part dependent on CDK5-evoked PARP-1 phosphorylation on Ser782, Ser785 or Ser786 [118]. Inhibition of CDK5 by roscovitine was shown to prevent pro-inflammatory signaling by inhibition of the transcriptional activity of NF-κB, and depletion of CDK5 resulted in an increase of PAR formation [124]. It seems that CDK5-catalyzed phosphorylation-dependent PARP-1 inhibition may lead to a reduction of the PAR level which, in consequence, should increase the transcriptional activity of several transcription factors (e.g., AP2, B-MYB, TEF-1/Max, Oct-1, p53, NF-κB, HSF1), and in this manner should affect pro-inflammatory signaling.

Conclusion

Systemic inflammatory response (SIR) activates a cascade of molecular events within the brain that includes alterations of gene expression and free radical levels, thus leading to oxidative/nitrosative stress, mitochondria failure, DNA damage and PARP-1 overactivation (Figure 9). Moreover, changes in the ultrastructure of the neurons and glia cells were observed in the brain. On the basis of our results we suggest that inhibition of PARP-1 activity should be considered as a promising therapeutic strategy in conditions of severe SIR.

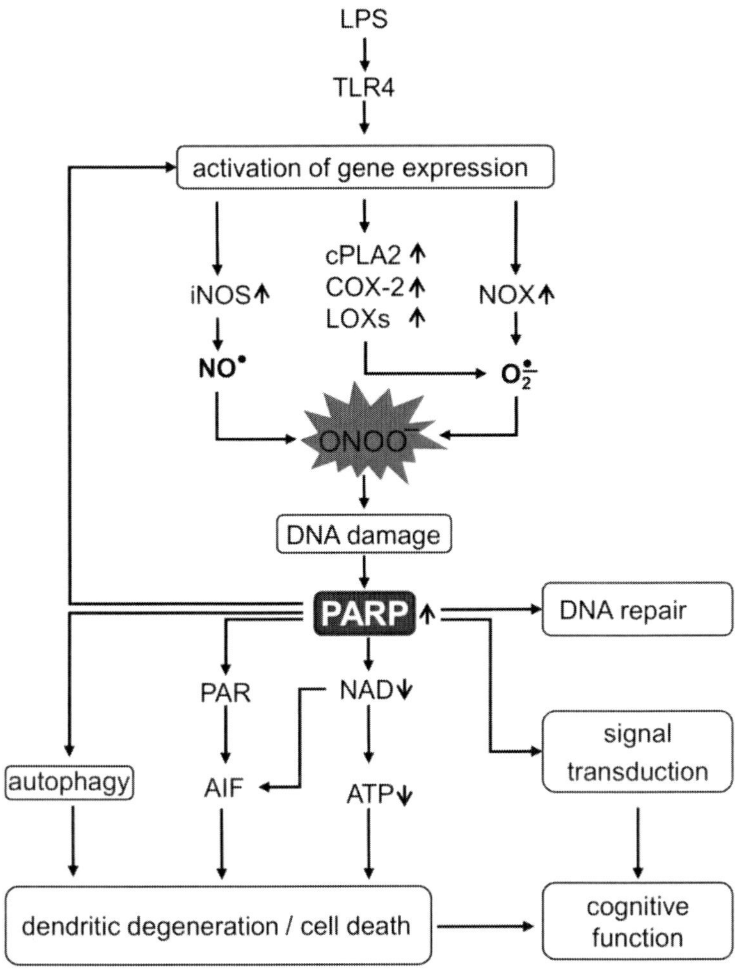

Figure 9. Systemic inflammatory reaction and pathophysiological alteration in the brain –the role of PARP.

ACKNOWLEDGMENT

This work was supported by grant from The National Science Centre 2011/03/B/NZ3/04549. The authors declare no conflicts of interest.

REFERENCES

[1] Dantzer, R; O'Connor, JC; Freund, GG; et al. From inflammation to sickness and depression: when the immune system subjugates the brain. *Nat Rev Neurosci.*, 2008, 9(1), 46-56.

[2] Sprung, CL; Peduzzi, PN; Shatney, CH; et al. Impact of encephalopathy on mortality in the sepsis syndrome. The Veterans Administration Systemic Sepsis Cooperative Study Group. *Crit Care Med.*, 1990, 18(8), 801-806.

[3] Zampieri, FG; Park, M; Machado, FS; Azevedo, LC. Sepsis-associated encephalopathy: not just delirium. *Clinics (Sao Paulo)*, 2011, 66(10), 1825-1831.

[4] Hopkins, RO; Weaver, LK; Chan, KJ; Orme, JF Jr. Quality of life, emotional, and cognitive function following acute respiratory distress syndrome. *J Int Neuropsychol Soc.*, 2004, 10(7), 1005-1017.

[5] Iwashyna, TJ; Ely, EW; Smith, DM; Langa, KM. Long-term cognitive impairment and functional disability among survivors of severe sepsis. *JAMA.*, 2010, 304(16), 1787-1794.

[6] Lamar, CD; Hurley, RA; Taber, KH. Sepsis-associated encephalopathy: review of the neuropsychiatric manifestations and cognitive outcome. *J Neuropsychiatry Clin Neurosci.*, 2011, 23(3), 237-241.

[7] Iwashyna, TJ; Cooke, CR; Wunsch, H; Kahn, JM. Population burden of long-term survivorship after severe sepsis in older Americans. *J Am Geriatr Soc.*, 2012, 60(6), 1070-1077.

[8] Stahl, O; Löffler, B; Haier, J; et al. Mimicry of human sepsis in a rat model--prospects and limitations. *J Surg Res.*, 2013, 179(1), e167-175.

[9] Bsibsi, M; Ravid, R; Gveric, D; van Noort, JM. Broad expression of Toll-like receptors in the human central nervous system. *J Neuropathol Exp Neurol.*, 2002, 61(11), 1013-1021.

[10] Rolls, A; Shechter, R; London, A; et al. Toll-like receptors modulate adult hippocampal neurogenesis. *Nat Cell Biol.*, 2007, 9(9), 1081-1088.

[11] Tang, SC; Arumugam, TV; Xu, X; et al. Pivotal role for neuronal Toll-like receptors in ischemic brain injury and functional deficits. *Proc Natl Acad Sci U S A.*, 2007, 104(34), 13798-13803.

[12] Mallard, C. Innate immune regulation by toll-like receptors in the brain. *ISRN Neurol.*, 2012, 2012, 701950.

[13] da Silva Correia, J; Soldau, K; Christen, U; et al. Lipopolysaccharide is in close proximity to each of the proteins in its membrane receptor

complex. transfer from CD14 to TLR4 and MD-2. *J Biol Chem.*, 2001, 276(24), 21129-21135.

[14] Dantzer, R. Cytokine, sickness behavior, and depression. *Immunol Allergy Clin North Am.*, 2009, 29(2), 247-264.

[15] Galea, I; Felton, LM; Waters, S; et al. Immune-to-brain signalling: The role of cerebral CD163-positive macrophages. *Neurosci Lett.*, 2008, 448(1), 41-46.

[16] Banks, WA; Robinson, SM. Minimal penetration of lipopolysaccharide across the murine blood-brain barrier. *Brain Behav Immun.*, 2010, 24(1), 102-109.

[17] Chakravarty, S; Herkenham, M. Toll-like receptor 4 on nonhematopoietic cells sustains CNS inflammation during endotoxemia, independent of systemic cytokines. *J Neurosci.*, 2005, 25(7), 1788-1796.

[18] Chen, Z; Jalabi, W; Shpargel, KB; et al. Lipopolysaccharide-induced microglial activation and neuroprotection against experimental brain injury is independent of hematogenous TLR4. *J Neurosci.*, 2012, 32(34), 11706-11715.

[19] Pan, W; Kastin, AJ. Interactions of cytokines with the blood-brain barrier: implications for feeding. *Curr Pharm Des.*, 2003, 9(10), 827-831.

[20] Murray, CL; Skelly, DT; Cunningham, C. Exacerbation of CNS inflammation and neurodegeneration by systemic LPS treatment is independent of circulating IL-1β and IL-6. *J Neuroinflammation.*, 2011, 8, 50.

[21] Czapski, GA; Cakała, M; Kopczuk, D; et al. Inhibition of nitric oxide synthase prevents energy failure and oxidative damage evoked in the brain by lipopolysaccharide. *Pol J Pharmacol.*, 2004, 56(5), 643-646.

[22] Czapski, GA; Cakala, M; Gajkowska, B; Strosznajder, JB. Poly(ADP-ribose) polymerase-1 inhibition protects the brain against systemic inflammation. *Neurochem Int.*, 2006, 49(8), 751-755.

[23] Czapski, GA; Cakała, M; Kopczuk, D; et al. Inhibition of nitric oxide synthase prevents energy failure and oxidative damage evoked in the brain by lipopolysaccharide. *Pol J Pharmacol.*, 2004, 56(5), 643-646.

[24] Czapski, GA; Gajkowska, B; Strosznajder, JB. Systemic administration of lipopolysaccharide induces molecular and morphological alterations in the hippocampus. *Brain Res.*, 2010, 1356, 85-94.

[25] Czapski, GA; Adamczyk, A; Strosznajder, RP; Strosznajder, JB. Expression and activity of PARP family members in the hippocampus

during systemic inflammation: their role in the regulation of prooxidative genes. *Neurochem Int.*, 2013, 62(5), 664-673.

[26] Jacewicz, M; Czapski, GA; Katkowska, I; Strosznajder, RP. Systemic administration of lipopolysaccharide impairs glutathione redox state and object recognition in male mice. The effect of PARP-1 inhibitor. *Folia Neuropathol.*, 2009, 47(4), 321-328.

[27] Hauss-Wegrzyniak, B; Dobrzanski, P; Stoehr, JD; Wenk, GL. Chronic neuroinflammation in rats reproduces components of the neurobiology of Alzheimer's disease. *Brain Res.*, 1998, 780(2), 294-303.

[28] Lynch, MA. Interleukin-1 beta exerts a myriad of effects in the brain and in particular in the hippocampus: analysis of some of these actions. *Vitam Horm.*, 2002, 64, 185-219.

[29] Semmler, A; Okulla, T; Sastre, M; et al. Systemic inflammation induces apoptosis with variable vulnerability of different brain regions. *J Chem Neuroanat.*, 2005, 30(2-3), 144-157.

[30] Semmler, A; Hermann, S; Mormann, F; et al. Sepsis causes neuroinflammation and concomitant decrease of cerebral metabolism. *J Neuroinflammation.*, 2008, 5, 38.

[31] Young, GB; Bolton, CF; Austin, TW; et al. The encephalopathy associated with septic illness. *Clin Invest Med.*, 1990, 13(6), 297-304.

[32] Layé, S; Parnet, P; Goujon, E; Dantzer, R. Peripheral administration of lipopolysaccharide induces the expression of cytokine transcripts in the brain and pituitary of mice. *Brain Res Mol Brain Res.*, 1994, 27(1), 157-162.

[33] Layé, S; Bluthé, RM; Kent, S; et al. Subdiaphragmatic vagotomy blocks induction of IL-1 beta mRNA in mice brain in response to peripheral LPS. *Am J Physiol.*, 1995, 268(5 Pt 2), R1327-1331.

[34] Hansen, MK; Nguyen, KT; Goehler, LE; et al. Effects of vagotomy on lipopolysaccharide-induced brain interleukin-1beta protein in rats. *Auton Neurosci.*, 2000, 85(1-3), 119-126.

[35] Dantzer, R; Bluthé, RM; Gheusi, G; et al. Molecular basis of sickness behavior. *Ann N Y Acad Sci.*, 1998, 856, 132-138.

[36] Won, JS; Im, YB; Khan, M; et al. Involvement of phospholipase A2 and lipoxygenase in lipopolysaccharide-induced inducible nitric oxide synthase expression in glial cells. *Glia.*, 2005, 51(1), 13-21.

[37] Dal-Pizzol, F; Ritter, C; Cassol-Jr, OJ; et al. Oxidative mechanisms of brain dysfunction during sepsis. *Neurochem Res.*, 2010, 35(1), 1-12.

[38] Halliwell, B. Oxidative stress and neurodegeneration: Where are we now? *J Neurochem*, 2006, 97, 1634–1658.

[39] Steckert, AV; Comim, CM; Mina, F; et al. Late brain alterations in sepsis-survivor rats. *Synapse*, 2013, 67(11), 786-793.
[40] Hassa, PO; Haenni, SS; Elser, M; Hottiger, MO. Nuclear ADP-ribosylation reactions in mammalian cells: where are we today and where are we going? *Microbiol Mol Biol Rev.*, 2006, 70(3), 789-829.
[41] Zong, WX; Ditsworth, D; Bauer, DE; et al. Alkylating DNA damage stimulates a regulated form of necrotic cell death. *Genes Dev.*, 2004, 18(11), 1272-1282.
[42] Diaz-Hernandez, JI; Moncada, S; Bolaños, JP; Almeida, A. Poly(ADP-ribose) polymerase-1 protects neurons against apoptosis induced by oxidative stress. *Cell Death Differ.*, 2007, 14(6), 1211-1221.
[43] Siegel, C; McCullough, LD. NAD+ depletion or PAR polymer formation: which plays the role of executioner in ischaemic cell death? *Acta Physiol (Oxf)*, 2011, 203(1), 225-234.
[44] Yu, SW; Wang, H; Poitras, MF; et al. Mediation of poly(ADP-ribose) polymerase-1-dependent cell death by apoptosis-inducing factor. *Science*, 2002, 297(5579), 259-263.
[45] Yu, SW; Andrabi, SA; Wang, H; et al. Apoptosis-inducing factor mediates poly(ADP-ribose) (PAR) polymer-induced cell death. *Proc Natl Acad Sci U S A.*, 2006, 103(48), 18314-18319.
[46] Vahsen, N; Candé, C; Brière, JJ; et al. AIF deficiency compromises oxidative phosphorylation. *EMBO J.*, 2004, 23(23), 4679-4689.
[47] Sevrioukova, IF. Apoptosis-inducing factor: structure, function, and redox regulation. *Antioxid Redox Signal.*, 2011, 14(12), 2545-2579.
[48] Alano, CC; Garnier, P; Ying, W; et al. NAD+ depletion is necessary and sufficient for poly(ADP-ribose) polymerase-1-mediated neuronal death. *J Neurosci.*, 2010, 30(8), 2967-2978.
[49] Nolan, Y; Vereker, E; Lynch, AM; Lynch, MA. Evidence that lipopolysaccharide-induced cell death is mediated by accumulation of reactive oxygen species and activation of p38 in rat cortex and hippocampus. *Exp Neurol.*, 2003, 184(2), 794-804.
[50] Lee, JW; Lee, YK; Yuk, DY; Choi, DY; et al. Neuro-inflammation induced by lipopolysaccharide causes cognitive impairment through enhancement of beta-amyloid generation. *J Neuroinflammation.*, 2008, 5, 37.
[51] Strosznajder, RP; Gadamski, R ; Czapski, GA; et al. Poly(ADP-ribose) polymerase during reperfusion after transient forebrain ischemia: its role in brain edema and cell death. *J Mol Neurosci.*, 2003, 20(1), 61-72.

[52] Strosznajder, R; Gajkowska, B. Effect of 3-aminobenzamide on Bcl-2, Bax and AIF localization in hippocampal neurons altered by ischemia-reperfusion injury. the immunocytochemical study. *Acta Neurobiol Exp (Wars)*, 2006, 66(1), 15-22.
[53] Hamby, AM; Suh, SW; Kauppinen, TM; Swanson, RA. Use of a poly(ADP-ribose) polymerase inhibitor to suppress inflammation and neuronal death after cerebral ischemia-reperfusion. *Stroke*, 2007, 38(2 Suppl), 632-636.
[54] O'Callaghan, EK; Anderson, ST; Moynagh, PN; Coogan, AN. Long-lasting effects of sepsis on circadian rhythms in the mouse. *PLoS One*, 2012, 7(10), e47087.
[55] Weberpals, M; Hermes, M; Hermann, S; et al. NOS2 gene deficiency protects from sepsis-induced long-term cognitive deficits. *J Neurosci.*, 2009, 29(45), 14177-14184.
[56] d'Avila, JC; Santiago, AP; Amâncio, RT; et al. Sepsis induces brain mitochondrial dysfunction. *Crit Care Med.*, 2008, 36(6), 1925-1932.
[57] Richwine, AF; Parkin, AO; Buchanan, JB; et al. Architectural changes to CA1 pyramidal neurons in adult and aged mice after peripheral immune stimulation. *Psychoneuroendocrinology*, 2008, 33(10), 1369-1377.
[58] Arimoto, T; Bing, G. Up-regulation of inducible nitric oxide synthase in the substantia nigra by lipopolysaccharide causes microglial activation and neurodegeneration. *Neurobiol Dis.*, 2003, 12(1), 35-45.
[59] Milatovic, D; Zaja-Milatovic, S; Montine, KS; et al. Pharmacologic suppression of neuronal oxidative damage and dendritic degeneration following direct activation of glial innate immunity in mouse cerebrum. *J Neurochem.*, 2003, 87(6), 1518-1526.
[60] Chavan, SS; Huerta, PT; Robbiati, S; et al. HMGB1 mediates cognitive impairment in sepsis survivors. *Mol Med.*, 2012, 18, 930-937.
[61] Young, GB. Sparing brain damage in severe sepsis: a beginning. *Crit Care*, 2010, 14(3), 159.
[62] Sharshar, T; Annane, D; de la Grandmaison, GL; et al. The neuropathology of septic shock. *Brain Pathol.*, 2004, 14(1), 21-33.
[63] Sharshar, T; Gray, F; Poron, F; Raphael, JC; Gajdos, P; Annane, D. Multifocal necrotizing leukoencephalopathy in septic shock. *Crit Care Med.*, 2002, 30(10), 2371-2375.
[64] Nguyen, DN; Spapen, H; Su, F; et al. Elevated serum levels of S-100beta protein and neuron-specific enolase are associated with brain

injury in patients with severe sepsis and septic shock. *Crit Care Med.*, 2006, 34(7), 1967-1974.

[65] Piazza, O; Russo, E; Cotena, S; et al. Elevated S100B levels do not correlate with the severity of encephalopathy during sepsis. *Br J Anaesth.*, 2007, 99(4), 518-521.

[66] Amé, JC; Spenlehauer, C; de Murcia, G. The PARP superfamily. *Bioessays*, 2004, 26(8), 882-893.

[67] Otto, H; Reche, PA; Bazan, F; et al. In silico characterization of the family of PARP-like poly(ADP-ribosyl)transferases (pARTs). *BMC Genomics*, 2005, 6, 139.

[68] Pieper, AA; Blackshaw, S; Clements, EE; et al. Poly(ADP-ribosyl)ation basally activated by DNA strand breaks reflects glutamate-nitric oxide neurotransmission. *Proc Natl Acad Sci U S A*, 2000, 97(4), 1845-1850.

[69] Smith, S. The world according to PARP. *Trends Biochem Sci.*, 2001, 26, 174-179.

[70] Strosznajder, RP; Jesko, H; Adamczyk, A. Poly(ADP-ribose) polymerase-1 is a novel nuclear target for cholinergic receptor signaling in the hippocampus. *J Physiol Pharmacol.*, 2005, 56 Suppl 4, 209-213.

[71] Strosznajder, RP; Czubowicz, K; Jesko, H; Strosznajder, JB. Poly(ADP-ribose) metabolism in brain and its role in ischemia pathology. *Mol Neurobiol.*, 2010, 41(2-3), 187-196.

[72] Szabó, C. Poly(ADP-ribose) polymerase activation by reactive nitrogen species--relevance for the pathogenesis of inflammation. *Nitric Oxide*, 2006, 14(2), 169-179.

[73] Ba, X; Garg, NJ. Signaling mechanism of poly(ADP-ribose) polymerase-1 (PARP-1) in inflammatory diseases. *Am J Pathol.*, 2011, 178(3), 946-955.

[74] Chopra, A; Ferreira-Alves, DL; Sirois, P; Thirion, JP. Cloning of the guinea pig 5-lipoxygenase gene and nucleotide sequence of its promoter. *Biochem Biophys Res Commun.*, 1992, 185(2), 489-495.

[75] Arakawa, T; Nakamura, M; Yoshimoto, T; Yamamoto, S. The transcriptional regulation of human arachidonate 12-lipoxygenase gene by NF kappa B/Rel. *FEBS Lett.*, 1995, 363(1-2), 105-110.

[76] Yamamoto, S; Yamamoto, K; Kurobe, H; Yamashita, R; Yamaguchi, H; Ueda, N. Transcriptional regulation of fatty acid cyclooxygenases-1 and -2. *Int J Tissue React.*, 1998, 20(1), 17-22

[77] Oliver, FJ; Ménissier-de Murcia, J; Nacci, C; Decker, P; Andriantsitohaina, R; Muller, S; de la Rubia, G; Stoclet, JC; de Murcia, G. Resistance to endotoxic shock as a consequence of defective NF-

kappaB activation in poly (ADP-ribose) polymerase-1 deficient mice. *EMBO J.*, 1999, 18(16), 4446-4454.

[78] Hassa, PO; Covic, M; Hasan, S; et al. The enzymatic and DNA binding activity of PARP-1 are not required for NF-kappa B coactivator function. *J Biol Chem.*, 2001, 276(49), 45588-45597.

[79] Hassa, PO; Hottiger, MO. The functional role of poly(ADP-ribose)polymerase 1 as novel coactivator of NF-kappaB in inflammatory disorders. *Cell Mol Life Sci.*, 2002, 59(9), 1534-1553.

[80] Genovese, T; Mazzon, E; Muià, C; et al. Inhibitors of poly(ADP-ribose) polymerase modulate signal transduction pathways and secondary damage in experimental spinal cord trauma. *J Pharmacol Exp Ther.*, 2005, 312(2), 449-457.

[81] Geraets, L; Moonen, HJ; Brauers, K; et al. Flavone as PARP-1 inhibitor: its effect on lipopolysaccharide induced gene-expression. *Eur J Pharmacol.*, 2007, 573(1-3), 241-8.

[82] Le Page, C; Sanceau, J; Drapier, JC; Wietzerbin, J. Inhibitors of ADP-ribosylation impair inducible nitric oxide synthase gene transcription through inhibition of NF kappa B activation. *Biochem Biophys Res Commun.*, 1998, 243(2), 451-457.

[83] Olszanecki, R; Gebska, A; Jawień, J; et al. Inhibition of NOS-2 induction in LPS-stimulated J774.2 cells by 1, 5-isoquinolinediol, an inhibitor of PARP. *J Physiol Pharmacol.*, 2006, 57(1), 109-117.

[84] Veres, B; Gallyas, F; Jr. Varbiro, G; et al. Decrease of the inflammatory response and induction of the Akt/protein kinase B pathway by poly-(ADP-ribose) polymerase 1 inhibitor in endotoxin-induced septic shock. *Biochem Pharmacol.*, 2003, 65(8), 1373-1382.

[85] Veres, B; Radnai, B; Gallyas, F; Jr. et al. Regulation of kinase cascades and transcription factors by a poly(ADP-ribose) polymerase-1 inhibitor, 4-hydroxyquinazoline, in lipopolysaccharide-induced inflammation in mice. *J Pharmacol Exp Ther.*, 2004, 310(1), 247-255.

[86] Buss, H; Dörrie, A; Schmitz, ML; et al. Phosphorylation of serine 468 by GSK-3beta negatively regulates basal p65 NF-kappaB activity. *J Biol Chem.*, 2004, 279(48), 49571-49574.

[87] Demarchi, F; Bertoli, C; Sandy, P; Schneider, C. Glycogen synthase kinase-3 beta regulates NF-kappa B1/p105 stability. *J Biol Chem.*, 2003, 278(41), 39583-39590

[88] Songin, M; Jeśko, H; Czapski, G; et al. GSK-3beta and oxidative stress in aged brain. Role of poly(ADP- -ribose) polymerase-1. *Folia Neuropathol.*, 2007, 45(4), 220-229.

[89] Kraus, WL. Transcriptional control by PARP-1: chromatin modulation, enhancer-binding, coregulation, and insulation. *Curr. Opin. Cell Biol.*, 2008, 20, 294-302.
[90] Oei, SL; Shi, Y. Poly(ADP-ribosyl)ation of transcription factor Yin Yang 1 under conditions of DNA damage. *Biochem Biophys Res Commun.*, 2001, 285(1), 27-31.
[91] Pleschke, JM; Kleczkowska, HE; Strohm, M; Althaus, FR. Poly(ADP-ribose) binds to specific domains in DNA damage checkpoint proteins. *J Biol Chem.*, 2000, 275(52), 40974-40980.
[92] Smith, HM; Grosovsky, AJ. PolyADP-ribose-mediated regulation of p53 complexed with topoisomerase I following ionizing radiation. *Carcinogenesis*, 1999, 20(8), 1439-1443.
[93] Hassa, PO; Hottiger, MO. The diverse biological roles of mammalian PARPS, a small but powerful family of poly-ADP-ribose polymerases. *Front Biosci.*, 2008, 13, 3046-3082.
[94] Phulwani, NK; Kielian, T. Poly (ADP-ribose) polymerases (PARPs) 1-3 regulate astrocyte activation. *J Neurochem.*, 2008, 106(2), 578-590.
[95] Boehler, C; Gauthier, LR; Mortusewicz, O; et al. Poly(ADP-ribose) polymerase 3 (PARP3), a newcomer in cellular response to DNA damage and mitotic progression. *Proc Natl Acad Sci U S A*, 2011, 108(7), 2783-2788.
[96] de la Lastra, CA; Villegas, I; Sánchez-Fidalgo, S. Poly(ADP-ribose) polymerase inhibitors: new pharmacological functions and potential clinical implications. *Curr Pharm Des.*, 2007, 13(9), 933-962.
[97] Rouleau, M; McDonald, D; Gagné, P; et al. PARP-3 associates with polycomb group bodies and with components of the DNA damage repair machinery. *J Cell Biochem.*, 2007, 100(2), 385-401.
[98] Rulten, SL; Fisher, AE; Robert, I; et al. PARP-3 and APLF function together to accelerate nonhomologous end-joining. *Mol Cell*, 2011, 41(1), 33-45.
[99] Pines, A; Mullenders, LH; van Attikum, H; Luijsterburg, MS. Touching base with PARPs: moonlighting in the repair of UV lesions and double-strand breaks. *Trends Biochem Sci.*, 2013, 38(6), 321-330.
[100] Loseva, O; Jemth, AS; Bryant, HE; et al. PARP-3 is a mono-ADP-ribosylase that activates PARP-1 in the absence of DNA. *J Biol Chem.*, 2010, 285(11), 8054-8060.
[101] A Angelov, D; Molla, A; Perche, PY; et al. The histone variant macroH2A interferes with transcription factor binding and SWI/SNF nucleosome remodeling. *Mol Cell*, 2003, 11(4), 1033-1041.

[102] Nusinow, DA; Hernández-Muñoz, I; Fazzio, TG; et al. Poly(ADP-ribose) polymerase 1 is inhibited by a histone H2A variant, MacroH2A, and contributes to silencing of the inactive X chromosome. *J Biol Chem.*, 2007, 282(17), 12851-91285.

[103] Ouararhni, K; Hadj-Slimane, R; Ait-Si-Ali, S; et al. The histone variant mH2A1.1 interferes with transcription by down-regulating PARP-1 enzymatic activity. *Genes Dev.*, 2006, 20(23), 3324-3336.

[104] Suzuki, K; Nakajima, H; Ikeda, K; et al. IL-4-Stat6 signaling induces tristetraprolin expression and inhibits TNF-alpha production in mast cells. *J Exp Med.*, 2003, 198(11), 1717-1727.

[105] Juszczynski, P; Kutok, JL; Li, C; Mitra, J; et al. BAL1 and BBAP are regulated by a gamma interferon-responsive bidirectional promoter and are overexpressed in diffuse large B-cell lymphomas with a prominent inflammatory infiltrate. *Mol Cell Biol.*, 2006, 26(14), 5348-5359.

[106] Mehrotra, P; Riley, JP; Patel, R; et al. PARP-14 functions as a transcriptional switch for Stat6-dependent gene activation. *J Biol Chem.*, 2011, 286(3), 1767-1776.

[107] Cho, SH; Ahn, AK; Bhargava, P; et al. Glycolytic rate and lymphomagenesis depend on PARP14, an ADP ribosyltransferase of the B aggressive lymphoma (BAL) family. *Proc Natl Acad Sci U S A*, 2011, 108(38), 15972-15977.

[108] Szabó, C. Role of poly(ADP-ribose)synthetase in inflammation. *Eur J Pharmacol.*, 1998, 350(1), 1-19.

[109] Giansanti, V; Donà, F; Tillhon, M; Scovassi, AI. PARP inhibitors: new tools to protect from inflammation. *Biochem Pharmacol.*, 2010, 80(12), 1869-1877.

[110] Soriano, FG; Liaudet, L; Szabó, E; et al. Resistance to acute septic peritonitis in poly(ADP-ribose) polymerase-1-deficient mice. *Shock*, 2002, 17(4), 286-292.

[111] Mabley, JG; Jagtap, P; Perretti, M; et al. Anti-inflammatory effects of a novel, potent inhibitor of poly (ADP-ribose) polymerase. *Inflamm Res.*, 2001, 50(11), 561-569.

[112] Tasatargil, A; Aksoy, NH; Dalaklioglu, S; Sadan, G. Poly (ADP-ribose) polymerase as a potential target for the treatment of acute renal injury caused by lipopolysaccharide. *Ren Fail*, 2008, 30(1), 115-120.

[113] Kang, X; Kim, HJ; Ramirez, M; Salameh, S; Ma, X. The septic shock-associated IL-10 -1082 A > G polymorphism mediates allele-specific transcription via poly(ADP-Ribose) polymerase 1 in macrophages engulfing apoptotic cells. *J Immunol*, 2010, 184(7), 3718-3724.

[114] Homburg, S; Visochek, L; Moran, N; et al. A fast signal-induced activation of Poly(ADP-ribose) polymerase: a novel downstream target of phospholipase c. *J Cell Biol.*, 2000, 150(2), 293-307.

[115] Hassa, PO; Haenni, SS; Buerki, C; et al. Acetylation of poly(ADP-ribose) polymerase-1 by p300/CREB-binding protein regulates coactivation of NF-kappaB-dependent transcription. *J Biol Chem.*, 2005, 280(49), 40450-40464.

[116] Messner, S; Schuermann, D; Altmeyer, M; et al. Sumoylation of poly(ADP-ribose) polymerase 1 inhibits its acetylation and restrains transcriptional coactivator function. *FASEB J.*, 2009, 23(11), 3978-3989.

[117] Martin, N; Schwamborn, K; Schreiber, V; et al. PARP-1 transcriptional activity is regulated by sumoylation upon heat shock. *EMBO J.*, 2009, 28(22), 3534-3548.

[118] Gagné, JP; Moreel, X; Gagné, P; et al. Proteomic investigation of phosphorylation sites in poly(ADP-ribose) polymerase-1 and poly(ADP-ribose) glycohydrolase. *J Proteome Res.*, 2009, 8(2), 1014-1029.

[119] Turner, NC; Lord, CJ; Iorns, E; et al. A synthetic lethal siRNA screen identifying genes mediating sensitivity to a PARP inhibitor. *EMBO J.*, 2008, 27(9), 1368-7137.

[120] Kauppinen, TM; Chan, WY; Suh, SW; et al. Direct phosphorylation and regulation of poly(ADP-ribose) polymerase-1 by extracellular signal-regulated kinases 1/2. *Proc Natl Acad Sci U S A*, 2006, 103(18), 7136-7141.

[121] Zhang, S; Lin, Y; Kim, YS; et al. c-Jun N-terminal kinase mediates hydrogen peroxide-induced cell death via sustained poly(ADP-ribose) polymerase-1 activation. *Cell Death Differ*, 2007, 14(5), 1001-1010.

[122] Du, J; Wei, N; Guan, T; et al. Inhibition of CDKS by roscovitine suppressed LPS-induced *NO production through inhibiting NFkappaB activation and BH4 biosynthesis in macrophages. *Am J Physiol Cell Physiol.*, 2009, 297(3), C742-749.

[123] Arif, A; Jia, J; Moodt, RA; et al. Phosphorylation of glutamyl-prolyl tRNA synthetase by cyclin-dependent kinase 5 dictates transcript-selective translational control. *Proc Natl Acad Sci U S A*, 2011, 108(4), 1415-1420.

[124] Bolin, C; Boudra, MT; Fernet, M; et al. The impact of cyclin-dependent kinase 5 depletion on poly(ADP-ribose) polymerase activity and responses to radiation. *Cell Mol Life Sci.*, 2012, 69(6), 951-962.

In: Neuro-Immune Interactions …
Editor: Oscar González-Pérez
ISBN: 978-1-62948-646-8

Chapter 3

Contribution of the Nervous System in the Pathogenesis and Morbidity in Rheumatoid Arthritis

Cesar Ramos-Remus[1,2]* and Jose Dionisio Castillo-Ortiz[1]

[1]Unidad de Investigación en Enfermedades Crónico-Degenerativas. Guadalajara, México

[2]Hospital General Regional 45, Instituto Mexicano del Seguro Social, Guadalajara, México

Abstract

The nervous system participates not only in the pathogenesis of RA, but it may also be damaged by the disease itself or its treatment, and produce a myriad of neurologic symptoms and signs ranging from numbness in a hand to sudden death. Nervous system involvement is associated with significant morbidity, may indicate heightened disease activity, and in some cases, reduced life span. Central and peripheral neurologic manifestations may arise from structural damage produced by RA in diarthroidal joints, by the systemic inflammatory process of the disease itself or by the drugs used to treat it. Neurologic syndromes may appear suddenly or developed slowly through months, and emerge early

* Corresponding author: Cesar Ramos-Remus, MD, Colomos 2292, Providencia, Guadalajara, 44620 Mexico, Email: rramos@cencar.udg.mx, Ph: +52 33 3817 0562, Fax: +52 33 3817 6335.

or after years of having RA. Neurologic manifestations may be easily overlooked or incorrectly assigned to peripheral arthritis unless the attending physician is aware of these complications. In this article, we review the contribution of the nervous system in the pathogenesis and morbidity in RA.

Keywords: Rheumatoid arthritis, entrapment neuropathies, compression neuropathies, dysautonomia, noncompressive neuropathies, drug toxicity

ACRONYMS LIST

RA	Rheumatoid Arthritis
SNS	Sympathetic Nervous System
IL	Interleukin
TNF	Tumor Necrosis Factor
Th	T helper
CNS	Central Nervous System
NP	Neuropsychiatric
SLE	Systemic lupus erythematosus
PNS	Peripheral Nervous System
ANS	Autonomic Nervous System
CRP	C-reactive protein
AAS	Atlantoaxial subluxation
CT	Computed tomography
MRI	Magnetic resonance image
DAS-28	Disease activity score -28 joints-
CTS	Carpal tunnel syndrome
PIN	Posterior interosseous nerve
NSAIDs	Non-steroid anti-inflammatory drugs
MTX	Methotrexate
HCQ	Hydroxychloroquine
CQ	Chloroquine
DMARD	Disease modifying anti-rheumatic drugs
CsA	Cyclosporin A
MS	Multiple Sclerosis
FDA	Food and Drug Administration
PML	Progressive multifocal leucoencephalopathy
JCV	JC Polyomavirus

INTRODUCTION

Even though the clinical hallmark is arthritis, rheumatoid arthritis (RA) is a complex systemic disorder where the inflammatory process may persist active for decades [1] with a deleterious impact in every aspects of the daily living to the patient and family, and important societal costs [2]. The nervous system participates not only in the pathogenesis of RA, but it may also be damaged by the disease itself or its treatment, and produce a myriad of neurologic features involving both the central and peripheral nervous system, and it is associated with significant morbidity and may indicate heightened disease activity.

Table 1. Neurological Syndromes Associated with Rheumatoid Arthritis

	Neurologic syndromes	Assigned Causes
Central nervous system	Cervical myelopathy Meningitis, focal neurological dysfunction, optic atrophy	Atlantoaxial subluxation Subaxial subluxation Vasculitis, rheumatoid nodules
Peripheral nervous system	Mononeuritis multiplex Distal symmetric sensory neuropathy Sensorimotor neuropathy Carpal tunnel syndrome Posterior interosseous nerve palsy Cubital tunnel syndrome Compression of radial nerve Tarsal tunnel syndrome Morton's neuroma	Vasculitis Unknown Unknown, Vasculitis? Compression neuropathies, local joint changes
Autonomic nervous system dysfunction	Diverse, related to dysautonomia	Unknown
Drug-related neurologic manifestations	Diverse, central and peripheral neurologic syndromes	Glucocorticoids NSAIDs* Methotrexate Antimalarials Sulphasalazine Leflunomide Penicillamine Gold salts Cyclosporin Anti-TNF† agents Rituximab

* NSAIDs, Non-Steroid Anti-inflammatory Drugs; †Anti-TNF, Anti-Tumor Necrosis Factor.

We review here the some aspects the nervous system participation in the pathogenesis of RA, and the neurologic manifestations associated with RA or its treatment (table 1) with emphasis on clinical manifestations and strategies for early detection.

Nervous System Participation in the Pathogenesis of RA

It is known that the nervous system has multiple anatomical and physiological connections with the immune system using neurotransmitters, cytokines and endocrine hormones [3]. Therefore, the nervous system is able to detect and regulate inflammation in peripheral tissues and is involved in maintaining immune homeostasis. Clinical observations published decades ago supported the concept that there are an interactions between the nervous system and inflammation not only in RA, but also other arthritis and are even in Heberden's node. For instance, it has been observed that hemiplegic patients who develop RA, psoriatic arthritis or Heberden's node do not develop arthritis or nodes on their hemiplegic (denervated) side [4,5].

The regulatory function of the sympathetic nervous system (SNS) includes monitoring and influencing immune homeostasis. During an immune response, peripherally secreted pro-inflammatory cytokines, such as interleukin (IL)-1, IL-6 and tumor necrosis factor (TNF)-alpha can signal to the brain, resulting in central activation of the SNS, which in turn, stimulates catecholamine production in the different lymphoid organs. Most evidence points toward the fact that SNS activity is able to inhibit the development of a T helper (Th)1 immune response and shift the Th1/Th2 balance toward a Th2 immune response. The SNS is involved in the regulation of leukocyte trafficking to sites of inflammation [6]. The number of sympathetic nerve fibers in the joitns of RA patients is reduced significantly, coinciding with an increased degree of inflammation, but also with more substance P –positive nerve fibers and augmented norepinephrine production by synovial cells [6]. In longstanding RA, a marked loss of sympathetic nerve fibers can be found, but the synovial tissue itself has a role in producing norepinephrine [7].

The synovium in RA is richly innervated with somatic afferent fibers, C-fibers that detect pain, and sympathetic neurons. In addition to providing information to the central nervous system (CNS) on the state of the synovium, peripheral nerves profoundly influence synovial inflammatory responses. For instance, neuropeptides such as substance P and vasoactive intestinal peptide can activate macrophages, increase vascular permeability, and modulate T cell phenotype. Sympathetic fibers can enhance or suppress inflammation depending on the site and timing of stimulation by modulating adrenergic tone. Although vagal branches have not been detected, their primary neurotransmitter acetylcholine is detected in tissues and can suppress synoviocyte cytokine production through the α7 nicotinic receptor. Also spinal cord circuits can directly modulate synovial inflammation [8].

Neurological Involvement in RA Patients

Neurological involvement may produce a myriad of symptoms and signs that may remain undetected or mistakenly assigned to peripheral arthritis unless the attending physician is aware of these complications. Moreover, some neurological manifestations are related to the drugs used to treat RA patients [9]. The reported frequency of neurologic involvement in RA patients depends on the used definitions, diagnostic methods, studied population and settings. For instance, Hanly JG et al. reported that cumulative neuropsychiatric (NP) syndromes were more frequently found in RA patients than in systemic lupus erythematosus (SLE) when using ACR nomenclature and standard definitions for NP-SLE [10].

For clarity purposes, we divided our discussion on neurological involvement in four sections: a) central nervous system (CNS) manifestations; b) peripheral nervous system (PNS) symptoms and signs; c) dysfunction of the autonomic nervous system (ANS) and d) drug related neurology involvement.

Central Nervous System (CNS) Involvement in RA Patients

There are several CNS syndromes associated with RA, including cervical myelopathy, vasculitis, meningitis, optic atrophy, and rheumatoid nodules (table 1). The prevalence of cervical involvement among those with RA varies with the patient subset studied ranging from 4 to 61% [11,12], and cervical myelopathy from either atlantoaxial subluxation or subaxial subluxation is the most frequent CNS involvement found in RA patients. An increased risk of radiographic cervical involvement has been associated with the presence of either rheumatoid factor or an elevated C-reactive protein level [13,14].

Atlantoaxial Subluxation (AAS)

AAS has been classified as congenital, traumatic, or spontaneous. Spontaneous AAS usually occurs in association with an infectious or inflammatory process, and has been described as a complication of various rheumatic conditions [15-26], including RA [27-31]. In one recent study AAS was found in 21% of 165 consecutive RA patients [32]; in other 68.7% [33], and in other study combining standard radiography, CT-scan and MRI, AAS was found in 45% of the patients (anterior in 25%, lateral in 15%, and vertical or rotatory in 10% each) [34].

AAS in RA is explained by inflammation of the synovial tissue. AAS can occur anteriorly, posteriorly, vertically, laterally and/or rotationally. Anterior AAS is characterized by an increase in the atlas-dens interval on a plain radiograph taken in the neutral position or with the neck flexed. There is no agreement on the definition of the minimal distance required to diagnose anterior AAS, but commonly a distance of more than 3 mm after the age of 44 and more than 4 mm in younger people should be considered [28], yet other definitions has been also proposed [35-38]. By other hand, Boden et al. found that the distance between the posterior margin of the odontoid and the anterior rim of the posterior arch of C1 (posterior atlas-odontoid interval) had stronger correlation with the risk of neurological compromise than the atlas-odontoid interval; all of their rheumatoid arthritis patients whose posterior atlas-odontoid interval was smaller than 14 mm had neurological abnormalities [39], and surgery should be considered promptly in these cases [40].

Superior migration of the odontoid process, or vertical AAS, is better assessed in lateral films taken in neutral position. Several measurements has been used to determine it, including Chamberlain's line, McRae's line, McGregor's line, Ranawat's method, Redlund's method and Sakaguchi-Kauppi method (reviewed in [41]). McRae and McGregor's lines may be both less sensitive if the apex of the odontoid is eroded. If the apex of the odontoid cannot be identified, these methods cannot be used. Ranawat's method has not gained wide acceptance because the radiological landmarks are difficult to define. Redlund's method is based on measurements of the distance from the endplate of the axis to the McGregor's line. Although these landmarks are easy to find and this is a good method to follow-up vertical AAS, unfortunately it is not satisfactory for screening because results depend on the height of the axis which has a wide distribution in healthy individuals [42]. For screening proposes we use the Sakaguchi-Kauppi method [41]; vertical AAS is diagnosed when the atlas falls around the axis; it is categorized into grades II, III, or IV [41].

AAS may produce a myriad of symptoms and signs that may range from neck pain on motion and occipital headache, to a broad range of neurologic or vascular manifestations, such as weakness (including quadriparesis), sphincter dysfunction, sensory deficits, pathologic reflexes, lower cranial nerve palsies, transient ischemic attacks with fluctuations of blood pressure and breathing. When is severe the clinical picture of AAS is characteristic, but in less severe degrees of displacement when the diagnosis is not to obvious, symptoms including those due to neurological changes may remain unexplained or mistakenly assigned to side effects of drugs or as a part of peripheral arthritis, unless this complication is considered. However, AAS may be present with no symptoms, so it is advisable to properly assess C1-2 stability in every patient with RA before undergoes surgical procedures to avoid damage to cervical cord or brainstem during intubation or as the patient is transferred while asleep [43,44].

Subaxial Subluxation

Translational displacement may occur at subaxial levels. It is named subaxial subluxation and may produce also pain, radicular pain, and myelopathy. Subaxial subluxation may be developed spontaneously or associated with AAS in approximately 10% [33,45] to 43% [32] of RA patients or as a complication after atlantoaxial transarticular screw fixation for AAS. In this last scenario, the increase of the atlantoaxial angle at the operation can lead to a decrease in the C2-C7 angle, followed by anterior subluxation of the upper cervical spine and possibly neurological deterioration [46,47].

Miscellaneous Conditions

There are rare conditions affecting CNS that may developed in RA patients, including vasculitis presenting with headache and gait disorders [48], meningitis and arteritis presenting with headaches, spells of focal neurological dysfunction and optic atrophy [49-52], and rheumatoid nodule formation [52]. Other unusual conditions reported in RA patients are aseptic pachymeningitis presented with aphasia and convulsions [53], normal pressure hydrocephalus with impaired mental status, urinary control and gait [54], cranial pachymeningitis with headache, hemiparesis, aphasia and confusion [55], and rheumatoid leptomeningitis with emotional lability, fever and myoclonic seizure [56].

Peripheral Neurologic Manifestations

Involvement of the peripheral nervous system is common in RA. Clinical neuropathy occurs in up to 20% of RA patients [57-60] and presents in the form of entrapment neuropathies, mononeuritis multiplex, distal sensory neuropathy and sensori-motor neuropathy [61] (table 1). Subclinical neuropathy has been reported to be prevalent in 65 to 85% of the RA patients [62,63]

Pallis et., described five patterns of peripheral neuropathy: a) upper limbs: major peripheral nerves (ulnar, median, terminal branches), b) upper limbs: digital neuropathy, with sensory symptoms, numbness, affecting one or more digits, c) lower limbs: major peripheral nerves, affecting lateral-popliteal nerve palsies, with symptoms of motor and sensory disturbances, d) lower limbs: producing distal numbness, affecting toes and variable proportions of the foot, with loss of vibration sense and abnormalities of the reflex pattern, and e) distal sensori-motor polyneuropathy of upper and lower limbs, presenting with symmetrical affection resembled polyneuritis of infective or toxic origin [60]. Nevertheless, peripheral neuropathy is divided in two groups: those with non-compressive affection and those with compressive symptoms and characteristic changes in electrophysiology.

Non-Compressive Neuropathies

Non-compressive neuropathies in RA patients may be asymptomatic in the early stages of the disease or may present with a variety of symptoms including pain, parenthesisparesthesia, and muscle weakness. These symptoms may mimic or overlap with those of arthritis. Yet the presence of non-compressive neuropathies increases the morbidity in RA patients [64].

Non-compressive neuropathies include mononeuritis multiplex and distal symmetric sensory or sensorimotor neuropathy [65]. Mononeuritis multiplex is a painful asymmetric asynchronous sensory and motor peripheral neuropathy involving isolated damage of at least two separate nerve areas [66,67]. It results from necrotizing or occlusive vasculitis of the vasa nervorum producing axonal degeneration [62,68]. The most common manifestations are foot and wrist drop [69,70]. Mononeuritis multiplex occurring in a patient with longstanding RA is considered diagnostic of systemic vVasculitis [64].

Primarily sensory neuropathy may present as axonal degeneration and demyelinization that affects the lower extremities in a symmetrical way. It is characterized by paresthesias, numbness, burning pain, and sometimes motor deficits. Electromyography can be used to confirm the neuropathy, but in doubtful cases a sural nerve biopsy is indicated [57]. Recently, Bayarak et al. described that 10 out of 60 patients with RA had electrophysiologically changes compatible with polyneuropathy, the most common finding was mild symmetric sensoriomotor axonal polyneuropathy. RA disease duration and DAS-28 were associated with a four- and three-fold increase in the risk of polyneuropathy [71]. Vasculitis, especially of the epineurial and endoneural arteries, is observed in the sural nerve biopsy [72]. Alternatively, an indirect confirmation of the vasculitic origin of the neuropathy may be obtained by detecting vasculitis in other tissues, such as skin or skeletal muscle [64,73].

Necrotizing vasculitis is responsible for the different patterns of non-compressive neuropathies in RA. Most common findings in the involved peripheral nerve are: fibrinoid necrosis of the media with infiltration by polymorphonuclear leukocytes, eosinophils, and mononuclear cells; perivascular infiltration with mononuclear cells; intimal proliferation with minimal cellular infiltrates and fibrosis. All these changes lead to vessel ischemia and subsequent axonal degeneration and neuronal demyelination [68].

Compression Neuropathies

Compression (entrapment) neuropathies are often found with early disease and associated with local joint changes. Carpal tunnel syndrome (CTS) is the most frequently encountered compression neuropathy in RA patients; its frequency varies from 23% to 69% depending on the diagnosis methods [74]. Carpal tunnel is the anatomic space borderer posteriorly by the carpal bones and anteriorly by the transverse carpal ligament. Tenosynovitis of the flexor tendons of the fingers, which also travel within the tunnels, is the probable cause of median nerve compression in RA patients. Patients complain of pain and paresthesia in one or both hands. Pain has a burning or stinging quality and is made worse by repetitive activities of the hand and at night. Sensory symptoms are usually limited to the median nerve territory (thenar area and palmar aspects of first four digits) [75]. However, these symptoms may involve forearm, upper arm and even the shoulder due to Martin-Gruber anastomosis (median-to-ulnar crossover) [76].

Symptoms arising from CTS may start at any time during the course of RA, or even before RA is clinically evident. There are two commonly used provocative tests useful as screening for CTS. The Tinel´s sign, light percussion at the flexor wrist triggers a shower of paresthesias down the involved fingers, and the Phalen's test, where the patient is asked to hold the forearms horizontally allowing the hands to drop into complete flexion at the wrist for 60 seconds; paresthesias in the median territory indicate a positive response. Phalen´s test performs litter better, as it has a sensitivity of 64%, specificity of 75%, positive likelihood ratio of 2.54 and a negative likelihood ratio of 49% [77]. However, they may be found positive in asymptomatic individuals and in other local problems [78]. CTS may coexist with additional impingement(s) on the nerve, whether at the proximal forearm in the pronator syndrome or in the neck. Multiple compressions (double crush syndromes) are responsible for some of the treatment failures of carpal tunnel release. RA patients with suspected CTS should have image studies such as ultrasound or MRI, and electrodiagnostic testing before deciding conservative or surgical treatment.

There are few reports of posterior interosseous nerve (PIN) palsy, cubital tunnel syndrome and compression neuropathy of the deep branch of the radial nerve in RA patients. PIN palsy presents with inability to extend the fingers, whereas wrist extension is normal. The mechanism of nerve impingement is an anterior synovial bulge due to synovitis of the elbow joint [79]. Differential diagnosis of PIN includes extensor tendon rupture, metacarpophalangeal joint dislocation and cervical neuropathy [74]. Cubital (ulnar) nerve palsy results when the ulnar nerve is compressed at the medial elbow. An early complaint is waking up with paresthesias in the ulnar portion of the hand (4th and 5th digits). Symptoms are promptly relieved by extending the extremity. Sensory loss, weakness of intrinsic muscles, and muscle atrophy are markers of late disease [75]. Compression neuropathy of the deep branch of the radial nerve is a rare condition. Symptoms include shooting paresthesias up and down the course of the radial nerve for several days or weeks followed by paresis of extensor digitorum communis and extensor carpi ulnaris [75]. There is an inability to extend the index, long, ring, and little fingers. Wrist dorsiflexion is weak and results in dorsoradial deviation. This clinical picture may be confused as extensor tendon rupture. Passive flexion of the wrist by automatically extending the fingers (tenodesis effect) rules out tendon rupture.

RA patients may have major structural changes in the midfoot and foot due to combination of chronic synovitis and weight bearing. Tarsal tunnel syndrome and Morton's neuroma may develop in these patients. Tarsal tunnel syndrome refers to the entrapment of posterior tibial nerve resulting from tenosynovitis of the tibialis posterior, flexor digitorum longus, and flexor hallucis longus. It is characterized by dysesthetic pain in the toes, sole, and heel. Tinel sign posterior to the medial malleolus may be present [75]. Morton's neuroma is a tender thickening of the digital nerve between the third and fourth toes or the second and third toes, causes forefoot pain. Two finger compression (one dorsal and one plantar) at the symptomatic intermetatarsal space may suggest Morton's neuroma, and may be felt as a tender fusiform swelling under the plantar skin [75]. Clinical assessment may perform better than ultrasonography and MR imaging in the preoperative evaluation of Morton´s neuroma [80].

AUTONOMIC NERVOUS SYSTEM DYSFUNCTION:

The autonomic nervous system (ANS) includes nerves that regulate bodily functions; it comprised sympathetic and parasympathetic nerves. Symptoms associated with autonomic dysfunction are unspecific, with affection of different systems as cardiovascular, neurological, or gastrointestinal [81]. Autonomic nervous system dysfunction or dysautonomia has been reported in several non-rheumatic and rheumatic conditions. It is manifested by a variety of symptoms that may occur in isolation or in various combinations and related to abnormalities of blood pressure regulation, thermoregulatory-thermoregulation, gastroin-testinal function, sweating, sexual function, sphincter control, ocular function and respiration. The characteristic imbalances in autonomic nervous system in RA patients consists imbalance in autonomic nervous system in RA patients consists in a reduced parasympathetic and increased sympathetic tone;, these this autonomic dysfunction may be due to vasculitis of vasa vasorum and secondary amyloidosis [82]. It has been suggested that sympathoneural and adrenomedullary systems are impaired in patients with RA, as a consequence these patients may alter sympatic response to orthostasis [83].

The dysfunction of the autonomic nervous system in RA patients has been recognized for almost 50 years [46] [29]. Most of the reports are cross-sectional studies with small samples, using heterogeneous methods to assess it, and including patients with no specific neurologic symptoms. For instance, Bidkar et al., reported a sympatethic dysfunction in 26% in a RA patients using standard tests [84];, in accordance Evrengül H. et al. [85], showed an increased sympathetic activity in patients with RA using the time-domain frequency to assess heart rate variability, reporting an increased ratio between low and high frequencies in the spectral measurement. Although dysautonomia has been well characterized and associated with short-term mortality in diseases such as Diabetes Mellitus, its frequency, clinical features, pathogenic mechanisms, treatment and prognosis in RA patients remain largely unknown.

Drug Related Neurologic Involvement in RA Patients

A number of drugs used in RA patients are associated with a wide range of neurological side effects (Table 2). A full drug history, including the use of non-conventional remedies [86,87], is essential in any RA patients with a neurologic syndrome since drug-related neurological symptoms and signs may mimic and/or overlap RA associated neurological problems. Drug-related neurological manifestations may be as simple as a common headache or as complicated as progressive multifocal leucoencephalopathy. We present a review of the principal drugs used in the treatment of RA patients and the reported neurological effects.

Corticosteroids

It is well known that glucocorticoid drugs may produce psychiatric symptoms such as hypomania, mania, depression, mood disturbances, psychosis and cognitive dysfunction [88-910] [89-91]. While certain clinical groups may be at greater risk of corticosteroid-induced psychiatric effects, toxicity is remarkably unpredictable [91,92]. Although high levels of endogenous glucocorticoids secreted during prolonged stress may induce hippocampus atrophy [93,94], it is possible that glucocorticoid drugs may produce neuronal degeneration and reactive gliosis [95,96].

Table 2. Drug Related Neurologic Involvement in Rheumatoid Arthritis Patients

Drugs	Side-effects
Corticosteroids	Hypomania, mania, depression, and psychosis. Myopathy
NSAIDs*	Aseptic meningitis, psychosis, and cognitive dysfunction
Methotrexate	Headache and impaired ability to concentrate
Antimalarials	Retinopathy. Ototoxicity: sensorineural hearing loss, tinnitus, cochleovestibular manifestations. Headaches, lightheadedness. Myopathy
Sulphasalazine	Headache, peripheral neuropathy and vertigo
Leflunomide	Peripheral neuropathy and headache
Penicillamine	Myopathy
Gold salts	Peripheral neuropathy, Guillain-Barré-type syndrome, cranial nerve palsies, and encephalopathy
Cyclosporin A	Tremor and headache. Myopathy. Leukoencephalopathy, cerebellar syndrome, extrapyramidal syndrome, and pyramidal weakness
Anti-TNF†	Guillain-Barré syndrome, Miller Fisher syndrome, chronic inflammatory demyelinating polyneuropathy, multifocal motor neuropathy, mononeuropathy multiplex, and axonal sensorimotor polyneuropathies
Rituximab	Progressive multifocal leucoencephalopathy

* NSAIDs, Non-Steroid Anti-inflammatory Drugs; †Anti-TNF, Anti-Tumor Necrosis Factor.

Non-Steroid Anti-Inflammatory Drugs (NSAIDs)

These drugs may cause serious adverse events, including neurologic syndromes, such as aseptic meningitis, psychosis, and cognitive dysfunction [97-99]. Psychosis and cognitive impairment are more prevalent in elderly patients, particularly with the use of indomethacin. Aseptic meningitis seems to be more prevalent in patients with systemic lupus erythematosus but cases are reported in RA patients who are treated with ibuprofen [100]. High doses of salicylates have been associated with tinnitus [99], although it can occur with all of the available NSAIDs.

Methotrexate (MTX)

MTX associate neurological toxicity includes headache, fatigue, or impaired ability to concentrate. It has been suggested that the neurotoxicity of MTX may be related to the accumulation of adenosine due to the inhibition of purine synthesis [101]. Nonspecific neurological symptoms has been reported after low doses of MTX intake (loss of recent memory, homonymus hemianopsia, dysarthria, weakness of lower limbs).Yokoo H et al. [102], reported an autopsy of RA female patient who developed a rapidly progressing leukoencephalopathy during low-dose oral MTX. The autopsy revealed uninterrupted severe demyelinating, partially liquefactive necrosis-like in the white matter. Other rare complication, aseptic meningitis, has been reported in a RA patient using intramuscular MTX [103].

Antimalarials

Hydroxychloroquine (HCQ) and chloroquine (CQ) are used as disease modifying anti-rheumatic drugs (DMARD) in the treatment of RA; CQ is claimed to be more toxic than HCQ, although the evidence is scarce. HCQ and CQ may be more toxic in patients with renal and/or liver insufficiency; therefore these medications should be used with caution in patients with renal/liver failure.

Retinopathy is the most important ophthalmologic complication of antimalarial therapy. Antimalarials bind to melanin in the pigmented epithelial layer of the retina that may damage rods and cones and lead to permanent vision loss. The exact incidence of retinopathy is unknown but it probably occurs in about 3 to 4 percent of patients taking HCQ and up to 10 percent taking CQ after 10-years of use [104,105].

Both HCQ and CQ use has been also associated with ototoxicity [106,107]. Some reports have described sensorineural hearing loss, tinnitus, sense of imbalance, and cochleovestibular manifestations. CQ ototoxicity results from variable injuries such as decrease in neuronal cells, loss of supporting hair cells, and atrophy of stria vascularis [108]. Brain-evoked response audiometry seems to be the most sensitive test in detecting early manifestations of cochlear injury caused by CQ when still in a reversible stage [109]. The reversibility of CQ ototoxicity has been controversial, but it may reverse if the drug is stopped. Other manifestations are headaches, lightheadedness [110], insomnia, nervousness, psychosis and convulsions; the last two in the context of malaria treatment [111].

Myopathy is a rare complication of antimalarial drugs; one study estimated the incidence to be 1 in 100 patient-years [112]. HCQ causes a vacuolar myopathy that is usually of mild to moderate severity. HCQ neuromyotoxicity is a rare complication characterized by proximal muscle weakness, normal creatinine kinase levels, and characteristic ultrastructural changes on muscle biopsy of curvilinear body formation. Casado E et al. [113], evaluated the prevalence of antimalarial myopathy in a cohort of 119 patients with rheumatic diseases and found a higher prevalence of myopathy than previously recognized when muscle enzyme determination is used as a screening method.

Leflunomide

Cases of toxic neuropathy have been observed in RA patients treated with leflunomide. Richards et al. reported, in a cohort of RA patients, an association between the use of leflunomide with an increase in the clinical symptoms of peripheral neuropathy; electromyographic studies showed an axonal, predominantly sensory or sensorimotor, polyneuropathy [114]. Antonio-Valdiviezo A. et al. reported segmental demyelination polyneuropathy and retrograde axonal degeneration with predominance of the thoracic members in a patient with rheumatoid arthritis and diabetes mellitus treated with leflunomide [115]. Case reports suggest that early discontinuation (within 30 days of the onset of symptoms) is associated with a better outcome than stopping at a later time [116], and symptomatic improvement follows after discontinuation of the drug [117-119].

Gold Salts

Gold therapy is responsible for many neurological complications [120]. Diagnostic confusion may arise because the neuropathy induced by gold can resemble some features of rheumatoid neuropathy. Typical findings include peripheral neuropathy, a Guillain-Barré-type syndrome, cranial nerve palsies including ophthalmoplegia, and, in rare cases, encephalopathy [121]. Neurologic toxicity arises after three months of weekly injections; myokymia (irregular muscle twitching) is a characteristic clinical sign. Neurologic complications of gold therapy are rare and reversible. Petiot P et al. reported a case of neuromyotonia, polyradiculoneuritis and Morvan's fibrillary chorea [122].

Cyclosporin A (CsA)

CsA induces neurological side effects in up to 40% of patients. Most common side effects are tremor and headache. Neurotoxicity is more frequent with high CsA blood levels. Dose reduction or withdrawal of CsA usually results in resolution of clinical symptoms. Adverse reactions involving skeletal muscle are not uncommon, and sometimes myopathy may occur requiring discontinuation of the drug [123-125]. A reversible posterior leukoencephalopathy syndrome is the most serious complication [126]. Symptoms include headache, altered mental functioning, seizures, and cortical. Neuroimaging studies show white matter changes in the posterior regions of the brain. Other neurological side effects of CsA include cerebellar syndrome, extrapyramidal syndrome, and pyramidal weakness. Hypertension, hypomagnesemia, hypocholesteremia, and the vasoactive agent endothelin may all play a role in the pathogenesis of CsA neurotoxicty [127].

Anti-Tumor Necrosis Factor (TNF)-Alpha Agents

TNF-alpha antagonists such as infliximab, etanercept and adalimumab are indicated for the treatment of some RA patients. Anti-TNF drugs may produce increasing of autoimmunity as a consequence of blocking the normal effect of TNF in the immune response; it has been hypothesized that the inhibition of TNF impedes the normal repair process of TNF of the remyelination of neurons [128]. Since the approval of anti TNF agents for the treatment of AR patients, it has been reported several neurological side effects that may be grouped in four: a) exacerbation of Multiple Sclerosis (MS), b) new diagnosis of MS, c) acute mental state changes as encephalopathy, and d) miscellaneous neurological manifestations [129]. Case-reports and case-series report the association between anti-TNF-alpha treatment and various disorders such as Guillain-Barré syndrome (acute immune-mediated polyneuropathy characterized by progressive, symmetric muscle weakness accompanied by absent or depressed deep tendon reflexes), Miller Fisher syndrome (ophthalmoplegia with ataxia and areflexia), chronic inflammatory demyelinating polyneuropathy, multifocal motor neuropathy, mononeuropathy multiplex, progressive multifocal leukoencephalopathy [130] and axonal sensorimotor polyneuropathies [131-135]. Demyelinating disease´s symptoms included confusion, ataxia, dysesthesia and paresthesia [136].

The United States Food and Drug Administration (FDA) Adverse Events Reporting system found 17 cases of demyelinating disease that occurred in patients receiving etanercept from 1998 to 2000 [132] . During that time, 77,152 patients received etanercept therapy. The incidence of demyelinating disease reported was of 31 per 100,000 patients per year of exposure. This prevalence appears to be higher than in the general population (4 to 6 per 100,000 per year). The proposed pathogeneses of TNF-alpha-associated neuropathies include both a T-cell and humoral immune attack against peripheral nerve myelin, vasculitis-induced nerve ischemia, and inhibition of signaling support for axons. Most neuropathies improve over a period of months by withdrawal of the TNF-alpha antagonist, with or without additional immune-modulating treatment. Preliminary observations suggest that TNF-alpha antagonists may be useful as an antigen-nonspecific treatment approach to immune-mediated neuropathies but further studies are required.

Also, central nervous system is affected is through a cerebral tuberculoma described in a patient treated with adalimumab [137].

Rituximab

Rituximab has been recently licensed for RA patients failing initial TNF inhibitor therapy. Progressive multifocal leucoencephalopathy (PML) is a rare and often fatal opportunistic infection that has been well reported in patients with diverse rheumatic diseases. The predisposing factors such as underlying disease and immunosuppressive drug selection are incompletely understood but it would appear that patients with systemic lupus erythematosus (SLE) may be at highest risk [138]. On December 18th 2006, the FDA in conjunction with Genentech and BiogenIdec issued a warning to health care providers and consumers, informing that 2 patients receiving rituximab for the treatment of SLE (an unapproved indication) had developed PML [139]. Additionally, in September, 2008, a second letter was issued describing a patient with RA who died from PML 18 months after receiving rituximab, corticosteroids, and methotrexate therapy [140].

PML is a demyelinating disease of the CNS that occurs almost exclusively in immunosuppressed individuals. This disease is caused by a reactivation of the polyomavirus JC (JCV), usually manifests with subacute neurologic deficits including altered mental status, motor deficits (hemiparesis or monoparesis), limb ataxia, gait ataxia, and visual symptoms such as hemianopia and diplopia. Although PML lesions are located in the white matter, symptoms may be mistaken for a cortical disorder. Seizures are usually thought to be a manifestation of cortical injury rather than white matter disease, they occur in up to 18 percent of patients with PML [141].

Other drugs used in RA may also produce neurological symptoms. For instance sulphasalazine has been associated with headache in up to 30%, and in rare cases with peripheral neuropathy and vertigo [142]. D-Penicillamine myopathy has been observed in 1.2 percent of treated RA patients [143,144]. The development of myositis appears not been related to either dose or the duration of therapy [143,145]. Affected patients present with symmetric proximal muscle weakness, muscle enzymes are elevated, and muscle biopsy reveals perifasicular cellular infiltrates and muscle fiber necrosis and regeneration [145,146]. Muscle weakness resolves and muscle enzymes return to normal within a few weeks after stopping the drug but some cases require treatment with corticosteroids.

CONCLUSION

RA patients may develop several neurological syndromes, either by the structural damage to the joints, by the systemic inflammatory process of the disease itself, or as consequence of the drugs used to treat it. In some cases, neurological involvement is associated with high morbidity and even be life-threatening. Early assessment and a high index of suspicion for recognized complications are essential in managing such patients.

REFERENCES

[1] Ramos-Remus, C., Sierra-Jimenez, G., Skeith, K., Aceves-Avila, F. J., Russell, A. S., Offer, R., Olguin-Redes, J. E., Homik, J., Sanchez, L., Sanchez-Ortiz, A. & Navarro-Cano, G. (2007). Latitude gradient influences the age of onset in rheumatoid arthritis patients. *Clin Rheumatol*, *26* (10), 1725-1728. doi:10.1007/s10067-007-0666-2

[2] Badley, E. M. (2008). Rheumatic diseases, the unnoticed elephant in the room. *J Rheumatol*, *35* (1), 6-7

[3] Steinman, L. (2004). Elaborate interactions between the immune and nervous systems. *Nat Immunol*, *5* (6), 575-581. doi:10.1038/ni1078

[4] Thompson, M. & Bywaters, E. G. (1962). Unilateral rheumatoid arthritis following hemiplegia. *Ann Rheum Dis*, *21*, 370-377

[5] Francon, F. (1963). [Some recent work on Heberden's nodes with a personal case of limitation of the articular lesions to the healthy side in a spasmodic hemiplegic]. *Prog Med (Paris)*, *91*, 183-189

[6] Koopman, F. A., Stoof, S. P., Straub, R. H., Van Maanen, M. A., Vervoordeldonk, M. J. & Tak, P. P. (2011). Restoring the balance of the autonomic nervous system as an innovative approach to the treatment of rheumatoid arthritis. *Mol Med*, *17* (9-10), 937-948. doi:10.2119/molmed. 2011.00065

[7] Miller, L. E., Justen, H. P., Scholmerich, J. & Straub, R. H. (2000). The loss of sympathetic nerve fibers in the synovial tissue of patients with rheumatoid arthritis is accompanied by increased norepinephrine release from synovial macrophages. *Faseb J*, *14* (13), 2097-2107. doi:10.1096/ fj.99-1082com

[8] Firestein, G. S. (2012). *Etiology and Pathogenesis of Rheumatoid Arthritis*. In: Kelleys Textbbok of Rheumatology.

[9] Lee, D. M. & Weinblatt, M. E. (2001). Rheumatoid arthritis. *Lancet*, *358*, (9285), 903-911. doi:10.1016/S0140-6736(01)06075-5

[10] Hanly, J. G., Fisk, J. D., McCurdy, G., Fougere, L. & Douglas, J. A. (2005). Neuropsychiatric syndromes in patients with systemic lupus erythematosus and rheumatoid arthritis. *J Rheumatol*, *32* (8), 1459-1456

[11] Collins, D. N., Barnes, C. L. & FitzRandolph, R. L. (1991). Cervical spine instability in rheumatoid patients having total hip or knee arthroplasty. *Clin Orthop Relat Res*, *(272)*, 127-135

[12] Neva, M. H., Kaarela, K. & Kauppi, M. (2000). Prevalence of radiological changes in the cervical spine--a cross sectional study after 20 years from presentation of rheumatoid arthritis. *J Rheumatol*, *27* (1), 90-93

[13] Paimela, L., Laasonen, L., Kankaanpaa, E. & Leirisalo-Repo, M. (1997). Progression of cervical spine changes in patients with early rheumatoid arthritis. *J Rheumatol*, *24* (7), 1280-1284

[14] Fujiwara, K., Fujimoto, M., Owaki, H., Kono, J., Nakase, T., Yonenobu, K. & Ochi, T. (1998). Cervical lesions related to the systemic

progression in rheumatoid arthritis. *Spine (Phila Pa 1976)*, *23*(19), 2052-2056

[15] Babini, S. M., Cocco, J. A., Babini, J. C., de la Sota, M., Arturi, A. & Marcos, J. C. (1990). Atlantoaxial subluxation in systemic lupus erythematosus: further evidence of tendinous alterations. *J Rheumatol*, *17* (2), 173-177

[16] Stuart, R. A. & Maddison, P. J. (1991). Atlantoaxial subluxation in a patient with mixed connective tissue disease. *J Rheumatol*, *18* (10), 1617-1620

[17] Laiho, K. & Kauppi, M. (2002). The cervical spine in patients with psoriatic arthritis. *Ann Rheum Dis*, *61* (7), 650-652

[18] Fox, B., Sahuquillo, J., Poca, M. A., Huguet, P. & Lience, E. (1997). Reactive arthritis with a severe lesion of the cervical spine. *Br J Rheumatol*, *36* (1), 126-129

[19] Jordan, J. M., Obeid, L. M. & Allen, N. B. (1986). Isolated atlantoaxial subluxation as the presenting manifestation of inflammatory bowel disease. *Am J Med*, *80* (3), 517-520

[20] Daumen-Legre, V., Lafforgue, P., Champsaur, P., Chagnaud, C., Pham, T., Kasbarian, M. & Acquaviva, P. C. (1999). Anteroposterior atlantoaxial subluxation in cervical spine osteoarthritis, case reports and review of the literature. *J Rheumatol*, *26* (3), 687-691

[21] Takasita, M., Matsumoto, H., Uchinou, S., Tsumura, H. & Torisu, T. (2000). Atlantoaxial subluxation associated with ossification of posterior longitudinal ligament of the cervical spine. *Spine (Phila Pa 1976)*, *25* (16), 2133-2136

[22] Herzka, A., Sponseller, P. D. & Pyeritz, R. E. (2000). Atlantoaxial rotatory subluxation in patients with Marfan syndrome. A report of three cases. *Spine (Phila Pa 1976)*, *25*(4), 524-526

[23] Shewell, P. C. & Thompson, A. G. (1996). Atlantoaxial instability in Lesch-Nyhan syndrome. *Spine (Phila Pa 1976)*, *21* (6), 757-762

[24] Coutts, M. B. (1934). Atlanto-epistropheal subluxation. *Arch Surg*, *29*, 14

[25] Verdone, F. (1999). Anterior atlantoaxial subluxation in a patient with DISH. *J Rheumatol*, *26* (7), 1639-1640

[26] Koss, J. C. & Dalinka, M. K. (1980). Atlantoaxial subluxation in Behcet's syndrome. *AJR Am J Roentgenol*, *134* (2), 392-393. doi:10.2214/ ajr.134.2.392

[27] Bland, J. H. (1990). Rheumatoid subluxation of the cervical spine. *J Rheumatol*, *17* (2), 134-137

[28] Sharp, J. & Purser, D. W. (1961). Spontaneous Atlanto-Axial Dislocation in Ankylosing Spondylitis and Rheumatoid Arthritis. *Ann Rheum Dis*, *20* (1), 47-77

[29] Martel, W. (1961). The occipito-atlanto-axial joints in rheumatoid arthritis and ankylosing spondylitis. *Am J Roentgenol Radium Ther Nucl Med*, *86*, 223-240

[30] Castro, S., Verstraete, K., Mielants, H., Vanderstraeten, G., de Reuck, J. & Veys, E. M. (1994). Cervical spine involvement in rheumatoid arthritis, a clinical, neurological and radiological evaluation. *Clin Exp Rheumatol*, *12* (4), 369-374

[31] Komusi, T., Munro, T. & Harth, M. (1985). Radiologic review: the rheumatoid cervical spine. *Semin Arthritis Rheum*, *14* (3), 187-195

[32] Zikou, A. K., Alamanos, Y., Argyropoulou, M. I., Tsifetaki, N., Tsampoulas, C., Voulgari, P. V., Efremidis, S. C. & Drosos, A. A. (2005). Radiological cervical spine involvement in patients with rheumatoid arthritis, a cross sectional study. *J Rheumatol*, *32* (5), 801-806

[33] Pisitkun, P., Pattarowas, C., Siriwongpairat, P., Totemchokchyakarn, K., Nantiruj, K. & Janwityanujit, S. (2004). Reappraisal of cervical spine subluxation in Thai patients with rheumatoid arthritis. *Clin Rheumatol*, *23* (1), 14-18. doi:10.1007/s10067-003-0782-6

[34] Younes, M., Belghali, S., Kriaa, S., Zrour, S., Bejia, I., Touzi, M., Golli, M., Gannouni, A. & Bergaoui, N. (2009). Compared imaging of the rheumatoid cervical spine: prevalence study and associated factors. *Joint Bone Spine*, *76* (4), 361-368. doi:10.1016/j.jbspin.2008.10.010

[35] Jackson, H. (1950). The diagnosis of minimal atlanto-axial subluxation. *Br J Radiol*, *23* (275), 672-674

[36] Hinck, V. C. & Hopkins, C. E. (1960). Measurement of the atlanto-dental interval in the adult. *Am J Roentgenol Radium Ther Nucl Med*, *84*, 945-951

[37] Ramos-Remus, C., Gomez-Vargas, A., Guzman-Guzman, J. L., Jimenez-Gil, F., Gamez-Nava, J. I., Gonzalez-Lopez, L., Farrera-Gamboa, H., Maksymowych, W. P. & Suarez-Almazor, M. E. (1995). Frequency of atlantoaxial subluxation and neurologic involvement in patients with ankylosing spondylitis. *J Rheumatol*, *22* (11), 2120-2125

[38] Ramos-Remus, C., Gomez-Vargas, A., Hernandez-Chavez, A., Gamez-Nava, J. I., Gonzalez-Lopez, L. & Russell, A. S. (1997). Two year followup of anterior and vertical atlantoaxial subluxation in ankylosing spondylitis. *J Rheumatol*, *24* (3), 507-510

[39] Boden, S. D., Dodge, L. D., Bohlman, H. H. & Rechtine, G. R. (1993). Rheumatoid arthritis of the cervical spine. A long-term analysis with predictors of paralysis and recovery. *J Bone Joint Surg Am*, *75*(9), 1282-1297

[40] Kim, D. H. & Hilibrand, A. S. (2005). Rheumatoid arthritis in the cervical spine. *J Am Acad Orthop Surg*, *13* (7), 463-474

[41] Kauppi, M., Sakaguchi, M., Konttinen, Y. T. & Hamalainen, M. (1990). A new method of screening for vertical atlantoaxial dislocation. *J Rheumatol*, *17* (2), 167-172

[42] Eulderink, F. & Meijers, K. A. (1976). Pathology of the cervical spine in rheumatoid arthritis, a controlled study of 44 spines. *J Pathol*, *120*(2), 91-108. doi:10.1002/path.1711200205

[43] Neva, M. H., Hakkinen, A., Makinen, H., Hannonen, P., Kauppi, M. & Sokka, T. (2006). High prevalence of asymptomatic cervical spine subluxation in patients with rheumatoid arthritis waiting for orthopaedic surgery. *Ann Rheum Dis*, *65* (7), 884-888. doi:10.1136/ard.2005.042135

[44] Lopez-Olivo, M. A., Andrabi, P. R., Palla, S. L. & Suarez-Almazor, M. E. (20112). Use of cervical spine radiographs in patients with rheumatoid arthritis undergoing general anesthesia. J *Clin Rheumatol,18(2):61-6.* [In press]

[45] Zikou, A. K., Argyropoulou, M. I., Voulgari, P. V., Xydis, V. G., Nikas, S. N., Efremidis, S. C. & Drosos, A. A. (2006). Magnetic resonance imaging quantification of hand synovitis in patients with rheumatoid arthritis treated with adalimumab. *J Rheumatol*, *33* (2), 219-223

[46] Ito, H., Neo, M., Sakamoto, T., Fujibayashi, S., Yoshitomi, H. & Nakamura, T. (2009). Subaxial subluxation after atlantoaxial transarticular screw fixation in rheumatoid patients. *Eur Spine J*, *18* (6), 869-876. doi:10.1007/s00586-009-0945-5

[47] Mukai, Y., Hosono, N., Sakaura, H., Fujii, R., Iwasaki, M., Fuchiya, T., Fujiwara, K., Fuji, T. & Yoshikawa, H. (2007). Sagittal alignment of the subaxial cervical spine after C1-C2 transarticular screw fixation in rheumatoid arthritis. *J Spinal Disord Tech*, *20* (6), 436-441

[48] Mrabet, D., Meddeb, N., Ajlani, H., Sahli, H. & Sellami, S. (2007). Cerebral vasculitis in a patient with rheumatoid arthritis. *Joint Bone Spine*, *74* (2), 201-204. doi:10.1016/j.jbspin.2006.08.004

[49] Chowdhry, V., Kumar, N., Lachance, D. H., Salomao, D. R. & Luthra, H. S. (2005). An unusual presentation of rheumatoid meningitis. *J Neuroimaging*, *15* (3), 286-288. doi:10.1177/1051228405275201

[50] Markenson, J. A., McDougal, J. S., Tsairis, P., Lockshin, M. D. & Christian, C. L. (1979). Rheumatoid meningitis, a localized immune process. *Ann Intern Med*, *90* (5), 786-789
[51] Bathon, J. M., Moreland, L. W. & DiBartolomeo, A. G. (1989). Inflammatory central nervous system involvement in rheumatoid arthritis. *Semin Arthritis Rheum*, *18* (4), 258-266
[52] Jackson, C. G., Chess, R. L. & Ward, J. R. (1984). A case of rheumatoid nodule formation within the central nervous system and review of the literature. *J Rheumatol*, *11* (2), 237-240
[53] Schmid, L., Muller, M., Treumann, T., Arnold, W., Moller, B., Aeberli, D. & Villiger, P. M. (2009). Induction of complete and sustained remission of rheumatoid pachymeningitis by rituximab. *Arthritis Rheum*, *60* (6), 1632-1634. doi:10.1002/art.24577
[54] Catananti, C., Mastropaolo, S., Calabrese, C., Silveri, M. C. & Onder, G. (2010). A case of normal-pressure hydrocephalus associated with rheumatoid arthritis. *Aging Clin Exp Res*, *22* (2), 189-191
[55] Bruggemann, N., Gottschalk, S., Holl-Ulrich, K., Stewen, J., Heide, W. & Seidel, G. (2010). Cranial pachymeningitis: a rare neurological syndrome with heterogeneous aetiology. *J Neurol Neurosurg Psychiatry*, *81* (3), 294-298. doi:10.1136/jnnp.2008.160457
[56] Ikeda, K., Takazawa, T., Ito, H., Ishikawa, Y., Miura, K., Yoshii, Y., Kawabe, K. & Iwasaki, Y. (2010). Rheumatoid leptomeningitis: radiological alteration of cerebral hypoperfusion and subarachnoid lesions. *Intern Med*, *49* (17), 1911-1916
[57] Agarwal, V., Singh, R., Wiclaf, Chauhan, S., Tahlan, A., Ahuja, C. K., Goel, D. & Pal, L. (2008). A clinical, electrophysiological, and pathological study of neuropathy in rheumatoid arthritis. *Clin Rheumatol*, *27* (7), 841-844. doi:10.1007/s10067-007-0804-x
[58] Steinberg, V. L. (1960). Neuropathy in rheumatoid disease. *Br Med J*, *1* (5186), 1600-1603
[59] Weller, R. O., Bruckner, F. E. & Chamberlain, M. A. (1970). Rheumatoid neuropathy, a histological and electrophysiological study. *J Neurol Neurosurg Psychiatry*, *33* (5), 592-604
[60] Pallis, C. A. & Scott, J. T. (1965). Peripheral Neuropathy in Rheumatoid Arthritis. *Br Med J*, *1* (5443), 1141-1147
[61] Chamberlain, M. A. & Bruckner, F. E. (1970). Rheumatoid neuropathy. Clinical and electrophysiological features. *Ann Rheum Dis*, *29* (6), 609-616

[62] Lanzillo, B., Pappone, N., Crisci, C., di Girolamo, C., Massini, R. & Caruso, G. (1998). Subclinical peripheral nerve involvement in patients with rheumatoid arthritis. *Arthritis Rheum*, *41* (7), 1196-1202. doi:10.1002/1529-0131(199807)41:7<1196::AID-ART8>3.0.CO;2-R

[63] Good, A. E., Christopher, R. P., Koepke, G. H., Bender, L. F. & Tarter, M. E. (1965). Peripheral Neuropathy Associated with Rheumatoid Arthritis. A Clinical and Electrodiagnostic Study of 70 Consecutive Rheumatoid Arthritis Patients. *Ann Intern Med*, *63*, 87-99

[64] Genta, M. S., Genta, R. M. & Gabay, C. (2006). Systemic rheumatoid vasculitis, a review. *Semin Arthritis Rheum*, *36* (2), 88-98. doi:10.1016/j.semarthrit.2006.04.006

[65] Singhal, B. S., Khadilkar, S. V., Gursahani, R. D. & Surya, N. (1995). Vasculitic neuropathy: profile of twenty patients. *J Assoc Physicians India*, *43* (7), 459-461

[66] Richter, C., Wanke, L., Steinmetz, J., Reinhold-Keller, E. & Gross, W. L. (2000). Mononeuritis secondary to rheumatoid arthritis responds to etanercept. *Rheumatology (Oxford)*, *39* (12), 1436-1437

[67] Mayer, D. F. & Matteson, E. L. (2004). Testicular involvement in rheumatoid vasculitis. *Clin Exp Rheumatol*, *22* (6 Suppl 36), S62-64

[68] Puechal, X., Said, G., Hilliquin, P., Coste, J., Job-Deslandre, C., Lacroix, C. & Menkes, C. J. (1995). Peripheral neuropathy with necrotizing vasculitis in rheumatoid arthritis. A clinicopathologic and prognostic study of thirty-two patients. *Arthritis Rheum*, *38* (11), 1618-1629

[69] Chatterjee, S. & Kupsky, W. J. (2005). Severe proximal myopathy and mononeuritis multiplex in rheumatoid arthritis: manifestations of rheumatoid vasculitis. *J Clin Rheumatol*, *11* (1), 50-55

[70] Armstrong, D. J., McCarron, M. T. & Wright, G. D. (2005). Successful treatment of rheumatoid vasculitis-associated foot-drop with infliximab. *J Rheumatol*, *32* (4), 759; author reply 759-760

[71] Bayrak, A. O., Durmus, D., Durmaz, Y., Demir, I., Canturk, F. & Onar, M. K. (2010). Electrophysiological assessment of polyneuropathic involvement in rheumatoid arthritis, relationships among demographic, clinical and laboratory findings. *Neurol Res*, *32* (7), 711-714. doi:10.1179/016164109X12581096870195

[72] Conn, D. L., McDuffie, F. C. & Dyck, P. J. (1972). Immunopathologic study of sural nerves in rheumatoid arthritis. *Arthritis Rheum*, *15* (2), 135-143

[73] Scott, D. G., Bacon, P. A. & Tribe, C. R. (1981). Systemic rheumatoid vasculitis, a clinical and laboratory study of 50 cases. *Medicine (Baltimore)*, *60* (4), 288-297

[74] Muramatsu, K., Tanaka, H. & Taguchi, T. (2008). Peripheral neuropathies of the forearm and hand in rheumatoid arthritis: diagnosis and options for treatment. *Rheumatol Int*, *28* (10), 951-957. doi:10.1007/s00296-008-0630-8

[75] Canoso, J. J. & Alvarez-Nemegyei, J. (2006). Soft Tissue Rheumatology. In: Lahita RG WA, eds (ed) *Educational Review Manual in Rheumatology*. 3 edn., New York: Castle Connolly Graduate Medical,

[76] Cardenaz-Diaz, R. I., Hernandez-Hernandez, M. & Ramos-Remus, C. (1994). Anastomosis de Martin-Gruber: Estudio electrofisiológico. *Rev Mex Reumatol*, *9*, 5

[77] Boland, R. A. & Kiernan, M. C. (2009). Assessing the accuracy of a combination of clinical tests for identifying carpal tunnel syndrome. *J Clin Neurosci*, *16* (7), 929-933. doi:10.1016/j.jocn.2008.09.004

[78] El Miedany, Y., Ashour, S., Youssef, S., Mehanna, A. & Meky, F. A. (2008). Clinical diagnosis of carpal tunnel syndrome: old tests-new concepts. *Joint Bone Spine*, *75* (4), 451-457. doi:10.1016/j.jbspin. 2007.09.014

[79] Ogawa, H., Akaike, A., Ishimaru, D., Yamada, K., Shimizu, T., Koyama, Y. & Hori, H. (2007). Posterior interosseous nerve palsy related to rheumatoid synovitis of the elbow. *Mod Rheumatol*, *17* (4), 327-329. doi:10.1007/s10165-007-0586-7

[80] Sharp, R. J., Wade, C. M., Hennessy, M. S. & Saxby, T. S. (2003). The role of MRI and ultrasound imaging in Morton's neuroma and the effect of size of lesion on symptoms. *J Bone Joint Surg Br*, *85* (7), 999-1005

[81] Stojanovich, L. (2009). Autonomic dysfunction in autoimmune rheumatic disease. Autoimmun Rev 8 (7), 569-572. doi:10.1016/j.autrev. 2009.01.018

[82] Saraswathi, P. V., Neelambikai, N., Mahesh, A. & Govindarajan, K. (2013). Cardiovascular parasympathetic nervous system dysfunction in female rheumatoid arthritis patients. *Indian J Physiol Pharmacol*, *57*, (1), 23-30

[83] Vlcek, M., Rovensky, J., Eisenhofer, G., Radikova, Z., Penesova, A., Kerlik, J. & Imrich, R. (2012). Autonomic nervous system function in rheumatoid arthritis. *Cell Mol Neurobiol*, *32* (5), 897-901. doi:10.1007/s10571-012-9805-7

[84] Bidikar, M. P. & Ichaporia, R. B. (2010). Autonomic (sympathetic) nervous system involvement in rheumatoid arthiritis patients. *Indian J Physiol Pharmacol*, *54* (1), 73-79

[85] Evrengul, H., Dursunoglu, D., Cobankara, V., Polat, B., Seleci, D., Kabukcu, S., Kaftan, A., Semiz, E. & Kilic, M. (2004). Heart rate variability in patients with rheumatoid arthritis. *Rheumatol Int*, *24* (4), 198-202. doi:10.1007/ s00296-003-0357-5

[86] Schilling, U., Muck, R. & Heidemann, E. (2004). [Lead poisoning after ingestion of ayurvedic drugs]. *Med Klin (Munich)*, *99* (8), 476-480. doi:10.1007/s00063-004-1072-2

[87] Karri, S. K., Saper, R. B. & Kales, S. N. (2008). Lead encephalopathy due to traditional medicines. *Curr Drug Saf*, *3* (1), 54-59

[88] Benyamin, R. M., Vallejo, R., Kramer, J. & Rafeyan, R. (2008). Corticosteroid induced psychosis in the pain management setting. *Pain Physician*, *11* (6), 917-920

[89] Perantie, D. C. & Brown, E. S. (2002). Corticosteroids, immune suppression, and psychosis. *Curr Psychiatry Rep*, *4* (3), 171-176

[90] Wolkowitz, O. M., Lupien, S. J., Bigler, E., Levin, R. B. & Canick, J. (2004). The "steroid dementia syndrome": an unrecognized complication of glucocorticoid treatment. *Ann N Y Acad Sci*, *1032*, 191-194. doi:10.1196/annals.1314.018

[91] Patten, S. B. & Neutel, C. I. (2000). Corticosteroid-induced adverse psychiatric effects: incidence, diagnosis and management. *Drug Saf*, *22* (2), 111-122

[92] Brown, E. S. & Chandler, P. A. (2001). Mood and Cognitive Changes During Systemic Corticosteroid Therapy. *Prim Care Companion J Clin Psychiatry*, *3* (1), 17-21

[93] Sapolsky, R. M. (1996). Stress, Glucocorticoids, and Damage to the Nervous System: The Current State of Confusion. *Stress*, *1* (1), 1-19

[94] Alderson, A. L. & Novack, T. A. (2002). Neurophysiological and clinical aspects of glucocorticoids and memory: a review. *J Clin Exp Neuropsychol*, *24* (3), 335-355. doi:10.1076/jcen.24.3.335.987

[95] Gonzalez-Perez, O., Ramos-Remus, C., Garcia-Estrada, J. & Luquin, S. (2001). Prednisone induces anxiety and glial cerebral changes in rats. *J Rheumatol*, *28* (11), 2529-2534

[96] Ramos-Remus, C., Gonzalez-Castaneda, R. E., Gonzalez-Perez, O., Luquin, S. & Garcia-Estrada, J. (2002). Prednisone induces cognitive dysfunction, neuronal degeneration, and reactive gliosis in rats. *J Investig Med*, *50* (6), 458-464

[97] Hoppmann, R. A., Peden, J. G. & Ober, S. K. (1991). Central nervous system side effects of nonsteroidal anti-inflammatory drugs. Aseptic meningitis, psychosis, and cognitive dysfunction. *Arch Intern Med, 151*, (7), 1309-1313

[98] Rodriguez, S. C., Olguin, A. M., Miralles, C. P. & Viladrich, P. F. (2006). Characteristics of meningitis caused by Ibuprofen: report of 2 cases with recurrent episodes and review of the literature. *Medicine (Baltimore), 85* (4), 214-220. doi:10.1097/01.md.0000229757.78057.50

[99] Simon, L. S. & Mills, J. A. (1980). Drug therapy: nonsteroidal antiinflammatory drugs (first of two parts). *N Engl J Med, 302* (21), 1179-1185. doi:10.1056/NEJM198005223022105

[100] Horn, A. C. & Jarrett, S. W. (1997). Ibuprofen-induced aseptic meningitis in rheumatoid arthritis. *Ann Pharmacother, 31* (9), 1009-1011

[101] Quinn, C. T. & Kamen, B. A. (1996). A biochemical perspective of methotrexate neurotoxicity with insight on nonfolate rescue modalities. *J Investig Med, 44* (9), 522-530

[102] Yokoo, H., Nakazato, Y., Harigaya, Y., Sasaki, N., Igeta, Y. & Itoh, H. (2007). Massive myelinolytic leukoencephalopathy in a patient medicated with low-dose oral methotrexate for rheumatoid arthritis: an autopsy report. *Acta Neuropathol, 114* (4), 425-430. doi:10.1007/s00401-007-0214-9

[103] Hawboldt, J. & Bader, M. (2007). Intramuscular methotrexate-induced aseptic meningitis. *Ann Pharmacother, 41*(11), 1906-1911. doi:10.1345/aph.1K308

[104] Rynes, R. I. (1997). Antimalarial drugs in the treatment of rheumatological diseases. *Br J Rheumatol, 36* (7), 799-805

[105] Rynes, R. I. (1996). Ophthalmologic considerations in using antimalarials in the United States. *Lupus, 5* Suppl 1, S73-74

[106] Seckin, U., Ozoran, K., Ikinciogullari, A., Borman, P. & Bostan, E. E. (2000). Hydroxychloroquine ototoxicity in a patient with rheumatoid arthritis. *Rheumatol Int, 19* (5), 203-204

[107] Johansen, P. B. & Gran, J. T. (1998). Ototoxicity due to hydroxychloroquine, report of two cases. *Clin Exp Rheumatol, 16* (4), 472-474

[108] Hadi, U., Nuwayhid, N. & Hasbini, A. S. (1996). Chloroquine ototoxicity, an idiosyncratic phenomenon. *Otolaryngol Head Neck Surg, 114* (3), 491-493

[109] Bernard, P. (1985). Alterations of auditory evoked potentials during the course of chloroquine treatment. *Acta Otolaryngol*, *99* (3-4), 387-392

[110] Scherbel, A. L., Harrison, J. W. & Atdjian, M. (1958). Further observations on the use of 4-aminoquinoline compounds in patients with rheumatoid arthritis or related diseases. *Cleve Clin Q*, *25* (2), 95-111

[111] Meier, C. R., Wilcock, K. & Jick, S. S. (2004). The risk of severe depression, psychosis or panic attacks with prophylactic antimalarials. *Drug Saf*, *27* (3), 203-213

[112] Avina-Zubieta, J. A., Johnson, E. S., Suarez-Almazor, M. E. & Russell, A. S. (1995) Incidence of myopathy in patients treated with antimalarials. A report of three cases and a review of the literature. *Br J Rheumatol*, *34* (2), 166-170

[113] Casado, E., Gratacos, J., Tolosa, C., Martinez, J. M., Ojanguren, I., Ariza, A., Real, J., Sanjuan, A. & Larrosa, M. (2006). Antimalarial myopathy: an underdiagnosed complication? Prospective longitudinal study of 119 patients. *Ann Rheum Dis*, *65* (3), 385-390. doi:10.1136/ard.2004.023200

[114] Richards, B. L., Spies, J., McGill, N., Richards, G. W., Vaile, J., Bleasel, J. F. & Youssef, P. P. (2007). Effect of leflunomide on the peripheral nerves in rheumatoid arthritis. *Intern Med J*, *37* (2), 101-107. doi:10.1111/j.1445-5994.2007.01266.x

[115] Antonio-Valdiviezo, A., Pena-Santos, G. & Martinez-Torres, J. (2010). [Peripheral neuropathy caused by leflunomide. A case reported with a brief review]. *Rev Med Inst Mex Seguro Soc*, *48* (5), 567-570

[116] Bonnel, R. A. & Graham, D. J. (2004). Peripheral neuropathy in patients treated with leflunomide. *Clin Pharmacol Ther*, *75* (6), 580-585. doi:10.1016/j.clpt.2004.01.016

[117] Martin, K., Bentaberry, F., Dumoulin, C., Longy-Boursier, M., Lifermann, F., Haramburu, F., Dehais, J., Schaeverbeke, T., Begaud, B. & Moore, N. (2005). Neuropathy associated with leflunomide: a case series. *Ann Rheum Dis*, *64* (4), 649-650. doi:10.1136/ard.2004.027193

[118] Bharadwaj, A. & Haroon, N. (2004). Peripheral neuropathy in patients on leflunomide. *Rheumatology (Oxford)*, *43* (7), 934. doi:10.1093/ rheumatology/keh191

[119] Martin, K., Bentaberry, F., Dumoulin, C., Miremont-Salame, G., Haramburu, F., Dehais, J. & Schaeverbeke, T. (2007). Peripheral neuropathy associated with leflunomide: is there a risk patient profile? *Pharmacoepidemiol Drug Saf*, *16* (1), 74-78. doi:10.1002/pds.1282

[120] Tilelli, J. A. & Heinrichs, M. M. (1997). Adverse reactions to parenteral gold salts. *Lancet*, *349* (9055), 853. doi:10.1016/S0140-6736(05)61757-6

[121] Fam, A. G., Gordon, D. A., Sarkozi, J., Blair, G. R., Cooper, P. W., Harth, M. & Lewis, A. J. (1984). Neurologic complications associated with gold therapy for rheumatoid arthritis. *J Rheumatol*, *11* (5), 700-706

[122] Petiot, P., Charles, N., Vial, C., McGregor, B., Aimard, G., Trillet, M. & Bady, B. (1993). [Neurological complications caused by gold salts. Nosologic report apropos of a case]. *Rev Neurol (Paris)*, *149* (10), 562-565

[123] Noppen, M., Velkeniers, B., Dierckx, R., Bruyland, M. & Vanhaelst, L. (1987). Cyclosporine and myopathy. *Ann Intern Med*, *107* (6), 945-946

[124] Owczarek, J., Jasinska, M. & Orszulak-Michalak, D. (2005). Drug-induced myopathies. An overview of the possible mechanisms. *Pharmacol Rep*, *57* (1), 23-34

[125] Goy, J. J., Stauffer, J. C., Deruaz, J. P., Gillard, D., Kaufmann, U., Kuntzer, T. & Kappenberger, L. (1989). Myopathy as possible side-effect of cyclosporin. *Lancet*, *1* (8652), 1446-1447

[126] Schwartz, R. B., Bravo, S. M., Klufas, R. A., Hsu, L., Barnes, P. D., Robson, C. D. & Antin, J. H. (1995). Cyclosporine neurotoxicity and its relationship to hypertensive encephalopathy: CT and MR findings in 16 cases. *AJR Am J Roentgenol*, *165* (3), 627-631. doi:10.2214/ajr.165.3.7645483

[127] Gijtenbeek, J. M., van den Bent, M. J. & Vecht, C. J. (1999). Cyclosporine neurotoxicity, a review. *J Neurol*, *246* (5), 339-346

[128] Lee, S. J. & Kavanaugh, A. (2005). Adverse reactions to biologic agents: focus on autoimmune disease therapies. *J Allergy Clin Immunol*, *116* (4), 900-905. doi:10.1016/j.jaci.2005.03.028

[129] Robinson, W. H., Genovese, M. C. & Moreland, L. W. (2001). Demyelinating and neurologic events reported in association with tumor necrosis factor alpha antagonism: by what mechanisms could tumor necrosis factor alpha antagonists improve rheumatoid arthritis but exacerbate multiple sclerosis? *Arthritis Rheum*, *44* (9), 1977-1983. doi:10.1002/1529-0131(200109)44:9<1977::AID-ART345>3.0.CO;2-6

[130] Kumar, D., Bouldin, T. W. & Berger, R. G. (2010). A case of progressive multifocal leukoencephalopathy in a patient treated with infliximab. *Arthritis Rheum*, *62* (11), 3191-3195. doi:10.1002/art.27687

[131] Lozeron, P., Denier, C., Lacroix, C. & Adams, D. (2009). Long-term course of demyelinating neuropathies occurring during tumor necrosis

factor-alpha-blocker therapy. *Arch Neurol*, *66* (4), 490-497. doi:10.1001/archneurol.2009.11

[132] Mohan, N., Edwards, E.. T., Cupps, T. R., Oliverio, P. J., Sandberg, G., Crayton, H., Richert, J. R. & Siegel, J. N. (2001). Demyelination occurring during anti-tumor necrosis factor alpha therapy for inflammatory arthritides. *Arthritis Rheum*, *44* (12), 2862-2869

[133] Kur-Zalewska, J., Swarowska-Knap, J. & Tlustochowicz, W. (2008). Neurological disorders with demyelinating brain white matter lesions in a patient with rheumatoid arthritis treated with etanercept. *Pol Arch Med Wewn*, *118* (4), 234-237

[134] Shin, I. S., Baer, A. N., Kwon, H. J., Papadopoulos, E. J. & Siegel, J. N. (2006). Guillain-Barre and Miller Fisher syndromes occurring with tumor necrosis factor alpha antagonist therapy. *Arthritis Rheum*, *54* (5), 1429-1434. doi:10.1002/art.21814

[135] Alshekhlee, A., Basiri, K., Miles, J. D., Ahmad, S. A. & Katirji, B. (2010). Chronic inflammatory demyelinating polyneuropathy associated with tumor necrosis factor-alpha antagonists. *Muscle Nerve*, *41* (5), 723-727. doi:10.1002/mus.21584

[136] Bosch, X., Saiz, A. & Ramos-Casals, M. (2011). Monoclonal antibody therapy-associated neurological disorders. *Nat Rev Neurol*, *7* (3), 165-172. doi:10.1038/nrneurol.2011.1

[137] Lynch, K. & Farrell, M. (2010). Cerebral tuberculoma in a patient receiving anti-TNF alpha (adalimumab) treatment. *Clin Rheumatol*, *29* (10), 1201-1204. doi:10.1007/s10067-010-1466-7

[138] Calabrese, L. H. & Molloy, E. S. (2008). Progressive multifocal leucoencephalopathy in the rheumatic diseases: assessing the risks of biological immunosuppressive therapies. *Ann Rheum Dis*, *67* Suppl 3, iii64-65. doi:10.1136/ard.2008.097972

[139] Food and Drug Administration. (2009). http://www.fda.gov/Safety/MedWatch/SafetyInformation/SafetyAlertsforHumanMedicalProducts/ucm150747.htm. Accessed 06/August/2009 2009

[140] Carson, K.. R., Focosi, D., Major, E. O., Petrini, M., Richey, E. A., West, D. P. & Bennett, C. L. (2009). Monoclonal antibody-associated progressive multifocal leucoencephalopathy in patients treated with rituximab, natalizumab, and efalizumab: a Review from the Research on Adverse Drug Events and Reports (RADAR) Project. *Lancet Oncol*, *10* (8), 816-824. doi:10.1016/S1470-2045(09)70161-5

[141] Lima, M. A., Drislane, F. W. & Koralnik, I. J. (2006). Seizures and their outcome in progressive multifocal leukoencephalopathy. *Neurology*, *66* (2), 262-264. doi:10.1212/01.wnl.0000194227.16696.11

[142] Alloway, J. A. & Mitchell, S. R. (1993). Sulfasalazine neurotoxicity: a report of aseptic meningitis and a review of the literature. *J Rheumatol*, *20* (2), 409-411

[143] Takahashi, K., Ogita, T., Okudaira, H., Yoshinoya, S., Yoshizawa, H. & Miyamoto, T. (1986). D-penicillamine-induced polymyositis in patients with rheumatoid arthritis. *Arthritis Rheum*, *29* (4), 560-564

[144] Chappel, R. & Willems, J. (1996). D-penicillamine-induced myositis in rheumatoid arthritis. *Clin Rheumatol*, *15* (1), 86-87

[145] Carroll, G. J., Will, R. K., Peter, J. B., Garlepp, M. J. & Dawkins, R. L. (1987). Penicillamine induced polymyositis and dermatomyositis. *J Rheumatol*, *14* (5), 995-1001

[146] Halla, J. T., Fallahi, S. & Koopman, W. J. (1984). Penicillamine-induced myositis. Observations and unique features in two patients and review of the literature. *Am J Med*, *77* (4), 719-722

In: Neuro-Immune Interactions …
Editor: Oscar González-Pérez
ISBN: 978-1-62948-646-8

Chapter 4

MESENCHYMAL STEM CELLS AS ALTERNATIVE THERAPY FOR BRAIN DISORDERS AND THEIR INTERACTION WITH THE IMMUNE SYSTEM

Qian Li[1,2], Kaisorn L. Chaichana[2], Julio J. Rodarte[2], Alfredo Quiñones-Hinojosa[2] and Hugo Guerrero-Cazares[2,*]

[1]Department of Biochemistry and Molecular Biology, Louis University School of Medicine, St. Louis, Missouri, US

[2]Department of Neurosurgery and Oncology, Johns Hopkins University School of Medicine, Baltimore, Maryland, US

ABSTRACT

Mesenchymal stem cells (MSCs) are cells that have the ability to maintain, self-renew, and give rise to different stromal cell types. These cells can be obtained from a variety of sources that includes bone marrow and adipose tissue. MSCs have an intrinsic tropism towards inflammation and tumor tissues, which makes them an attractive candidate for cellular-based therapies.

* Corresponding Author: Hugo Guerrero-Cazares M.D., Ph.D. Johns Hopkins University School of Medicine, Neurosurgery, CRB-II Rm 272, 1550 Orleans St, Baltimore, MD 21231. Phone: 410-502-8776, Fax: 410-502-7995.

This chapter summarizes the properties of different sources of MSCs, their potential therapeutic use for brain tumor and other brain disorders, and their interaction with immune system cells. Ultimately, MSCs represent a promising new cellular therapy paradigm where these cells can be used as delivery vehicles for therapeutic molecules or serve as a source of replacement cells in degenerative diseases.

INTRODUCTION

Mesenchymal Stem Cell Properties

Mesenchymal stem cells (MSCs), also known as mesenchymal stromal cells (Friedenstein, Chailakhyan et al., 1974), are cells that are generated from peripheral tissues with the ability to maintain, self-renew, and differentiate into skeletal tissues such as bone, cartilage, and fat. Unlike embryonic stem cells (ESCs), MSCs are not totipotent as they do not have the potential to differentiate into all the cell types that comprise an organism, which includes hematopoetic cells, neural cells, and stromal cells, among others. MSCs were first isolated in the 1970s by Friedenstein and colleagues, where they isolated them from bone marrow using *in vitro* conditions (Friedenstein, Chailakhyan et al., 1974). MSCs can also be harvested from other sources besides bone marrow including adipose tissue, adult muscle, corneal stroma, and placental tissue, among others. MSCs, regardless of source, share basic characteristics which are used to isolate them in culture. These common features include: 1) MSCs have spindle-shaped, fibroblast-like morphology, and are adherent to plastic under standard tissue culture conditions; 2) MSCs express certain stem cell surface markers (CD73, CD90, and CD105), but notably absent are hematopoietic surface antigens (CD31 and CD45) (Pendleton, Li et al., 2013); 3) MSCs are capable of self-renewal and are able to maintain their stem-ness for several passages (until P5-P15); 4) Under certain stimuli, MSCs are able to differentiate into adipocyte, osteocyte, and chondrocyte (Rogers, Young et al., 1995), which can be identified using Oil Red O, Alizarin Red S, and Collagen II staining (Pendleton, Li et al., 2013), respectively.

MSCs can be isolated form a variety of sources. MSCs can be successfully isolated from bone marrow (BM-MSC) (Sale and Storb 1983; Sparks, Seibel-Ross et al., 1986; Bruder, Jaiswal et al., 1997; Pittenger, Mackay et al., 1999), adipose tissue (AMSC) (Zuk, Zhu et al., 2001; Zuk, Zhu et al., 2002), skeletal muscle (Uezumi, Ojima et al., 2006), umbilical cord (UMSC) (Erices, Conget et al., 2000; Covas, Siufi et al., 2003; Uezumi, Ojima et al., 2006), Wharton's jelly (Wang, Hung et al., 2004), synovium (De Bari, Dell'Accio et al., 2001), and deciduous dental pulp (Pierdomenico, Bonsi et al., 2005; Kerkis and Caplan 2012). However, some of the characteristics observed in MSCs are specific to the source. MSCs from muscles and adipose tissue have a slightly lower proliferation potential than those derived from bone marrow since muscles and adipose tissue have a lower turnover rate than cells within the bone marrow (Sakaguchi, Sekiya et al., 2005).

Furthermore, the age of the donor and the culture conditions that are used also affect the rate and persistence of MSC proliferation (Reyes, Lund et al., 2001; Via, Frizziero et al., 2012). Besides proliferation, the differentiation potential of MSCs is also different depending on their source.

MSCs isolated from adipose tissue are only able to differentiate into osteoblasts, chondrocytes, and adipocytes (Huibregtse, Johnstone et al., 2000; Sakaguchi, Sekiya et al., 2005; Danisovic, Varga et al., 2009); while BM-MSCs are also able to differentiate into tenocyte and vascular smooth muscle cells (Delorme, Ringe et al., 2009; Violini, Ramelli et al., 2009).

Stem-like cells derived from muscular tissue only have the ability to become skeletal muscle cells (Relaix and Marcelle 2009), while MSCs from umbilical cord blood have a broader differentiation potential and can differentiate into neuron, cardiomyocytes-like cells, endothelial cells, and skeletal muscle cells, besides the traditional three classic cell types (adipocytes, chondroctyes, osteocytes) (Conconi, Burra et al., 2006; Wu, Zhou et al., 2007) (Figure 1).

MSCs are particularly attractive as a therapeutic agent due to their intrinsic tropism towards inflammation and tumor cells. MSCs have been determined to target cancer cells from brain, breast, colon, and prostate (Nakamura, Ito et al., 2004; Nakamizo, Marini et al., 2005; Sasportas, Kasmieh et al., 2009; Alieva, Bago et al., 2012).

Although some studies have suggested that MSCs have an anti-tumor effect for certain cancers, these findings remain controversial (Nakamura, Ito et al., 2004; Nakamizo, Marini et al., 2005; Sasportas, Kasmieh et al., 2009; Alieva, Bago et al., 2012). For brain tumors, some *in vitro* and *in vivo* findings suggest that MSCs also have the ability to penetrate the blood-brain barrier (BBB), which is a common obstacle for chemotherapeutic drugs (Liu, Eckert et al., 2013).

Due to their potential use as therapeutic vehicles and/or replacement cells for damaged tissue, inflammation sites, and tumor tissue, MSCs are being actively studied in translational researches.

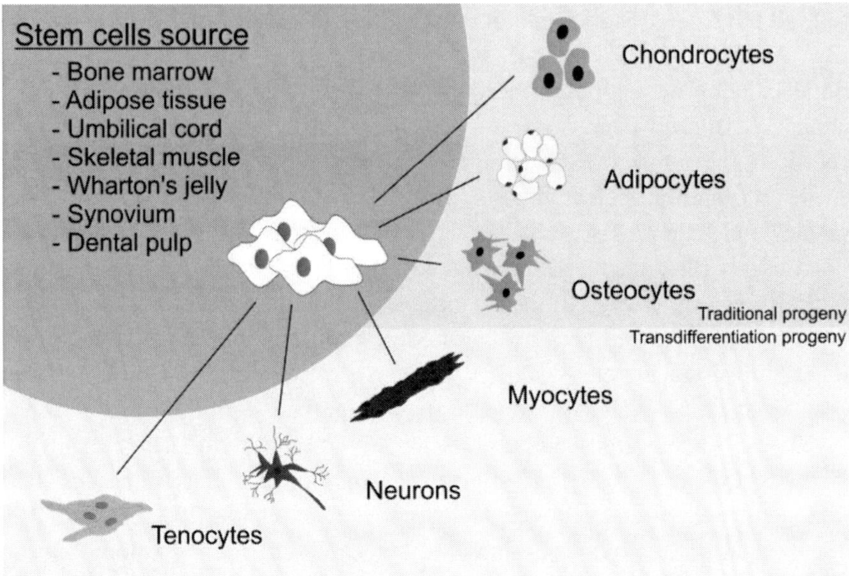

Figure 1. Tissue sources for mesenchymal stem cells (MSCs) and their progeny. MSCs can be isolated form a variety of sources: bone marrow, adipose tissue, umbilical cord, skeletal muscle, Wharton's jelly, synovium, and dental pulp. The differentiation potential of MSCs is different depending on their source. Most sources of MSCs are able to differentiate into chondrocytes, adipocytes, and osteoblasts, while some are also able to become myocytes, neurons, and tenocytes.

Among MSC sources, one of the most attractive is adipose tissue. The potential of human AMSCs has created a lot of enthusiasm over other sources because adipose tissue is easier to obtain and more readily available.

Moreover, cells from adipose tissue are genetically and morphologically more stable in long-term culture, have a lower senescence ratio, and have a greater proliferative capacity (Deng, Makizumi et al., 2007; Lamfers, Idema et al., 2009; Ikegame, Yamashita et al., 2011; Guo, Huang et al., 2012; Strioga, Viswanathan et al., 2012; Pendleton, Li et al., 2013).

Due to these properties, these cells are attractive candidates for cell-based treatment (Strioga, Viswanathan et al., 2012).

These properties make them suitable for different clinical applications from inflammatory disorders including stroke, brain tumors such as glioblastoma, and neurodegenerative diseases including Parkinson’s disease.

Mesenchymal Stem Cells and the Immune System

The use of MSCs as cell replacement therapy or delivery vehicles of therapeutic proteins for different pathologies will have an implication on the patient's immune system (Figure 2).

MSCs have generated considerable interest in the fields of immune modulation (English 2013). They have an intriguing capacity to modulate the immune response whereby they have the potential to suppress T-cell proliferation *in vitro* and prolong survival of allogeneic skin grafts *in vivo* (Bartholomew, Sturgeon et al., 2002; Di Nicola, Carlo-Stella et al., 2002). A number of *in vitro* studies has provided insight into the effects that MSCs have on both innate and adaptive immune responses (English 2013).

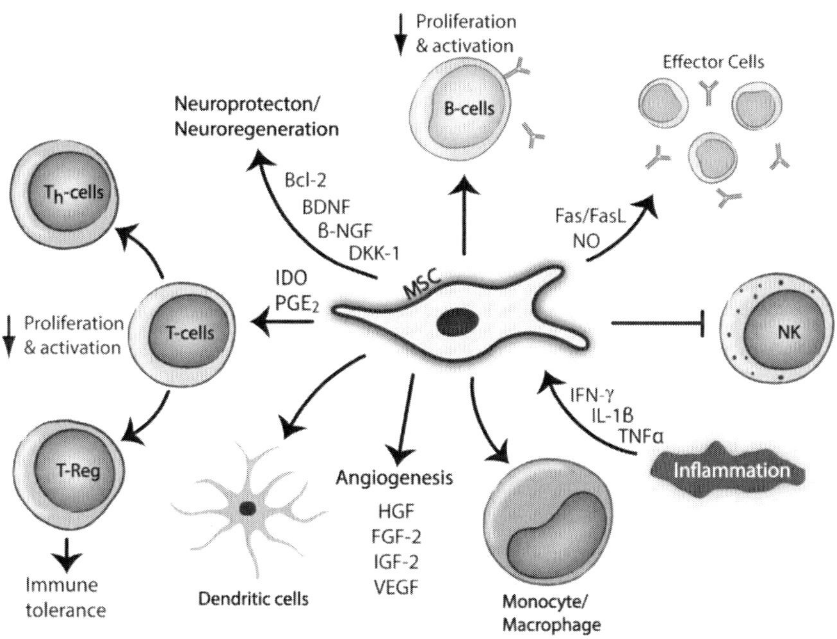

Figure 2. Immune modulation by MSCs. MSCs can be activated by various inflammatory factors. MSCs can then modulate immune system cells via different secreted factors and intercellular signaling pathways. Generally, MSCs can blunt the immune response by inhibiting the proliferation and activation of T-cells and B-cells, as well as suppressing Natural Killer (NK) cells. In addition, MSCs can also provide neuro-protection and augment the vascular response by promoting angiogenesis.

Specifically, MSCs have the capacity to interfere with many components of the innate immune system including complement, Toll-like receptor (TLR) signaling, macrophages, dendritic cells, neutrophils, mast cells, and natural killer cells (Spaggiari, Capobianco et al., 2006; English, Barry et al., 2008; Kim and Hematti 2009; Nemeth, Leelahavanichkul et al., 2009; Cutler, Limbani et al., 2010; Choi, Lee et al., 2011). In regard to the adaptive immune response, MSCs can also directly inhibit T-cell function, shift the T-helper lymphocyte balance, induce functional regulatory T cells (Tregs), and may also modulate B-cell proliferation and function (Comoli, Ginevri et al., 2008; Kong, Sun et al., 2009; Ge, Jiang et al., 2010; Akiyama, Chen et al., 2012).

As mentioned previously, MSCs can migrate to inflammatory sites in response to the release of pro-inflammatory cytokines and chemokines (Medzhitov 2010). They can also recruit innate immune cells such as neutrophils and macrophages to these same sites (Medzhitov 2010).

After migrating to these inflammatory sites, MSCs are "activated" by interferon (IFN)-g, TNF-α or IL-1β. This activation is required for MSCs to modulate immune responses and, more specifically, repress immune effects (Ren, Zhang et al., 2008). Once MSCs have attracted immune cells such as effector T cells, MSCs can facilitate the direct immunomodulation of T cells via either direct contact of production of molecules including NO or FAS/FASL (Fas ligand)-induced apoptosis (Ren, Zhang et al., 2008; Akiyama, Chen et al., 2012).

Furthermore, MSCs can interact, modify, and activate monocyte/macrophages functions (Cutler, Limbani et al., 2010; Choi, Lee et al., 2011). Besides activating these immune cells that modify the immune response, MSCs also play a role in the modification of immunosuppressive soluble factors (English 2013). However, these factors are not secreted by MSCs directly, but are a consequence of activating MSCs under inflammation (English 2013). Some well-known soluble factors include indoleamine 2,3-dioxygenase (IDO) that enhance microbial clearance as well as inhibition of immune responses, prostaglandin E-2 (PGE-2) that suppresses T-cell activation and proliferation, TNF-α that stimulates gene/protein 6 (TSG-6) that inhibit the early inflammatory response include neutrophil infiltration and proinflammatory cytokines release, and nitric oxide (NO) that inhibits T-cell proliferation and induces T-cell apoptosis (English, Barry et al., 2007; Ren, Zhang et al., 2008; Lee, Pulin et al., 2009; Ge, Jiang et al., 2010). Besides all the mechanisms mentioned previously, MSCs can also alter the helper T cells balance, induce tolerogenic dendritic cells, and induce Tregs to enhance immune tolerance.

Despite these findings, there are still conflicting reports that suggest MSCs may not actually enhance immune cell survival and function (English 2013). It is therefore crucial that these disparate findings be evaluated to ensure that MSC therapy does not exacerbate inflammatory response that can interfere with their intended functions.

In addition, MSCs exert their anti-inflammatory effects on a number of *in vivo* models including graft versus host disease (GvHD), experimental autoimmune encephalomyelitis, inflammatory bowel disease, and allergic airway disease, among others (Polchert, Sobinsky et al., 2008; Ren, Zhang et al., 2008; Nemeth, Leelahavanichkul et al., 2009; Kavanagh and Mahon 2011; Akiyama, Chen et al., 2012).

Based on those *in vitro* and *in vivo* findings, MSCs have been used in clinical trials for the treatment of various inflammatory diseases like: Crohn's disease, Systemic Lupus Erythematosus, Multiple Sclerosis, and arthritis, among others (http://clinicaltrials.gov). Further research, however, is needed to define the influence of ongoing pathogenic infections that are prominent in diseases like GvHD and organ transplantation on MSC activation and function (English 2013).

Mesenchymal Stem Cells and Brain Diseases

Since 1995, there have been 352 clinical trials using MSCs (http://clinical trials.gov). Most of these trials aimed to treat bone/cartilage diseases because of the ability of MSCs to differentiate into mesenchymal type cells. However more recent data has opened the possibilities of using MSCs in a larger range of diseases (Table 1 and Figure 3).

MSCs in Brain Tumors

Brain tumors, especially glioblastoma (GBM, stage IV Glioma), have a propensity to recur despite aggressive local therapy because they are able to invade surrounding brain tissue and escape local therapy (Stupp, Mason et al., 2005; McGirt, Chaichana et al., 2008; Chaichana, Guerrero-Cazares et al., 2009; McGirt, Chaichana et al., 2009; Zaidi, Kosztowski et al., 2009). The median survival for patients with GBM is approximately 14.6 months, despite aggressive combinatorial treatment (resection plus chemotherapy and radio-therapy) (Stupp, Mason et al., 2005).

Table 1. Mesenchymal Stem Cell involved clinical trials

Category of disease	Examples
Cancers (34)	Acute lymphoblastic leukemia Bone cancer
Neurodegeneration diseases (6)	Parkinson's disease Alzheimer's Disease
Immune system diseases (62)	Acute graft versus host disease Autoimmune diseases Endocrine system diseases
Wounds and injuries (33)	Brain and spinal injuries Bone fractures Musculoskeletal diseases
Others (196)	Pain

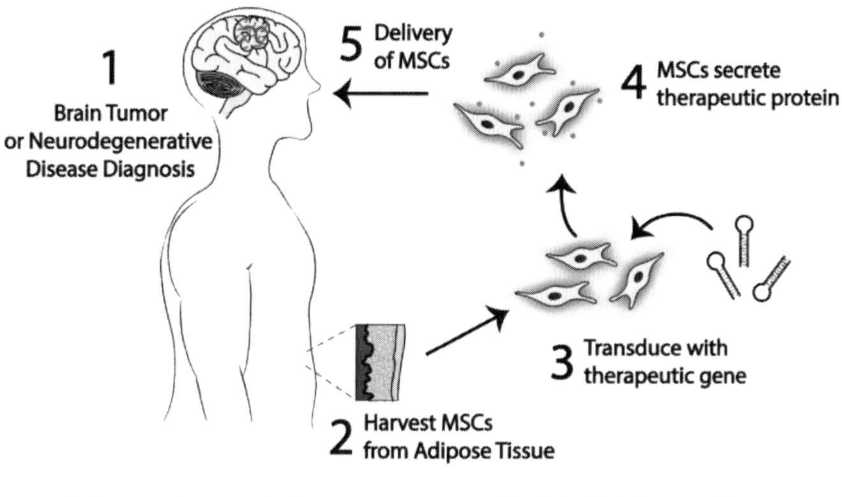

Figure 3. Therapeutic potential for autologous use of MSCs. MSCs would be harvested from patients suffering from brain tumors or neurodegenerative diseases, modified in vitro to produce therapeutic proteins and implanted into the same patient. The autologous MSCs implants would bypass immune reactions and act a delivery vehicle for therapeutic substances.

While more tumor resection is associated with prolonged time to recurrence and overall survival, nearly all patients will eventually have tumor recurrence and subsequently die (McGirt, Chaichana et al., 2008; McGirt, Chaichana et al., 2009; Chaichana, McGirt et al., 2010; Chaichana, Garzon-Muvdi et al., 2011; Chaichana, Zadnik et al., 2013).

A major part of the inefficacy of current treatment algorithms is that invading cells escape local treatment including radiation and chemotherapy (Bao, Wu et al., 2006; Rich 2007). Furthermore, GBMs have the property of inhibiting the host immune system, at the systemic (Dix, Brooks et al., 1999; Waziri 2010) and local (Yang, Han et al., 2010) levels. A curative approach therefore needs to target these invading cells that escape the tumor bulk (Rich 2007; Chesler, Berger et al., 2012; Guerrero-Cazares, Attenello et al., 2012). Cellular therapy, namely stem cell therapy, may be an effective treatment option because of the intrinsic ability of stem cells to home to cancer cells, both in the tumor bulk and periphery. Stem cells, including neural (NSCs) and MSCs, therefore represent an attractive potential treatment option for GBM. NSCs have been found to selectively migrate to GBM (Quinones-Hinojosa and Chaichana 2007; Tyler, Ulasov et al., 2009). However, human NSCs are limited in supply, challenging to obtain, and difficult to expand *ex vivo* (Parsons, Teng et al., 2011). These limitations make NSC auto-transplantation difficult and unreliable. This therefore makes MSCs a more promising source for clinical application.

Besides possessing an innate ability to home to cancer cells, MSCs can be engineered to serve as delivery vehicles. Human AMSCs, as well as with BM-MSC, can be engineered to deliver various anti-tumorigenic proteins (like TRAIL and IL12) to treat GBM cells both *in vitro* and *in vivo* (Table 2) (Nakamizo, Marini et al., 2005; Elzaouk, Moelling et al., 2006; Yuan, Hu et al., 2006; Kucerova, Matuskova et al., 2010; Matuskova, Hlubinova et al., 2010; Choi, Hwang et al., 2011).

Engineered MSCs could be delivered by intravenous (tail vain), intracardiac, intracarotid, intranasal, or intracranial injection. Antitumorigenic proteins could then be synthesized and secreted by MSCs, and provide a localized anti-tumor effect by affecting tumor cell proliferation and/or migration. Subsequently, GBM tumor-bearing animal models have been shown to have decreased tumor burden and a prolonged survival rate following engineered MSCs treatment (Nakamizo, Marini et al., 2005; Yuan, Hu et al., 2006).

Besides choosing the right source of MSCs, there are other factors that need to be addressed in preclinical studies. First, only 1% of systemically-injected MSCs reach the tumor bulk, where an overwhelming majority of them are trapped in peripheral organs including the lungs, liver, kidney, and skin (Deak, Seifried et al., 2010). Therefore, methods need to be developed to increase MSC tumor tropism and/or improve their ability to cross biological barriers.

Table 2. Mesenchymal Stem Cell Therapies for Gliomas

Application (specific use)	Reference
Chemotherapeutic vehicles	
HSV-thymidine kinase	Mietic et al., 2007
Viral delivery vehicles	
Adenovirus	Sonabend et al., 2008
Immunotherapeutic vehicles	
IL-2	Nakamura et al., 2004
IL-12	Ryu at al., 2011
IL-18	Xu et al., 2008
IL-23	Yuan et al., 2006
TRAIL	Choi et al., 2011; Kim et al., 2012
Interferon-α	Sato et al., 2005
Interferon-β	Nakamiza et al., 2005

In oncology, the tropism of MSCs depends on various ligand-receptors under different cancer circumstances. Some of the chemokine axes that are involved in this tropism of MSCs to brain tumor cells are: VEGF/VEGFR, PDGFBB/PDGFR, and SDF1α/CXCL12 (Wynn, Hart et al., 2004; Nakamizo, Marini et al., 2005; Elzaouk, Moelling et al., 2006; Xu, Cochran et al., 2006; Batchelor, Sorensen et al., 2007; Verhaak, Hoadley et al., 2010; Chaturvedi, Gilkes et al., 2013). More ligand-receptor signaling pathways still need to be explored and manipulated to enhance their tropism. In addition to these chemokine axes, cadherin adhesions increase MSC transmigration efficiency across blood vessels and boost their therapeutic effects. Additionally, preventing MSCs from being trapped in undesired organs would be ideal in order to minimize potential side effects that therapeutic proteins or chemical drugs may have on non-diseased organs. These concerns are important if these cells are to be used in various pathological conditions including brain tumors and other neurologic disorders including ischemic stroke and neurodegenerative diseases.

Hypoxic–Ischemic (HI) Conditions

Ischemic events occur when blood supply to the brain is interrupted. This leads to diminished delivery of oxygen and nutrients to brain tissue. When oxygen and glucose delivery become insufficient to meet the metabolic demands of the brain tissue, a sequence of biochemical events is triggered.

This includes intracellular calcium release, excito-toxicity, oxidative stress, inflammation and apoptosis, autophagy, and necrosis, which all contribute to global brain injury (Ferriero 2004; Northington, Chavez-Valdez et al., 2011; van Velthoven, Kavelaars et al., 2012). The key to stroke treatment is to commence treatment within a therapeutic time window, which is typically 6 hours after onset of the ischemia (van Velthoven, Kavelaars et al., 2012). The biggest limitation of this traditional treatment is that the 6-hour time frame is often too short to be able to start therapy. Moreover, once brain damage has become established, the resulting injured tissue is no longer amenable for neuroprotection (van Velthoven, Kavelaars et al., 2012). Therefore, a novel treatment aimed at improving existing brain damage is critical. Administration of MSCs 3 to 24 hours after stroke in adult animals reduces the number of apoptotic cells by approximately 50% in the ischemic boundary zone, which is accompanied by an increased expression of anti-apoptotic proteins including Bcl-2 and surviving (Okazaki, Magaki et al., 2008). These results indicate that transplantation of MSCs in the early phase after ischemic brain injury can be neuroprotective and thereby improves functional outcome (Okazaki, Magaki et al., 2008). Additionally, other studies have demonstrated that intranasal delivery of MSCs after neonatal HI resulted in reduced lesion volume and improved motor function (van Velthoven, Kavelaars et al., 2010). Besides their neuroprotective effects, MSCs harvested from bone marrow are able to secrete multiple angiogenic cytokines: HGF, FGF-2, IGF-I and VEGF, which contribute to improving brain function by stimulating angiogenesis (Joyce, Annett et al., 2010). These potential beneficial effects caused by MSC transplantation has been shown by several independent groups, where MSC were delivered by various methods including intravenous, intracardiac, intranasal, and intracranial delivery methods (Yasuhara, Matsukawa et al., 2006; Yasuhara, Hara et al., 2008; Lee, Kim et al., 2010; van Velthoven, Kavelaars et al., 2010; van Velthoven, Kavelaars et al., 2010; van Velthoven, Kavelaars et al., 2010).

Neurodegenerative Diseases

While MSC treatment for stoke is currently only at the preclinical phase, there are 16 human Phase I clinical trials that have used MSCs for neuro-degenerative diseases including Alzheimer's Disease, Parkinson's Disease, and amyotrophic lateral sclerosis, among others (http://clinicaltrials. gov).

Neurodegenerative diseases are characterized by the loss of neurons in the brain and/or spinal cord. In the brain, Alzheimer's disease (AD) and Huntington's disease (HD) result in widespread loss of neurons, whereas Parkinson's disease (PD) involves specific and localized loss of dopaminergic (DA) neurons in the substantia nigra (Lunn, Sakowski et al., 2011). There is a growing interest in using MSCs for the treatment of neurodegenerative diseases because they can provide neurotrophic factors to promote repair and, potentially, lead to new growth of neurons (Joyce, Annett et al., 2010).

Upon transplantation, MSCs in the brain promote endogenous neuronal growth, decrease apoptosis, and regulate inflammation primarily through the secretion of neurotrophic factors (Joyce, Annett et al., 2010).

MSCs can enhance endogenous neural regeneration and protection by mediating the microenvironment of the damaged area.

Other Uses of MSCs in the Nervous System

MSCs transplanted at sites of nerve injury have been demonstrated to promote functional recovery by producing trophic factors that induce survival and regeneration of host neurons (Crigler, Robey et al., 2006). Transplantation of human BM-MSCs into the brain of immunodeficient mice markedly increased the proliferation of endogenous neural stem cells (Munoz, Stoutenger et al., 2005). In an experimental allergic encephalomyelitis model of multiple sclerosis (MS), rodents that receive an intraventricular infusion of MSCs were found to have almost twice the number of axons as control animals (Kassis, Grigoriadis et al., 2008). MSCs can secrete brain-derived neurotrophic factor (BDNF), β-NGF, and Dkk-1, which both help generate new neurons and protect existing ones (Gregory, Singh et al., 2003; Etheridge, Spencer et al., 2004; Crigler, Robey et al., 2006; Endo, Beauchamp et al., 2008; Wilkins, Kemp et al., 2009). The ability of producing these neurotrophic factors makes MSCs an attractive candidate because they not only can serve as delivery vehicles of therapeutic molecules, but they also possess intrinsic therapeutic abilities themselves (Joyce, Annett et al., 2010).

Concerns about the Usage of MSCs

While there is a growing body of evidence supporting the use of MSCs for therapeutic treatments of various clinical conditions, other studies have suggested that MSCs can increase tumor cell growth and induce tumor angiogenesis (Hall, Dembinski et al., 2007; Mishra, Humeniuk et al., 2008; Spaeth, Dembinski et al., 2009; Akimoto, Kimura et al., 2013). It has also been proposed that cancer cells may be able to induce MSCs (reported on BM-MSCs) to form tumor associated fibroblasts (TAFs), which can then support and stimulate tumor growth and migration as well as promote a malignant phenotype (Hall, Dembinski et al., 2007; Mishra, Humeniuk et al., 2008; Mishra and Merlino 2008; Mishra, Glod et al., 2009; Spaeth, Dembinski et al., 2009).

The effects of MSCs on tumor cells *in vivo*, however, remain incompletely characterized, and seem to depend heavily on the cancer type and source of MSCs (Momin, Mohyeldin et al., 2010; Momin, Vela et al., 2010; Akimoto, Kimura et al., 2013). These concerns about the safety of using MSCs in the context of cancer need to be addressed before moving into pre-clinical and clinical trials.

Conclusion

Stem cell therapy has become a topic of interest for decades. However, due to ethical issues, limitation of current sources, and technical difficulties with Embryonic Stem Cells and induced Pluripotent Stem Cells usage, stem cell therapy has stalled. The therapeutic properties of MSCs include multipotency, immune suppression, and ability to act as therapeutic vehicles.

Another advantage of MSCs is the ease to harvest them, where they can be used in an autologous manner. Although most of the research is only at the preclinical/translational stages, a new era of treatment has opened and will likely involve MSCs.

References

Akimoto, K., K. Kimura, et al., (2013). "Umbilical Cord Blood-Derived Mesenchymal Stem Cells Inhibit, But Adipose Tissue-Derived Mesenchymal Stem Cells Promote, Glioblastoma Multiforme Proliferation." *Stem Cells Dev.*

Akiyama, K., C. Chen, et al., (2012). "Mesenchymal-stem-cell-induced immunoregulation involves FAS-ligand-/FAS-mediated T cell apoptosis." *Cell stem cell* 10(5): 544-555.

Alieva, M., J. R. Bago, et al., (2012). "Glioblastoma therapy with cytotoxic mesenchymal stromal cells optimized by bioluminescence imaging of tumor and therapeutic cell response." *PLoS One* 7(4): e35148.

Bao, S., Q. Wu, et al., (2006). "Glioma stem cells promote radioresistance by preferential activation of the DNA damage response." *Nature* 444(7120): 756-760.

Bartholomew, A., C. Sturgeon, et al., (2002). "Mesenchymal stem cells suppress lymphocyte proliferation in vitro and prolong skin graft survival in vivo." *Experimental hematology* 30(1): 42-48.

Batchelor, T. T., A. G. Sorensen, et al., (2007). "AZD2171, a pan-VEGF receptor tyrosine kinase inhibitor, normalizes tumor vasculature and alleviates edema in glioblastoma patients." *Cancer Cell* 11(1): 83-95.

Bruder, S. P., N. Jaiswal, et al., (1997). "Growth kinetics, self-renewal, and the osteogenic potential of purified human mesenchymal stem cells during extensive subcultivation and following cryopreservation." *Journal of cellular biochemistry* 64(2): 278-294.

Chaichana, K. L., T. Garzon-Muvdi, et al., (2011). "Supratentorial glioblastoma multiforme: the role of surgical resection versus biopsy among older patients." *Ann. Surg. Oncol.* 18(1): 239-245.

Chaichana, K. L., H. Guerrero-Cazares, et al., (2009). "Intra-operatively obtained human tissue: protocols and techniques for the study of neural stem cells." *J. Neurosci. Methods* 180(1): 116-125.

Chaichana, K. L., M. J. McGirt, et al., (2010). "Recurrence and malignant degeneration after resection of adult hemispheric low-grade gliomas." *J. Neurosurg.* 112(1): 10-17.

Chaichana, K. L., P. Zadnik, et al., (2013). "Multiple resections for patients with glioblastoma: prolonging survival." *J. Neurosurg.* 118(4): 812-820.

Chaturvedi, P., D. M. Gilkes, et al., (2013). "Hypoxia-inducible factor-dependent breast cancer-mesenchymal stem cell bidirectional signaling promotes metastasis." *J. Clin. Invest.* 123(1): 189-205.

Chesler, D. A., M. S. Berger, et al., (2012). "The potential origin of glioblastoma initiating cells." *Front Biosci. (Schol Ed.)* 4: 190-205.

Choi, H., R. H. Lee, et al., (2011). "Anti-inflammatory protein TSG-6 secreted by activated MSCs attenuates zymosan-induced mouse peritonitis by decreasing TLR2/NF-kappaB signaling in resident macrophages." *Blood* 118(2): 330-338.

Choi, S. A., S. K. Hwang, et al., (2011). "Therapeutic efficacy and safety of TRAIL-producing human adipose tissue-derived mesenchymal stem cells against experimental brainstem glioma." *Neuro Oncol.* 13(1): 61-69.

Comoli, P., F. Ginevri, et al., (2008). "Human mesenchymal stem cells inhibit antibody production induced in vitro by allostimulation." *Nephrology, dialysis, transplantation: official publication of the European Dialysis and Transplant Association - European Renal Association* 23(4): 1196-1202.

Conconi, M. T., P. Burra, et al., (2006). "CD105(+) cells from Wharton's jelly show in vitro and in vivo myogenic differentiative potential." *Int. J. Mol. Med.* 18(6): 1089-1096.

Covas, D. T., J. L. Siufi, et al., (2003). "Isolation and culture of umbilical vein mesenchymal stem cells." *Brazilian journal of medical and biological research = Revista brasileira de pesquisas medicas e biologicas / Sociedade Brasileira de Biofisica ... [et al.,]* 36(9): 1179-1183.

Crigler, L., R. C. Robey, et al., (2006). "Human mesenchymal stem cell subpopulations express a variety of neuro-regulatory molecules and promote neuronal cell survival and neuritogenesis." *Experimental neurology* 198(1): 54-64.

Cutler, A. J., V. Limbani, et al., (2010). "Umbilical cord-derived mesenchymal stromal cells modulate monocyte function to suppress T cell proliferation." *Journal of immunology* 185(11): 6617-6623.

Danisovic, L., I. Varga, et al., (2009). "Comparison of in vitro chondrogenic potential of human mesenchymal stem cells derived from bone marrow and adipose tissue." *Gen. Physiol. Biophys.* 28(1): 56-62.

De Bari, C., F. Dell'Accio, et al., (2001). "Multipotent mesenchymal stem cells from adult human synovial membrane." *Arthritis Rheum.* 44(8): 1928-1942.

Deak, E., E. Seifried, et al., (2010). "Homing pathways of mesenchymal stromal cells (MSCs) and their role in clinical applications." *International reviews of immunology* 29(5): 514-529.

Delorme, B., J. Ringe, et al., (2009). "Specific lineage-priming of bone marrow mesenchymal stem cells provides the molecular framework for their plasticity." *Stem Cells* 27(5): 1142-1151.

Deng, H., R. Makizumi, et al., (2007). "Bone morphogenetic protein-4 is overexpressed in colonic adenocarcinomas and promotes migration and invasion of HCT116 cells." *Exp. Cell Res.* 313(5): 1033-1044.

Di Nicola, M., C. Carlo-Stella, et al., (2002). "Human bone marrow stromal cells suppress T-lymphocyte proliferation induced by cellular or nonspecific mitogenic stimuli." *Blood* 99(10): 3838-3843.

Dix, A. R., W. H. Brooks, et al., (1999). "Immune defects observed in patients with primary malignant brain tumors." *J. Neuroimmunol.* 100(1-2): 216-232.

Elzaouk, L., K. Moelling, et al., (2006). "Anti-tumor activity of mesenchymal stem cells producing IL-12 in a mouse melanoma model." *Exp. Dermatol.* 15(11): 865-874.

Endo, Y., E. Beauchamp, et al., (2008). "Wnt-3a and Dickkopf-1 stimulate neurite outgrowth in Ewing tumor cells via a Frizzled3- and c-Jun N-terminal kinase-dependent mechanism." *Molecular and cellular biology* 28(7): 2368-2379.

English, K. (2013). "Mechanisms of mesenchymal stromal cell immunomodulation." *Immunology and cell biology* 91(1): 19-26.

English, K., F. P. Barry, et al., (2007). "IFN-gamma and TNF-alpha differentially regulate immunomodulation by murine mesenchymal stem cells." *Immunology letters* 110(2): 91-100.

English, K., F. P. Barry, et al., (2008). "Murine mesenchymal stem cells suppress dendritic cell migration, maturation and antigen presentation." *Immunology letters* 115(1): 50-58.

Erices, A., P. Conget, et al., (2000). "Mesenchymal progenitor cells in human umbilical cord blood." *British journal of haematology* 109(1): 235-242.

Etheridge, S. L., G. J. Spencer, et al., (2004). "Expression profiling and functional analysis of wnt signaling mechanisms in mesenchymal stem cells." *Stem cells* 22(5): 849-860.

Ferriero, D. M. (2004). "Neonatal brain injury." *The New England journal of medicine* 351(19): 1985-1995.

Friedenstein, A. J., R. K. Chailakhyan, et al., (1974). "Stromal cells responsible for transferring the microenvironment of the hemopoietic tissues. Cloning in vitro and retransplantation in vivo." *Transplantation* 17(4): 331-340.

Ge, W., J. Jiang, et al., (2010). "Regulatory T-cell generation and kidney allograft tolerance induced by mesenchymal stem cells associated with indoleamine 2,3-dioxygenase expression." *Transplantation* 90(12): 1312-1320.

Gregory, C. A., H. Singh, et al., (2003). "The Wnt signaling inhibitor dickkopf-1 is required for reentry into the cell cycle of human adult stem cells from bone marrow." *The Journal of biological chemistry* 278(30): 28067-28078.

Guerrero-Cazares, H., F. J. Attenello, et al., (2012). "Stem cells in gliomas." *Handb Clin. Neurol.* 104: 63-73.

Guo, D., J. Huang, et al., (2012). "Bone morphogenetic protein 4 (BMP4) is required for migration and invasion of breast cancer." *Mol. Cell Biochem.* 363(1-2): 179-190.

Hall, B., J. Dembinski, et al., (2007). "Mesenchymal stem cells in cancer: tumor-associated fibroblasts and cell-based delivery vehicles." *Int. J. Hematol.* 86(1): 8-16.

Huibregtse, B. A., B. Johnstone, et al., (2000). "Effect of age and sampling site on the chondro-osteogenic potential of rabbit marrow-derived mesenchymal progenitor cells." *J. Orthop. Res.* 18(1): 18-24.

Ikegame, Y., K. Yamashita, et al., (2011). "Comparison of mesenchymal stem cells from adipose tissue and bone marrow for ischemic stroke therapy." *Cytotherapy* 13(6): 675-685.

Joyce, N., G. Annett, et al., (2010). "Mesenchymal stem cells for the treatment of neurodegenerative disease." *Regenerative medicine* 5(6): 933-946.

Kassis, I., N. Grigoriadis, et al., (2008). "Neuroprotection and immunomodulation with mesenchymal stem cells in chronic experimental autoimmune encephalomyelitis." *Archives of neurology* 65(6): 753-761.

Kavanagh, H. and B. P. Mahon (2011). "Allogeneic mesenchymal stem cells prevent allergic airway inflammation by inducing murine regulatory T cells." *Allergy* 66(4): 523-531.

Kerkis, I. and A. I. Caplan (2012). "Stem cells in dental pulp of deciduous teeth." *Tissue engineering*. Part B, Reviews 18(2): 129-138.

Kim, J. and P. Hematti (2009). "Mesenchymal stem cell-educated macrophages: a novel type of alternatively activated macrophages." *Experimental hematology* 37(12): 1445-1453.

Kong, Q. F., B. Sun, et al., (2009). "Administration of bone marrow stromal cells ameliorates experimental autoimmune myasthenia gravis by altering the balance of Th1/Th2/Th17/Treg cell subsets through the secretion of TGF-beta." *Journal of neuroimmunology* 207(1-2): 83-91.

Kucerova, L., M. Matuskova, et al., (2010). "Tumor cell behaviour modulation by mesenchymal stromal cells." *Mol. Cancer* 9: 129.

Lamfers, M., S. Idema, et al., (2009). "Homing properties of adipose-derived stem cells to intracerebral glioma and the effects of adenovirus infection." *Cancer Lett.* 274(1): 78-87.

Lee, J. A., B. I. Kim, et al., (2010). "Mesenchymal stem-cell transplantation for hypoxic-ischemic brain injury in neonatal rat model." *Pediatric research* 67(1): 42-46.

Lee, R. H., A. A. Pulin, et al., (2009). "Intravenous hMSCs improve myocardial infarction in mice because cells embolized in lung are activated to secrete the anti-inflammatory protein TSG-6." *Cell stem cell* 5 (1): 54-63.

Liu, L., M. A. Eckert, et al., (2013). "From blood to the brain: can systemically transplanted mesenchymal stem cells cross the blood-brain barrier?" *Stem Cells Int.* 2013: 435093.

Lunn, J. S., S. A. Sakowski, et al., (2011). "Stem cell technology for neurodegenerative diseases." *Annals of neurology* 70(3): 353-361.

Matuskova, M., K. Hlubinova, et al., (2010). "HSV-tk expressing mesenchymal stem cells exert bystander effect on human glioblastoma cells." *Cancer Lett.* 290(1): 58-67.

McGirt, M. J., K. L. Chaichana, et al., (2008). "Extent of surgical resection is independently associated with survival in patients with hemispheric infiltrating low-grade gliomas." *Neurosurgery* 63(4): 700-707; author reply 707-708.

McGirt, M. J., K. L. Chaichana, et al., (2009). "Independent association of extent of resection with survival in patients with malignant brain astrocytoma." *J. Neurosurg.* 110(1): 156-162.

Medzhitov, R. (2010). "Inflammation 2010: new adventures of an old flame." *Cell* 140(6): 771-776.

Mishra, P. J., J. W. Glod, et al., (2009). "Mesenchymal stem cells: flip side of the coin." *Cancer Res.* 69(4): 1255-1258.

Mishra, P. J., R. Humeniuk, et al., (2008). "Carcinoma-associated fibroblast-like differentiation of human mesenchymal stem cells." *Cancer Res.* 68 (11): 4331-4339.

Mishra, P. J. and G. Merlino (2008). "A traitor in our midst: mesenchymal stem cells contribute to tumor progression and metastasis." *Future Oncol.* 4(6): 745-749.

Momin, E. N., A. Mohyeldin, et al., (2010). "Mesenchymal stem cells: new approaches for the treatment of neurological diseases." *Curr. Stem Cell Res. Ther.* 5(4): 326-344.

Momin, E. N., G. Vela, et al., (2010). "The Oncogenic Potential of Mesenchymal Stem Cells in the Treatment of Cancer: Directions for Future Research." *Curr. Immunol. Rev.* 6(2): 137-148.

Munoz, J. R., B. R. Stoutenger, et al., (2005). "Human stem/progenitor cells from bone marrow promote neurogenesis of endogenous neural stem cells in the hippocampus of mice." *Proceedings of the National Academy of Sciences of the United States of America* 102(50): 18171-18176.

Nakamizo, A., F. Marini, et al., (2005). "Human bone marrow-derived mesenchymal stem cells in the treatment of gliomas." *Cancer Res.* 65(8): 3307-3318.

Nakamura, K., Y. Ito, et al., (2004). "Antitumor effect of genetically engineered mesenchymal stem cells in a rat glioma model." *Gene Ther.* 11 (14): 1155-1164.

Nemeth, K., A. Leelahavanichkul, et al., (2009). "Bone marrow stromal cells attenuate sepsis via prostaglandin E(2)-dependent reprogramming of host macrophages to increase their interleukin-10 production." *Nature medicine* 15(1): 42-49.

Northington, F. J., R. Chavez-Valdez, et al., (2011). "Neuronal cell death in neonatal hypoxia-ischemia." *Annals of neurology* 69(5): 743-758.

Okazaki, T., T. Magaki, et al., (2008). "Intravenous administration of bone marrow stromal cells increases survivin and Bcl-2 protein expression and improves sensorimotor function following ischemia in rats." *Neuroscience letters* 430(2): 109-114.

Parsons, X. H., Y. D. Teng, et al., (2011). "Efficient derivation of human neuronal progenitors and neurons from pluripotent human embryonic stem cells with small molecule induction." *Journal of visualized experiments: JoVE*(56): e3273.

Pendleton, C., Q. Li, et al., (2013). "Mesenchymal stem cells derived from adipose tissue vs bone marrow: in vitro comparison of their tropism towards gliomas." *PloS one* 8(3): e58198.

Pierdomenico, L., L. Bonsi, et al., (2005). "Multipotent mesenchymal stem cells with immunosuppressive activity can be easily isolated from dental pulp." *Transplantation* 80(6): 836-842.

Pittenger, M. F., A. M. Mackay, et al., (1999). "Multilineage potential of adult human mesenchymal stem cells." *Science* 284(5411): 143-147.

Polchert, D., J. Sobinsky, et al., (2008). "IFN-gamma activation of mesenchymal stem cells for treatment and prevention of graft versus host disease." *European journal of immunology* 38(6): 1745-1755.

Quinones-Hinojosa, A. and K. Chaichana (2007). "The human subventricular zone: a source of new cells and a potential source of brain tumors." *Exp. Neurol.* 205(2): 313-324.

Relaix, F. and C. Marcelle (2009). "Muscle stem cells." *Curr. Opin. Cell Biol.* 21(6): 748-753.

Ren, G., L. Zhang, et al., (2008). "Mesenchymal stem cell-mediated immunosuppression occurs via concerted action of chemokines and nitric oxide." *Cell stem cell* 2(2): 141-150.

Reyes, M., T. Lund, et al., (2001). "Purification and ex vivo expansion of postnatal human marrow mesodermal progenitor cells." *Blood* 98(9): 2615-2625.

Rich, J. N. (2007). "Cancer stem cells in radiation resistance." *Cancer Res.* 67 (19): 8980-8984.

Rogers, J. J., H. E. Young, et al., (1995). "Differentiation factors induce expression of muscle, fat, cartilage, and bone in a clone of mouse pluripotent mesenchymal stem cells." *The American surgeon* 61(3): 231-236.

Sakaguchi, Y., I. Sekiya, et al., (2005). "Comparison of human stem cells derived from various mesenchymal tissues: superiority of synovium as a cell source." *Arthritis Rheum.* 52(8): 2521-2529.

Sale, G. E. and R. Storb (1983). "Bilateral diffuse pulmonary ectopic ossification after marrow allograft in a dog. Evidence for allotransplantation of hemopoietic and mesenchymal stem cells." *Experimental hematology* 11(10): 961-966.

Sasportas, L. S., R. Kasmieh, et al., (2009). "Assessment of therapeutic efficacy and fate of engineered human mesenchymal stem cells for cancer therapy." *Proc. Natl. Acad. Sci. US* 106(12): 4822-4827.

Spaeth, E. L., J. L. Dembinski, et al., (2009). "Mesenchymal stem cell transition to tumor-associated fibroblasts contributes to fibrovascular network expansion and tumor progression." *PLoS One* 4(4): e4992.

Spaggiari, G. M., A. Capobianco, et al., (2006). "Mesenchymal stem cell-natural killer cell interactions: evidence that activated NK cells are capable of killing MSCs, whereas MSCs can inhibit IL-2-induced NK-cell proliferation." *Blood* 107(4): 1484-1490.

Sparks, R. L., E. I. Seibel-Ross, et al., (1986). "Differentiation, dedifferentiation, and transdifferentiation of BALB/c 3T3 T mesenchymal stem cells: potential significance in metaplasia and neoplasia." *Cancer research* 46(10): 5312-5319.

Strioga, M., S. Viswanathan, et al., (2012). "Same or not the same? Comparison of adipose tissue-derived versus bone marrow-derived mesenchymal stem and stromal cells." *Stem cells and development* 21(14): 2724-2752.

Strioga, M., S. Viswanathan, et al., (2012). "Same or not the same? Comparison of adipose tissue-derived versus bone marrow-derived mesenchymal stem and stromal cells." *Stem Cells Dev.* 21(14): 2724-2752.

Stupp, R., W. P. Mason, et al., (2005). "Radiotherapy plus concomitant and adjuvant temozolomide for glioblastoma." *N. Engl. J. Med.* 352(10): 987-996.

Tyler, M. A., I. V. Ulasov, et al., (2009). "Neural stem cells target intracranial glioma to deliver an oncolytic adenovirus in vivo." *Gene Ther.* 16(2): 262-278.

Uezumi, A., K. Ojima, et al., (2006). "Functional heterogeneity of side population cells in skeletal muscle." *Biochem. Biophys. Res. Commun.* 341 (3): 864-873.

Van Velthoven, C. T., A. Kavelaars, et al., (2012). "Mesenchymal stem cells as a treatment for neonatal ischemic brain damage." *Pediatric research* 71(4 Pt 2): 474-481.

Van Velthoven, C. T., A. Kavelaars, et al., (2010). "Mesenchymal stem cell treatment after neonatal hypoxic-ischemic brain injury improves behavioral outcome and induces neuronal and oligodendrocyte regeneration." *Brain, behavior, and immunity* 24(3): 387-393.

Van Velthoven, C. T., A. Kavelaars, et al., (2010). "Nasal administration of stem cells: a promising novel route to treat neonatal ischemic brain damage." *Pediatric research* 68(5): 419-422.

Van Velthoven, C. T., A. Kavelaars, et al., (2010). "Repeated mesenchymal stem cell treatment after neonatal hypoxia-ischemia has distinct effects on formation and maturation of new neurons and oligodendrocytes leading to restoration of damage, corticospinal motor tract activity, and sensorimotor function." *The Journal of neuroscience: the official journal of the Society for Neuroscience* 30(28): 9603-9611.

Verhaak, R. G., K. A. Hoadley, et al., (2010). "Integrated genomic analysis identifies clinically relevant subtypes of glioblastoma characterized by abnormalities in PDGFRA, IDH1, EGFR, and NF1." *Cancer Cell* 17(1): 98-110.

Via, A. G., A. Frizziero, et al., (2012). "Biological properties of mesenchymal Stem Cells from different sources." *Muscles Ligaments Tendons J.* 2(3): 154-162.

Violini, S., P. Ramelli, et al., (2009). "Horse bone marrow mesenchymal stem cells express embryo stem cell markers and show the ability for tenogenic differentiation by in vitro exposure to BMP-12." *BMC Cell Biol.* 10: 29.

Wang, H. S., S. C. Hung, et al., (2004). "Mesenchymal stem cells in the Wharton's jelly of the human umbilical cord." *Stem Cells* 22(7): 1330-1337.

Waziri, A. (2010). "Glioblastoma-derived mechanisms of systemic immunosuppression." *Neurosurg. Clin. N. Am.* 21(1): 31-42.

Wilkins, A., K. Kemp, et al., (2009). "Human bone marrow-derived mesenchymal stem cells secrete brain-derived neurotrophic factor which promotes neuronal survival in vitro." *Stem cell research* 3(1): 63-70.

Wu, K. H., B. Zhou, et al., (2007). "In vitro and in vivo differentiation of human umbilical cord derived stem cells into endothelial cells." *J. Cell Biochem.* 100(3): 608-616.

Wynn, R. F., C. A. Hart, et al., (2004). "A small proportion of mesenchymal stem cells strongly expresses functionally active CXCR4 receptor capable of promoting migration to bone marrow." *Blood* 104(9): 2643-2645.

Xu, L., D. M. Cochran, et al., (2006). "Placenta growth factor overexpression inhibits tumor growth, angiogenesis, and metastasis by depleting vascular endothelial growth factor homodimers in orthotopic mouse models." *Cancer Res.* 66(8): 3971-3977.

Yang, I., S. J. Han, et al., (2010). "The role of microglia in central nervous system immunity and glioma immunology." *J. Clin. Neurosci.* 17(1): 6-10.

Yasuhara, T., K. Hara, et al., (2008). "Intravenous grafts recapitulate the neurorestoration afforded by intracerebrally delivered multipotent adult progenitor cells in neonatal hypoxic-ischemic rats." *Journal of cerebral blood flow and metabolism: official journal of the International Society of Cerebral Blood Flow and Metabolism* 28(11): 1804-1810.

Yasuhara, T., N. Matsukawa, et al., (2006). "Behavioral and histological characterization of intrahippocampal grafts of human bone marrow-derived multipotent progenitor cells in neonatal rats with hypoxic-ischemic injury." *Cell transplantation* 15(3): 231-238.

Yuan, X., J. Hu, et al., (2006). "Interleukin-23-expressing bone marrow-derived neural stem-like cells exhibit antitumor activity against intracranial glioma." *Cancer Res.* 66(5): 2630-2638.

Zaidi, H. A., T. Kosztowski, et al., (2009). "Origins and clinical implications of the brain tumor stem cell hypothesis." *J. Neurooncol.* 93(1): 49-60.

Zuk, P. A., M. Zhu, et al., (2002). "Human adipose tissue is a source of multipotent stem cells." *Molecular biology of the cell* 13(12): 4279-4295.

Zuk, P. A., M. Zhu, et al., (2001). "Multilineage cells from human adipose tissue: implications for cell-based therapies." *Tissue engineering* 7(2): 211-228.

In: Neuro-Immune Interactions … ISBN: 978-1-62948-646-8
Editor: Oscar González-Pérez

Chapter 5

NEURO-IMMUNE INTERACTIONS IN NEURAL STEM CELLS OF THE POSTNATAL SUBVENTRICULAR ZONE

Fernando Gutiérrez-Fernández, María Pinto-Gonzalez and Oscar Gonzalez-Perez*

Laboratory of Neuroscience, School of Psychology, University of Colima
Mexico, Colima, México

ABSTRACT

As described in this book, the interaction between the immune system and the brain can affect multiple cerebral functions, such as: neural remodeling, synaptic plasticity or neurotransmitter releasing. Neurogenic niches are not the exception, in fact, pro-inflammatory cytokines and chemokines exert a strong regulation in neural stem cells (NSCs) of the subventricular zone (SVZ) by interacting with cell membrane receptors and activating multiple downstream pathways. These neuro-immune interactions modulate quiescence, cell adhesion, migration, self-renewal, differentiation, cytoskeletal rearrangement, and cell survival. In this chapter, we describe the cellular composition and cytoarchitecture of the main neurogenic niche in the adult mammalian

* Corresponding author: Oscar Gonzalez-Perez, Laboratorio de Neurociencias, Facultad de Psicología, Universidad de Colima. Av. Universidad 333, Colima, COL 28040 Mexico, Email: osglez@ucol.mx.

brain: the SVZ. We also discuss the current evidence indicating that many immunological molecules can control the function of this neurogenic niche in the adult brain under both physiological and pathological conditions.

ACRONYMS

NSCs	Neural stem cells;
SVZ	subventricular zone;
CNS	central nervous system;
NPCs	neural precursor cells;
SGZ	subgranular zone;
OB	olfactory bulb;
RMS	rostral migratory stream;
EGF	epidermal growth factor;
bFGF or FGF-2	basic fibroblast growth factor;
PDGF	platelet derived growth factor;
BMP	bone morphogenetic protein;
Y (NPY)	erythropoietin, neuropeptide;
PLC	phospholipase C;
PKC	protein kinase C;
JAK/STAT	pathway, Janus kinase-signal transducer;
IL-1	interleukin-1;
IGF-1	interleukin-4 (IL-4); insulin growth factor-1;
IL-6	interleukin-6;
BMP	bone morphogenetic proteins;
TNF-α	Tumor necrosis factor-α;
IFN-γ	interferon-γ;
IL-10	interleukin-10;
Th2	T-helper lymphocyte type2;
CSF	cerebrospinal fluid;
IL-15	Interleukin-15;
LIF	leukemia inhibitory factor;
CNTF	ciliary neurotrophic factor;
CT-1	cardiotrophin-1;
CLC/CLF	cardotrophin-like cytokine/cytokine like factor-1;
TGF-β1	transforming growth factor-β1;
SDF-1α	stromal cell-derived factor-1;
IL-17	Interleukin-17

INTRODUCTION

The last century was a breaking era of many prevailing dogmas in neuroscience. Until the last decades of the twentieth century, it was believed that postnatal cell proliferation in the central nervous system (CNS) was limited to glial cells. Hence, from this traditional point of view, the loss of postnatal neurons was irreversible. In the 1960's, postnatal neurogenesis was first described by Joseph Altman [1]. However, in the 1980's and 1990′s the phenomenon of neurogenesis was totally demonstrated in the telencephalon of reptiles, birds and several mammalian species. This cell plasticity possibly occurs in the CNS of all vertebrate species. Nowadays, it's well accepted that there are brain-specific niches of multipotent neural stem cells (NSCs) that generate new neurons and oligodendrocytes. These novel cells help maintain tissue homeostasis of the gray and the white matter.

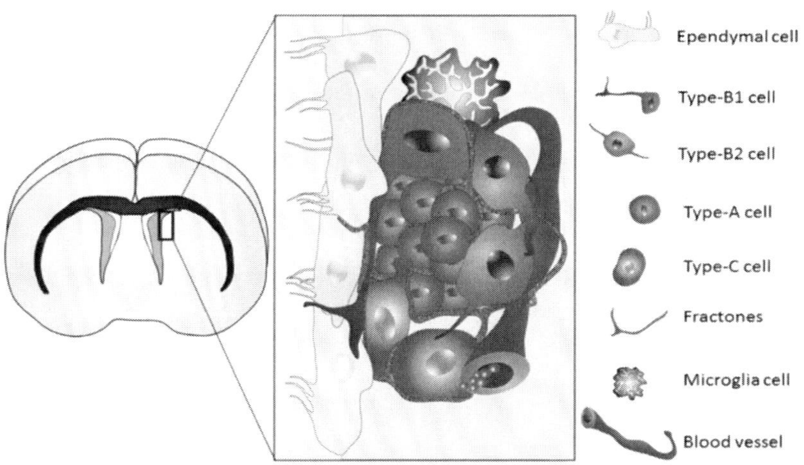

Figure 1. Mouse subventricular zone (SVZ). On the right: a coronal section of the mouse brain indicating a portion of adult SVZ. On the left: a magnified view of this germinal region. Within the SVZ there are *bona fide* neural stem cells (type B1 cells), which maintain a close contact to ventricular lumen, blood vessels and fractones. Microglia cells are commonly found near to type-B and type-C cells.

The postnatal sources of NSCs or neural precursor cells (NPCs) are two germinal niches in the brain: the subventricular zone (SVZ) and the subgranular zone (SGZ) [2, 3]. The largest germinal region in the adult brain is the SVZ, which contains NSCs with structural and molecular characteristics of astrocytes known as type-B1 cells (Figure 1). The mitotic division of type-B1 cell gives rise to intermediate neural progenitors, also known as transit amplifying progenitors or type-C cells, which in turn give rise to migrating neuroblasts (type–A cells) that migrate to the olfactory bulb. Subventricular NSCs also generate oligodendrocytes that populate the neighboring white matter of corpus callosum, fimbria and striatum [4-6].

Increasing evidence supports the existence of a bi-directional communication between the CNS and the immune system. Under physiological conditions a few immune cells (T lymphocytes, macrophages and dendritic cells) can penetrate the blood brain barrier. In contrast, neuroinflammation triggers the infiltration of macrophages and lymphocytes into the cerebral parenchyma, activating microglia and astrocytes that release anti- and pro-inflammatory cytokines, chemokines, neurotransmitters, reactive oxygen species (ROS), and surface receptors, such as: cytokine receptors and toll-like receptors [7-10]. This cellular and chemical interaction between the immune system and the brain can affect multiple cerebral functions, such as: neural remodeling, synaptic plasticity, neurotransmitter release and neurogenesis. A number of immunological cytokines and chemokines modulate the function of NSCs in the SVZ triggering a myriad of cellular effects, such as: quiescence, cell adhesion, migration, survival, differentiation, cytoskeletal rearrangement, self-renewal and cell survival [10-13]. To date, elucidating the regulatory factors that preserve the stem-cells homeostasis is one of the main goals for stem-cell-based therapies against a wide range of neurodegenerative diseases and/or psychiatric disorders.

THE SUBVENTRICULAR ZONE

The SVZ is the largest source of new neurons in the adult brain (Gonzalez-Pérez, 2011), which is adjacent to the lateral wall of lateral ventricles in all mammals. Interestingly, there are remarkable differences between the cytoarchitecture and cell composition between the human SVZ as compared to other animal species. Human SVZ consists of four layers with different cell composition (Figure 2) [14-16]. Layer I, adjacent to the lateral ventricle, is a monocellular layer, composed by non-mitotic multiciliated ependymal cells with cytoplasm expansions perpendicular to the ventricle surface. The layer II, also known as hypocellular layer, consists of ependymal cytoplasm expansions interconnected with astrocyte processes and less frequently with astrocytic and neuronal cell bodies. The layer II is thought to play a relevant role in development at embryonic stages, as a source of neurons for cortical and subcortical regions; other hypotheses propose that that the astrocytic and ependymal interconnections within this layer may regulate neuronal functions and metabolic homeostasis of the SVZ. Contiguous to the hypocellular layer, it is the III layer, a ribbon of cells comprised of astrocytes which show proliferative activity, olygodendrocytes, and small clusters of displaced ependymal cells. Astrocytes in the SVZ can be subdivided in three types: small astrocytes, found in the hypocellular layer; large astrocytes, located at the interface between Layer II and III and in the medial wall at the level of the body of the lateral ventricle; the third type of astrocytes are also large, and are primarily found in the ventral temporal horn overlying the hippocampus [14-16]. Current evidence indicates that one of these subtypes of astrocytes may be the *bona fide* NSCs in the adult SVZ. The Layer IV is formed by myelin tracts and is considered a transition zone between the astrocytic ribbon and the brain parenchyma [14, 17]. Migration of human SVZ NSCs to the olfactory bulb and prefrontal cortex has been recently described in early postnatal human brain [18].

The minor mammalians SVZ contains a slow primary dividing progeny (type-B cells) and fast dividing cell precursors (type-C cells). Type B-cells are a subclass of astrocytes which constitute the primary neural progenitors, and can be divided in Type-B1 and Type B2 astrocytes [19, 20]. Type-B1 astrocytes are polarized cells, where the ependymal side is associated with the ependymal layer, extending an apical process towards the ventricle, which terminus has a cilium that contacts the cerebrospinal fluid; whereas the parenchymal side, contacts the basal lamina and the blood vessel [21, 22]. In contrast Type-2 astrocytes are located near the brain parenchyma. Mitotic division of type-B1 cells gives rise to transit amplifying progenitors or type-C cells, which, in turn, generate migrating neuroblasts or type-A cells [19, 20].

NSCs from the subventricular zone migrate towards the olfactory bulb (OB) through the rostral migratory stream (RMS), forming chains of migratory cells [23-25]. Once in the core of the OB, NSCs disperse radially and complete their differentiation into glomerular and periglomerular GABAergic interneurons, and only a small percentage become dopaminergic, which seem to play a role in the olfaction process [26]. On the other hand, stem cell-derived olygodendrocytes are incorporated in the white matter of corpus callosum, fimbria and striatum as myelinating and non-myelinating oligodendrocytes [4-6]. Remarkably, oligodendrogenesis from the SVZ is significantly up-regulated during a demyelinating lesion [4-6]. Multiple proteins and chemical mediators regulate SVZ including: the epidermal growth factor (EGF), basic fibroblast growth factor (bFGF or FGF-2), platelet derived growth factor (PDGF), bone morphogenetic protein (BMP), erythropoietin, neuropeptide Y (NPY), noggin, prolactin, PACAP, Notch, , Sonic hedgehog and gp130 [27-33].

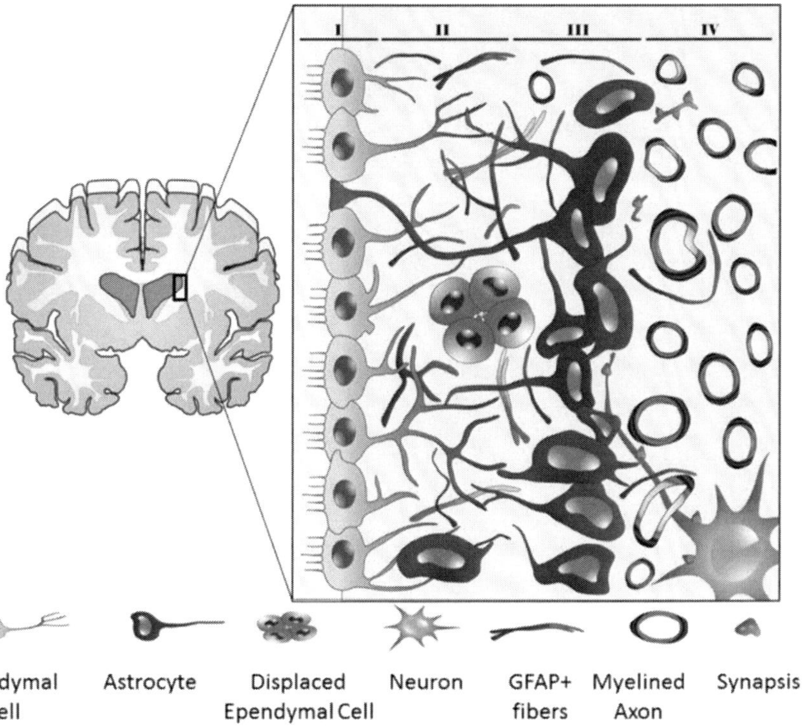

Figure 2. Human subventricular zone (hSVZ). On the right: a coronal section of the human brain indicating a portion of adult SVZ. On the left: a magnified view of this germinal region. Within the hSVZ there is a subpopulation of astrocytes (type B cells), which are comprised between the layers II and III. These cells are putative neural stem cells as demonstrated by their capacity to give rise to neurons, astrocytes and oligodendrocytes *in vitro*. Note the presence of displaced ependymal cells within the brain parenchyma and the ribbon of astrocytes, which are some of the distinctive characteristics of the human SVZ.

IMMUNOLOGICAL REGULATION OF NEURAL PRECURSOR CELLS IN THE SUBVENTRICULAR ZONE

In the brain, an inflammatory process triggers a cascade of molecular and transcriptional events that conclude in a massive production of cytokines from local microglia and parenchymal cell infiltration by neutrophils, monocytes and lymphocytes. Microglia is abundant along the wall of the ventricles, which suggest a local interaction between immune molecules and neural progenitors in the SVZ. Secreted cytokines initiate a myriad of effects in neural progenitor cells of the SVZ that depend on their molar concentration, length of inflammatory stimuli, brain region involved and neural progenitor subtypes (Figure 3). Microglial modulation of NSCs is mediated by the phospholipase C (PLC)/protein kinase C (PKC) and Janus kinase-signal transducer (JAK/STAT) pathways, mitogen activated PKC and phosphatidylinositol-3-kinase/Akt signaling pathways, [13, 34-36] Therefore, immunological modulation of NSCs is a very dynamic process and, so far, is not quite understood.

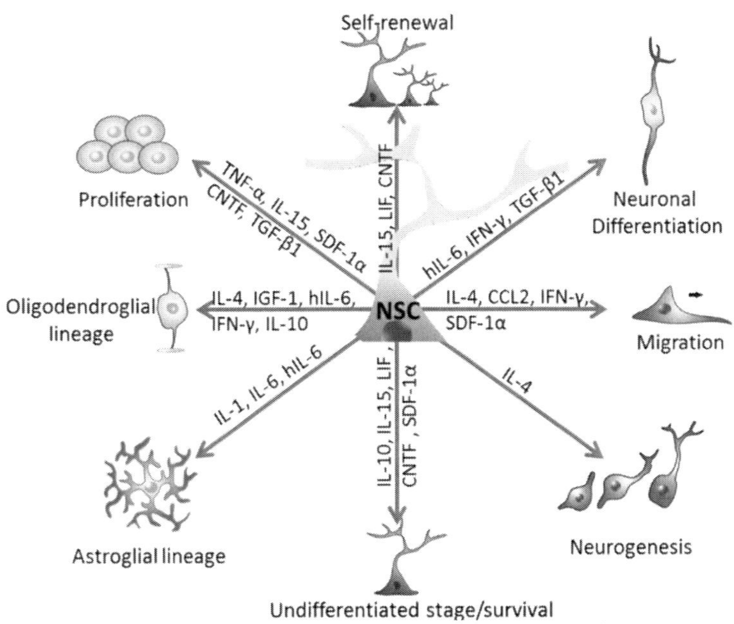

Figure 3. Effects of immunological cytokines on neural stem cells (NSCs). Cytokines derived from immune cells trigger a myriad of biological effects in the NSCs of the adult SVZ.

IL-1 Family

Interleukin-1family is a group of pro-inflammatory cytokines, consisting of three closely related proteins derived from distinct genes. IL-1α and IL-1β are agonists that exert similar actions and bind to a single cell surface receptor (IL-1R1), whereas the third member is an IL-1 receptor antagonist (IL-Ra), which blocks the actions of IL-1α and IL-1β [37, 38]. LPS stimulation of microglia, up regulates mature IL-1α and IL-1β levels. Preliminary experiments reported that IL-R1 was not expressed in the SVZ [37, 39, 40]. In contrast, recent reports demonstrate that IL-1R1 is expressed in SVZ NSCs. IL-1R1 activation by IL-1α enhances SVZ NSCs differentiation into astrocytes, without affecting cell viability or neuronal differentiation [38, 41].

IL-4

Interleukin-4 (IL-4) is an anti-inflammatory cytokine produced by Th2 cells, which extravasate through the endothelium of the choroid plexus towards the cerebrospinal fluid. This mechanism allows IL-4 to reach the NSCs of SVZ [42]. IL-4 has no direct effect on SVZ NSCs cultures [42]. Nevertheless, the interaction of IL-4 with microglia enhances neurogenesis and provides neuroprotection *in vitro*. These effects are thought to be mediated by indirect mechanisms. IL-4 enhances the production of insulin growth factor-1 (IGF-1) which, in turn, induces NSCs to differentiate into oligodendrocytic lineage [43]. It has also been reported that treatment of NSCs with IL-4 up regulates the expression of surface adhesion molecule LFA-1 (lymphocyte function associated antigen) and chemokine receptors CXCR4 and CCR5, leading to an enhanced chemotaxis of NSCs to RANTES (regulated on activation, normal T cells expressed and secreted, also known as CCL5), which suggests a role of IL-4 in the process of NSCs migration towards the site of damage [38, 44].

IL-6

Interleukin-6 (IL-6) is commonly considered a pro-inflammatory cytokine. However, according to its physiological role, IL-6 is better classified as a neurotrophic factor. IL-6 is produced by activated microglia [45]. IL-6 cannot target directly NSCs, because of the lacking expression of a functional receptor (IL-6R) in neural precursor cells. Instead, IL-6 couples to a soluble form of IL-6R (sIL-6R) that binds to gp-130, activating the JAK/STAT3 and the MAPK pathways [46, 47]. In the SVZ, IL-6 induces differentiation of NSCs into astrocytic lineage [47, 48]. Some reports suggest that IL-6 and bone morphogenetic proteins (BMP) family cytokines exert a synergic effect on neuroephitelial cells to induce astrocytic differentiation, via the formation of a complex between their downstream transcription factors, STAT3 and Smad1 respectively, which are linked by the transcriptional coactivator p300 [49]. The activation of this common transcriptional effector modifies methylation patterns, which are determinant in the regulation of astrocytogenesis [49]. Further evidence indicates that hyper IL-6, the active protein derived from IL-6/sIL-6R fusion, induces NSCs differentiation into glutamate-responsive neurons, oligodendroglia and astrocytes [47, 48]. Instead, IL-6 has also been reported as a contributor of the anti-neurogenic effects of lipopolysaccharides (**LPS**)-activated microglia.

TNF-α

Tumor necrosis factor-alpha (TNF-α) is a pro-inflammatory cytokine member of the TNF superfamily of ligands. TNF-α is produced by activated microglia, and seems to have both negative and positive effects on neurogenesis depending on the receptor activated: TNF-α binding to the TNFR1 receptor inhibits neurogenesis, unlike when it binds to the TNFR2 receptor NSCs survival and proliferation is increased [50, 51]. TNF-α increases the expression of MCP-1 (CCL2). This chemokine that induces NSCs migration, neuronal and oligodendroglial differentiation via the MCP-1 receptor CCR2 [36, 52-55]. MCP-1 appears to protect neurons against NMDA-mediated excitotoxicity [56]. In contrast, recent evidence suggests that TNF-α induces NSCs apoptosis via a mitochondrial pathway regulated by the Bcl-2 family protein Bax [51].

IFN-γ

Interferon-γ (IFN-γ) is a pro-inflammatory cytokine produced by activation of resident microglial cells, and exerts its effects on NSCs through its receptors (IFN-γR), which activation has been reported to have both pro and anti-neurogenic properties, depending on the particular experimental conditions [57]. IFN-γR activates STAT-1 signaling, reducing cell proliferation and survival [57]. Additionally, it has been reported that the decrease of NSCs proliferation induced by IFN-γ is mediated by overexpression of p21 (a gen regulator of the cell cycle); IFN-γ was also found to increase levels of the BH-3 only protein PUMA in the NPCs, which induces the mitochondrial pathway of cell death [57]. In contrast, other papers report that IFN-γ activated microglia enhances neurogenesis [42]. Besides, IFN-γ regulates the expression of cytokine and chemokine receptors such as MCP-1/CCL2 receptor (or CCR2), CXCR4 and CCR5, which expression has been proved in astrocytes, and in NSCs from the SVZ [12, 36]. CCR2 activation by its ligand MCP-1/CCL2 chemokine, promotes NSCs migration and both neuronal (probably via CXCL9) and oligodendroglial differentiation without affecting proliferation or survival [12, 54, 58]. Pro-neuronal differentiation induced by IFN-γ is mediated by the JNK pathways [59]. CXCR4 (CXCL12/SDF-1α receptor) activation promotes differentiation of oligodendrocyte precursor cells [55]; whereas CCR5 is a receptor activated by a wide range of ligands such as MCP-1/CCL2, CCL3/MIP-1α, and CCL5 or RANTES on NSCs.

IL-10

The anti-inflammatory cytokine interleukin-10 (IL-10) is a cytokine mainly produced by T-helper lymphocyte type2 (Th2) cells, and is present at low levels in circulating blood and the cerebrospinal fluid (CSF), moreover, neurons and glial cells are also able to produce IL-10; after inflammation or injury levels of this cytokine increase [60, 61]. IL-10 inhibits the activity of Th1 and Th17 lymphocytes, natural killer cells and macrophages, thus inhibiting the production of pro-inflammatory cytokines, such as TNFα, IL-1 and IFN-γ, and chemokines [61]. Recent reports have demonstrated the expression of the IL-10 receptor (IL-10R) in a group of nestin (an intermediate filament protein, used as a marker for NSCs) positive NSCs located in the dorsal SVZ, an immediate region to the RMS. IL-10 would act as a promoter of the undifferentiated stage, preventing neuronal differentiation [60]. Consistently, lacking of IL-10 enhances in vivo neuronal differentiation of SVZ NSCs and consequently, the incorporation of new neurons in the OB [60]. On the other hand, SVZ derived neurospheres treated with IL-10, upregulates the expression of the surface adhesion molecule LFA-1, and CXCR4, CCR5 chemokine receptors in the precursor cells, thus enhancing migration of NSCs to the inflammation site [44]. It has also been reported that transplanted SVZ NSCs engineered to produce IL-10, promote neuron survival, axonal growth, and remyelination of both transplanted and endogenous NSCs, in model of experimental autoimmune encephalitis [62].

IL-15

Interleukin-15 (IL-15) is a pleiotropic pro-inflammatory cytokine produced by microglial and astroglial cells, which up regulate IL-15 secretion after injury; moreover IL-15 and its receptor (IL-15R) is expressed in nestin-positive SVZ NSCs, the RMS and the developing mouse olfactory epithelium [50, 63]. NSCs and differentiating neurons, but not astrocytes or oligodendrocytes, express the IL-15Rα subunit of the IL-15 receptor, which in turn, up regulates neurogenesis. In addition, other papers report that IL-15Rα knockout mice have less olfactory neurons and proliferating cells, comparing with the wild type group [38, 63]. IL-15 enhances NSCs proliferation as reported in experiments using IL-15 knockout mice (IL-15$^{-/-}$). These animals have a reduced neurogenesis that can be reverted by IL-15 intraventricular administration. Wild type NSCs increase their proliferation and self-renewal when stimulated with recombinant IL-15 under non-proliferative cell-culture conditions. Consequently, the maintenance of the self-renewal consequently keeps NSCs in an undifferentiated stage [50, 64]. In contrast, IL-15$^{-/-}$ derived neurospheres showed diminished proliferation and self-renewal rate [50]. IL-15 exerts its action on NSCs, through the activation of the MAPK and JAK-1/STAT-3/5 signaling pathways, whereas IL-15 microglial stimulation activates both ERK and p38 MAPK pathways [50].

LIF, CNTF and CT-1

The leukemia inhibitory factor (LIF), ciliary neurotrophic factor (CNTF), cardiotrophin-1 (CT-1), and cardiotrophin-like cytokine/cytokine like factor-1 (CLC/CLF) belong to a group of structurally related cytokines, which is known as the neuropoietic cytokine family [34, 38]. These cytokines activate receptors that share similar signal-transducing subunits (gp130). Therefore they are called LIF-related cytokines [38]. Exogenous and endogenous application of CNTF has been shown to have positive effects on SVZ NSCs proliferation [65]. In contrast, Bauer and Patterson [66] reported diminished

NSC proliferation, when exogenous LIF was applied. Other studies have remarked the role of both LIF and CNTF in maintaining NSCs survival [67]. LIFR (leukemia inhibitor factor receptor)/gp130 mediated signaling promotes NSCs self-renewal by suppressing their lineage restriction to glial progenitor cells [38, 67]. Acute exposure to LIF or CNTF promotes SVZ NSCs amplification and self-renewal [66, 68], whereas chronic exposure to the same cytokines also promotes NSCs self-renewal, but alters the formation of NSCs progenies [34]. A role for LIF-related cytokines in NSCs differentiation has also been suggested. LIF and CNTF seem to induce astrocytic differentiation [38, 47]. Interestingly, in the peripheral nervous system, Schwann cell-derived CNTF, LIF and CT-1 exert a synergic effect on postnatal motoneuron survival and function. The whole effects of LIF-related cytokines are mainly mediated by the JAK/STAT pathway [34].

TGF-β1

Transforming growth factor-beta 1 (TGF-β1) is a cytokine present at low levels in health conditions but, after injury, TGF-β1 systemic levels rapidly raise. The main sources of TGF-β1 in the brain are astrocytes and microglia [69]. The role of TGF-β1 in SVZ NSCs regulation seems to depend on the physiological circumstances. In the SVZ, TGF-β1 transgenic expression or intraventricular injection results in a decrement of NSCs proliferation and null effects on neuronal differentiation [70]. However, if a stroke lesion occurs, TGF-β1 promotes NSCs proliferation and neuronal differentiation. Consistently, adenoviral-mediated delivery of TGF-β also increases NSCs proliferation and neuronal differentiation [69].

CXCL12/SDF-1α

CXCL12 or stromal cell-derived factor-1 (SDF-1α) is a chemokine that joins to its receptor CXCR4 promoting a wide range of effects. Some authors have reported its participation in the enhancement of NSCs migration, proliferation, quiescence as well in cell survival, but null effects on neural precursors differentiation [58, 71, 72]. In contrast, other reports remark the role of CXCR4 in olygodendrocyte precursor cells differentiation [73], and well as in neuronal differentiation of SVZ NSCs [58]. Finally, a recent report indicates that SDF-1α has an inhibitory role of in NSCs proliferation [36].

Other Cytokines and Chemokines

There are also important functions of another cytokines and chemokines in SVZ NSCs regulation. IL-17 is Interleukin-17 (IL-17), a pro-inflammatory cytokine generated by Th17 cells. Recent studies suggest that IL-17 plays a negative role in NSCs proliferation, differentiation and survival [74, 75]. IL-18 is a pro-inflammatory cytokine that exerts its action via the IL-18 receptor (IL-18R), a receptor of the interleukin 1 receptor/Toll like superfamily [76]. The effects of IL-18 in the developmental brain have been studied in rat neural progenitor cells. In this stage, IL-18 acts as an inhibitor of neuronal differentiation and induces neuronal cell death [77]. In the adult rodent brain, IL-18 expression has only been demonstrated in ependymal cells [78] and it has been proposed that IL-18 participates in the regulation of NSCs [76]. MIP-1α (macrophage inflammatory protein-1α or CCL3) and growth regulated oncogene-α (GRO-α o CXCL1) are both chemokines able to influence NSCs migration and differentiation as well as it has been found a positive effect on cell proliferation and survival [55]. CX_3CR1 is a pro-inflammatory leukocyte receptor and its ligand is the chemokine fractalkine. The expression of CX_3CR1 has been proved in SVZ-derived neurospheres and in the OB. Thus, it has been proposed that fractalkine guides the migration of SVZ-derived neuroblast toward the OB. CCL5 or RANTES (regulated on activation, normal T cells expressed and secreted) is a chemotactic chemokine possibly secreted by reactive astrocytes, microglia and activated lymphocytes that increases the proliferation of adult NSCs [79].

Conclusion

As described above, the cross-talk between immune system and NSCs can modify the efficacy of endogenous regenerative responses, as well as the cell fate and functional integration NSCs. In several experimental conditions, it has been shown that stimulation of endogenous SVZ progenitors with immunological cytokines appears to promote neural regeneration and act as local immunomodulators [64]. Nevertheless, the significance of the modulation of adult neurogenesis by immunological cytokines in neurological disorders is to be elucidated. Furthermore, pro- and anti-inflammatory cytokines may have both detrimental and beneficial effects on neural diseases.

Thus, more research is necessary before a stem-cell-based therapy is useful for human therapy.

ACKNOWLEDGMENTS

This work was financed by Fondo Ramon Alvarez-Buylla (FRABA 841/13) and Programa de Mejoramiento del Profesorado (PROMEP 103.5/12/4857)

REFERENCES

[1] Altman, J. Are new neurons formed in the brains of adult mammals? *Science*, 1962, 135, 1127-8.

[2] Kriegstein, A; Alvarez-Buylla, A. The glial nature of embryonic and adult neural stem cells. *Annu Rev Neurosci.*, 2009, 32, 149-84.

[3] Ming, GL; Song, H. Adult neurogenesis in the mammalian central nervous system. *Annu Rev Neurosci.*, 2005, 28, 223-50.

[4] Menn, B; Garcia-Verdugo, JM; Yaschine, C; Gonzalez-Perez, O; Rowitch, D; Alvarez-Buylla, A. Origin of oligodendrocytes in the subventricular zone of the adult brain. *J Neurosci.*, 2006, 26(30), 7907-18.

[5] Gonzalez-Perez, O; Alvarez-Buylla, A. Oligodendrogenesis in the subventricular zone and the role of epidermal growth factor. *Brain Res Rev.*, 2011, 67(1-2), 147-56.

[6] Gonzalez-Perez, O; Romero-Rodriguez, R; Soriano-Navarro, M; Garcia-Verdugo, JM; Alvarez-Buylla, A. Epidermal growth factor induces the progeny of subventricular zone type B cells to migrate and differentiate into oligodendrocytes. *Stem Cells*, 2009, 27(8), 2032-43.

[7] Hickey, WF. Leukocyte traffic in the central nervous system: the participants and their roles. *Semin Immunol.*, 1999,11(2), 125-37.

[8] Bonecchi, R; Galliera, E; Borroni, EM; Corsi, MM; Locati, M; Mantovani, A. Chemokines and chemokine receptors: an overview. *Front Biosci.*, 2009, 14, 540-51.

[9] Whitney, NP; Eidem, TM; Peng, H; Huang, Y; Zheng, JC. Inflammation mediates varying effects in neurogenesis: relevance to the pathogenesis of brain injury and neurodegenerative disorders. *J Neurochem.*, 2009, 108(6), 1343-59.

[10] Gonzalez-Perez, O; Gutierrez-Fernandez, F; Lopez-Virgen, V; Collas-Aguilar, J; Quinones-Hinojosa, A; Garcia-Verdugo, JM. Immunological regulation of neurogenic niches in the adult brain. *Neuroscience.*, 2012, 226, 270-81. Epub 2012/09/19.

[11] Gonzalez-Perez, O. Immunological regulation of the central nervous system: From physiological to pathological processes. *Current immunology reviews*, 2011, 6(3), 149.

[12] Das, S; Basu, A. Inflammation: a new candidate in modulating adult neurogenesis. *J Neurosci Res.*, 2008, 86(6), 1199-208.

[13] Miller, RJ; Rostene, W; Apartis, E; Banisadr, G; Biber, K; Milligan, ED; et al. Chemokine action in the nervous system. *J Neurosci.*, 2008, 28(46), 11792-5.

[14] Quinones-Hinojosa, A; Sanai, N; Soriano-Navarro, M; Gonzalez-Perez, O; Mirzadeh, Z; Gil-Perotin, S; et al. Cellular composition and cytoarchitecture of the adult human subventricular zone: a niche of neural stem cells. *J Comp Neurol.*, 2006, 494(3), 415-34.

[15] Quinones-Hinojosa, A; Sanai, N; Gonzalez-Perez, O; Garcia-Verdugo, JM. The human brain subventricular zone: stem cells in this niche and its organization. *Neurosurg Clin N Am.*, 2007, 18(1), 15-20, vii.

[16] Alvarez-Palazuelos, LE; Robles-Cervantes, MS; Castillo-Velazquez, G; Rivas-Souza, M; Gonzalez-Castaneda, RE; Luquin, S; et al. Regulation of neural stem cell in the human SVZ by trophic and morphogenic factors. *Curr Signal Transduct Ther.*, 2011, 6(3), 320-6.

[17] Sanai, N; Tramontin, AD; Quinones-Hinojosa, A; Barbaro, NM; Gupta, N; Kunwar, S; et al. Unique astrocyte ribbon in adult human brain contains neural stem cells but lacks chain migration. *Nature*, 2004, 427(6976), 740-4.

[18] Sanai, N; Nguyen, T; Ihrie, RA; Mirzadeh, Z; Tsai, HH; Wong, M; et al. Corridors of migrating neurons in the human brain and their decline during infancy. *Nature*, 2011, 478(7369), 382-6. Epub 2011/10/04.

[19] Doetsch, F; Garcia-Verdugo, JM; Alvarez-Buylla, A. Cellular composition and three-dimensional organization of the subventricular germinal zone in the adult mammalian brain. *J Neurosci*, 1997, 17, 5046-61.

[20] Doetsch, F; Caille, I; Lim, DA; García-Verdugo, JM; Alvarez-Buylla, A. Subventricular Zone Astrocytes Are Neural Stem Cells in the Adult mammalian Brain. *Cell*, 1999, 97, 1-20.

[21] Mirzadeh, Z; Merkle, FT; Soriano-Navarro, M; Garcia-Verdugo, JM; Alvarez-Buylla, A. Neural stem cells confer unique pinwheel

architecture to the ventricular surface in neurogenic regions of the adult brain. *Cell stem cell*, 2008, 3(3), 265-78.

[22] Mirzadeh, Z; Han, YG; Soriano-Navarro, M; Garcia-Verdugo, JM; Alvarez-Buylla, A. Cilia organize ependymal planar polarity. *J Neurosci.*, 2010, 30(7), 2600-10.

[23] Lois, C; Alvarez-Buylla, A. Long-distance neuronal migration in the adult mammalian brain. *Science*, 1994, 264(5162), 1145-8.

[24] Lois, C; Garcia-Verdugo, JM; Alvarez-Buylla, A. Chain migration of neuronal precursors. *Science*, 1996, 271, 978-81.

[25] Wichterle, H; Garcia-Verdugo, JM; Alvarez-Buylla, A. Direct evidence for homotypic, glia-independent neuronal migration. *Neuron*, 1997, 18, 779-91.

[26] Hack, MA; Saghatelyan, A; de Chevigny, A; Pfeifer, A; Ashery-Padan, R; Lledo, PM; et al. Neuronal fate determinants of adult olfactory bulb neurogenesis. *Nat Neurosci.*, 2005, 8(7), 865-72.

[27] Jackson, EL; Garcia-Verdugo, JM; Gil-Perotin, S; Roy, M; Quinones-Hinojosa, A; VandenBerg, S; et al. PDGFR alpha-positive B cells are neural stem cells in the adult SVZ that form glioma-like growths in response to increased PDGF signaling. *Neuron*, 2006, 51(2), 187-99.

[28] Galvao, RP; Garcia-Verdugo, JM; Alvarez-Buylla, A. Brain-derived neurotrophic factor signaling does not stimulate subventricular zone neurogenesis in adult mice and rats. *J Neurosci.*, 2008, 28(50), 13368-83.

[29] Gonzalez-Perez, O; Quinones-Hinojosa, A. Dose-dependent effect of EGF on migration and differentiation of adult subventricular zone astrocytes. *Glia.*, 2010, 58(8), 975-83.

[30] Aguirre, A; Dupree, JL; Mangin, JM; Gallo, V. A functional role for EGFR signaling in myelination and remyelination. *Nat Neurosci.*, 2007, 10(8), 990-1002.

[31] Lai, K; Kaspar, BK; Gage, FH; Schaffer, DV. Sonic hedgehog regulates adult neural progenitor proliferation in vitro and in vivo. *Nat Neurosci.*, 2003, 6(1), 21-7.

[32] Cooper, O; Isacson, O. Intrastriatal transforming growth factor alpha delivery to a model of Parkinson's disease induces proliferation and migration of endogenous adult neural progenitor cells without differentiation into dopaminergic neurons. *J Neurosci.*, 2004, 24(41), 8924-31.

[33] Machold, R; Hayashi, S; Rutlin, M; Muzumdar, MD; Nery, S; Corbin, JG; et al. Sonic hedgehog is required for progenitor cell maintenance in telencephalic stem cell niches. *Neuron*, 2003, 39(6), 937-50.

[34] Bauer, S. Cytokine control of adult neural stem cells. *Ann N Y Acad Sci.*, 2009, 1153, 48-56.

[35] Morgan, SC; Taylor, DL; Pocock, JM. Microglia release activators of neuronal proliferation mediated by activation of mitogen-activated protein kinase, phosphatidylinositol-3-kinase/Akt and delta-Notch signalling cascades. *J Neurochem.*, 2004, 90(1), 89-101.

[36] Leong, SY; Turnley, AM. Regulation of adult neural precursor cell migration. *Neurochemistry international*, 2011, 59(3), 382-93.

[37] Greco, SJ; Rameshwar, P. Enhancing effect of IL-1alpha on neurogenesis from adult human mesenchymal stem cells: implication for inflammatory mediators in regenerative medicine. *J Immunol.*, 2007, 179(5), 3342-50.

[38] Dooley, D; Vidal, P; Hendrix, S. Immunopharmacological intervention for successful neural stem cell therapy: New perspectives in CNS neurogenesis and repair. *Pharmacology & therapeutics*, 2013. Epub 2013/08/21.

[39] Ben-Hur, T; Ben-Menachem, O; Furer, V; Einstein, O; Mizrachi-Kol, R; Grigoriadis, N. Effects of proinflammatory cytokines on the growth, fate, and motility of multipotential neural precursor cells. *Mol Cell Neurosci.*, 2003, 24(3), 623-31.

[40] Koo, JW; Duman, RS. IL-1beta is an essential mediator of the antineurogenic and anhedonic effects of stress. *Proc Natl Acad Sci U S A*, 2008, 105(2), 751-6.

[41] Ajmone-Cat, MA; Cacci, E; Ragazzoni, Y; Minghetti, L; Biagioni, S. Pro-gliogenic effect of IL-1alpha in the differentiation of embryonic neural precursor cells in vitro. *J Neurochem.*, 2010, 113(4), 1060-72.

[42] Butovsky, O; Ziv, Y; Schwartz, A; Landa, G; Talpalar, AE; Pluchino, S; et al. Microglia activated by IL-4 or IFN-gamma differentially induce neurogenesis and oligodendrogenesis from adult stem/progenitor cells. *Mol Cell Neurosci.*, 2006, 31(1), 149-60.

[43] Ziv, Y; Avidan, H; Pluchino, S; Martino, G; Schwartz, M. Synergy between immune cells and adult neural stem/progenitor cells promotes functional recovery from spinal cord injury. *Proc Natl Acad Sci U S A*, 2006, 103(35), 13174-9.

[44] Guan, Y; Jiang, Z; Ciric, B; Rostami, AM; Zhang, GX. Upregulation of chemokine receptor expression by IL-10/IL-4 in adult neural stem cells.

Experimental and molecular pathology, 2008, 85(3), 232-6. Epub 2008/09/09.

[45] Spooren, A; Kolmus, K; Laureys, G; Clinckers, R; De Keyser, J; Haegeman, G; et al. Interleukin-6, a mental cytokine. *Brain Res Rev*, 2011, 67(1-2), 157-83.

[46] Dominguez, E; Rivat, C; Pommier, B; Mauborgne, A; Pohl, M. JAK/STAT3 pathway is activated in spinal cord microglia after peripheral nerve injury and contributes to neuropathic pain development in rat. *J Neurochem.*, 2008, 107(1), 50-60.

[47] Nakanishi, M; Niidome, T; Matsuda, S; Akaike, A; Kihara, T; Sugimoto, H. Microglia-derived interleukin-6 and leukaemia inhibitory factor promote astrocytic differentiation of neural stem/progenitor cells. *Eur J Neurosci.*, 2007, 25(3), 649-58. Epub 2007/03/03.

[48] Islam, O; Gong, X; Rose-John, S; Heese, K. Interleukin-6 and neural stem cells: more than gliogenesis. *Mol Biol Cell*, 2009, 20(1), 188-99.

[49] Taga, T; Fukuda, S. Role of IL-6 in the neural stem cell differentiation. *Clinical reviews in allergy & immunology*, 2005, 28(3), 249-56. Epub 2005/09/01.

[50] Gomez-Nicola, D; Valle-Argos, B; Pallas-Bazarra, N; Nieto-Sampedro, M. Interleukin-15 regulates proliferation and self-renewal of adult neural stem cells. *Mol Biol Cell*, 2011, 22(12), 1960-70.

[51] Guadagno, J; Xu, X; Karajgikar, M; Brown, A; Cregan, SP. Microglia-derived TNFalpha induces apoptosis in neural precursor cells via transcriptional activation of the Bcl-2 family member Puma. *Cell death & disease*, 2013, 4, e538. Epub 2013/03/16.

[52] Widera, D; Holtkamp, W; Entschladen, F; Niggemann, B; Zanker, K; Kaltschmidt, B; et al. MCP-1 induces migration of adult neural stem cells. *Eur J Cell Biol.*, 2004, 83(8), 381-7.

[53] Schwamborn, J; Lindecke, A; Elvers, M; Horejschi, V; Kerick, M; Rafigh, M; et al. Microarray analysis of tumor necrosis factor alpha induced gene expression in U373 human glioblastoma cells. *BMC Genomics*, 2003, 4(1), 46.

[54] Turbic, A; Leong, SY; Turnley, AM. Chemokines and inflammatory mediators interact to regulate adult murine neural precursor cell proliferation, survival and differentiation. *PLoS One*, 2011, 6(9), e25406.

[55] Gordon, RJ; Mehrabi, NF; Maucksch, C; Connor, B. Chemokines influence the migration and fate of neural precursor cells from the young

adult and middle-aged rat subventricular zone. *Exp Neurol.*, 2012, 233(1), 587-94.

[56] Eugenin, EA; D'Aversa, TG; Lopez, L; Calderon, TM; Berman, JW. MCP-1 (CCL2) protects human neurons and astrocytes from NMDA or HIV-tat-induced apoptosis. *J Neurochem.*, 2003, 85(5), 1299-311.

[57] Makela, J; Koivuniemi, R; Korhonen, L; Lindholm, D. Interferon-gamma produced by microglia and the neuropeptide PACAP have opposite effects on the viability of neural progenitor cells. *PLoS One*, 2010, 5(6), e11091.

[58] Liu, XS; Zhang, ZG; Zhang, RL; Gregg, SR; Wang, L; Yier, T; et al. Chemokine ligand 2 (CCL2) induces migration and differentiation of subventricular zone cells after stroke. *J Neurosci Res.*, 2007, 85(10), 2120-5.

[59] Kim, SJ; Son, TG; Kim, K; Park, HR; Mattson, MP; Lee, J. Interferon-gamma promotes differentiation of neural progenitor cells via the JNK pathway. *Neurochem Res.*, 2007, 32(8), 1399-406.

[60] Perez-Asensio, FJ; Perpina, U; Planas, AM; Pozas, E. Interleukin-10 regulates progenitor differentiation and modulates neurogenesis in adult brain. *J Cell Sci.*, 2013, 126(Pt 18), 4208-19. Epub 2013/07/12.

[61] Klose, J; Schmidt, NO; Melms, A; Dohi, M; Miyazaki, J; Bischof, F; et al. Suppression of experimental autoimmune encephalomyelitis by interleukin-10 transduced neural stem/progenitor cells. *Journal of neuroinflammation*, 2013, 10(1), 117. Epub 2013/09/24.

[62] Yang, J; Jiang, Z; Fitzgerald, DC; Ma, C; Yu, S; Li, H; et al. Adult neural stem cells expressing IL-10 confer potent immunomodulation and remyelination in experimental autoimmune encephalitis. *J Clin Invest.*, 2009, 119(12), 3678-91. Epub 2009/11/04.

[63] Pan, W; Wu, X; He, Y; Hsuchou, H; Huang, EY; Mishra, PK; et al. Brain interleukin-15 in neuroinflammation and behavior. *Neurosci Biobehav Rev.*, 2013, 37(2), 184-92. Epub 2012/12/04.

[64] Kokaia, Z; Martino, G; Schwartz, M; Lindvall, O. Cross-talk between neural stem cells and immune cells: the key to better brain repair? *Nat Neurosci.*, 2012, 15(8), 1078-87.

[65] Emsley, JG; Hagg, T. Endogenous and exogenous ciliary neurotrophic factor enhances forebrain neurogenesis in adult mice. *Exp Neurol.*, 2003, 183(2), 298-310. Epub 2003/10/14.

[66] Bauer, S; Patterson, PH. Leukemia inhibitory factor promotes neural stem cell self-renewal in the adult brain. *J Neurosci.*, 2006, 26(46), 12089-99.

[67] Shimazaki, T; Shingo, T; Weiss, S. The ciliary neurotrophic factor/leukemia inhibitory factor/gp130 receptor complex operates in the maintenance of mammalian forebrain neural stem cells. *J Neurosci.*, 2001, 21(19), 7642-53.

[68] Oshima, K; Teo, DT; Senn, P; Starlinger, V; Heller, S. LIF promotes neurogenesis and maintains neural precursors in cell populations derived from spiral ganglion stem cells. *BMC Dev Biol.*, 2007, 7, 112.

[69] Mathieu, P; Battista, D; Depino, A; Roca, V; Graciarena, M; Pitossi, F. The more you have, the less you get: the functional role of inflammation on neuronal differentiation of endogenous and transplanted neural stem cells in the adult brain. *J Neurochem.*, 2010, 112(6), 1368-85.

[70] Wachs, FP; Winner, B; Couillard-Despres, S; Schiller, T; Aigner, R; Winkler, J; et al. Transforming growth factor-beta1 is a negative modulator of adult neurogenesis. *J Neuropathol Exp Neurol.*, 2006, 65(4), 358-70. Epub 2006/05/13.

[71] Gong, X; He, X; Qi, L; Zuo, H; Xie, Z. Stromal cell derived factor-1 acutely promotes neural progenitor cell proliferation in vitro by a mechanism involving the ERK1/2 and PI-3K signal pathways. *Cell Biol Int.*, 2006, 30(5), 466-71.

[72] Filippo, TR; Galindo, LT; Barnabe, GF; Ariza, CB; Mello, LE; Juliano, MA; et al. CXCL12 N-terminal end is sufficient to induce chemotaxis and proliferation of neural stem/progenitor cells. *Stem cell research*, 2013, 11(2), 913-25. Epub 2013/07/16.

[73] Patel, JR; McCandless, EE; Dorsey, D; Klein, RS. CXCR4 promotes differentiation of oligodendrocyte progenitors and remyelination. *Proc Natl Acad Sci U S A*, 2010, 107(24), 11062-7. Epub 2010/06/11.

[74] Paintlia, MK; Paintlia, AS; Singh, AK; Singh, I. Synergistic activity of interleukin-17 and tumor necrosis factor-alpha enhances oxidative stress-mediated oligodendrocyte apoptosis. *J Neurochem.*, 2011, 116(4), 508-21. Epub 2010/12/15.

[75] Li, Z; Li, K; Zhu, L; Kan, Q; Yan, Y; Kumar, P; et al. Inhibitory effect of IL-17 on neural stem cell proliferation and neural cell differentiation. *BMC immunology*, 2013, 14, 20. Epub 2013/04/27.

[76] Alboni, S; Cervia, D; Sugama, S; Conti, B. Interleukin 18 in the CNS. *Journal of neuroinflammation*, 2010, 7, 9.

[77] Liu, YP; Lin, HI; Tzeng, SF. Tumor necrosis factor-alpha and interleukin-18 modulate neuronal cell fate in embryonic neural progenitor culture. *Brain Res.*, 2005, 1054(2), 152-8.

[78] Sugama, S; Cho, BP; Baker, H; Joh, TH; Lucero, J; Conti, B. Neurons of the superior nucleus of the medial habenula and ependymal cells express IL-18 in rat CNS. *Brain Res.*, 2002, 958(1), 1-9. Epub 2002/12/07.

[79] Krathwohl, MD; Kaiser, JL. HIV-1 promotes quiescence in human neural progenitor cells. *J Infect Dis.*, 2004, 190(2), 216-26.

In: Neuro-Immune Interactions ...
Editor: Oscar González-Pérez
ISBN: 978-1-62948-646-8

Chapter 6

THE ROLE OF CYTOKINES IN THE NEUROIMMUNOENDOCRINE NETWORK: THEIR PARTICIPATION IN NEUROTRANSMISSION AND REPRODUCTION

Karen E. Nava-Castro[1], Hugo Aguilar-Díaz[2], Marco A. Cerbón[2] and Jorge Morales-Montor[1]

[1]Departamento de Inmunología, Instituto de Investigaciones Biomédicas, Universidad Nacional Autónoma de México, Mexico City, Mexico.

[2]Facultad de Química, Departamento de Biología, Universidad Nacional Autónoma de México, Mexico City, Mexico.

ABSTRACT

Cytokines are inducible, secretory proteins that mediate intercellular communication in the immune system. They are grouped in families referred as tumour necrosis factors, interleukins, interferons and colony stimulating factors. In recent years, it is clear that some of these proteins and their receptors are also produced in the central nervous system (CNS) by specific neural cell lineages under physiological and pathological conditions. The data we have hitherto let us suggest that cytokines play an important role in the regulation of both excitatory and inhibitory neurotransmission in the CNS. Growing evidence indicates that, in addition to the hormones of hypothalamic, pituitary and gonadal origin, autocrine/paracrine regulators play important roles in the reproductive functions. Cytokines, originally known as immunoregulatory proteins, may affect the neuroendocrine events of reproduction, ovarian/testis function, endometrium, the developing embryo, placenta and parturition. Cytokines can modulate and mediate the actions of hormones at their target cells and, in the opposite way, hormones may regulate the production and action of cytokines at three different levels: cytokine secretion, cytokine receptor expression and cellular responses. Cytokines may also function in an endocrine manner affecting distant targets. In addition, many cells in the reproductive system also produce cytokines independently of the presence of leukocytes, thus reproductive tissues are sites of cytokine action and production. There is compelling evidence that cytokines, in fact, play an important regulatory role in the development and normal function of ovarian and testicular tissues, and are surveyed as the important regulators of steroidogenesis and gamete production. Cytokines interfere with steroidogenesis at the level of testes, and ovaries. For instance, secretory products of macrophages are involved in the regulation of steroidogenesis, Sertoli cell activity, and germ cell survival in the human testes. In conclusion, cytokines interact with steroidogenesis in a systemic and complex manner, influencing development, function, and hormone production of the testes, and ovaries. Thus a variety of clinical situations may be due to cytokine action in the gonads. Therapeutic manipulation of the immune system may affect reproductive function. The aim of this chapter is to provide a summary of the extensive literature dealing with cytokines in central nervous system function, and gonadal biology, and to follow this with some speculation concerning the significance of these molecules in interactions between the immune system and the neuroendocrine system. This knowledge could be fundamental for the proposal of new therapeutic approaches to neurological, psychiatric and reproductive disorders.

Introduction

In recent years, interest has grown regarding the interactions of an organism's systems that regulate its homeostasis. These interactions have currently been solidly documented, and they include the nervous, endocrine and immunological systems. Interactions are bidirectional and several molecules are known to be produced by the three systems and to act at target cell level through specific receptors, which are frequently common to different cell-types [1]. Among these soluble molecules, the nervous system secretes the classic neurotransmitters (such as histamine, dopamine, serotonin and enkephalins), which act at immunological cell level either stimulating or inhibiting specific functions. The immune system produces cytokines, which are soluble products generated by an array of immune cells, but mainly by lymphocytes and macrophages as a response to external stimuli. Cytokines in turn, modify nervous or endocrine system functions as a result of their autocrine, paracrine or endocrine action on diverse target tissues [1, 2]. The neuroendocrine system secretes two types of hormones, which have diverse effects on the immunologic system: peptide and steroid hormones [2]. These two hormone types have been amply studied and regulate cytokine secretion, antibody synthesis, immunoglobulin isotype changing, MHC antigen and TCR expression, T lymphocyte maturation and cell adhesion for cell communication [2-4].

Studies on neuroimmunoendocrine communication have led to the very interesting concept that the immunological system may be an internal sensor organ. The immune system may sense stimuli that are not recognized by the central and peripheral nervous system. These have been labeled non-cognitive stimuli and include phenomena (such as presence of bacteria, tumors, viruses and antigens) which could otherwise go unnoticed within the organism. Recognition of these non-cognitive stimuli by immune cells is then converted into information in the form of peptide hormones, steroid hormones, cytokines, neurotransmitters, which stimulate the neuroendocrine system and lead to physiological changes [2, 3]. On the other hand, the recognition of cognitive stimuli by the central and peripheral nervous system leads to neurohormonal information, which is recognized by immunocyte receptors, leading to immunological changes [3, 4]. Thus, the sensor function of the immune system mimics the neuroendocrine system in the sense that a given stimulus produces a particular hormone combination that leads to physiological responses and changes [4]. If this is the case, then the pathologies that are associated with a particular infectious agent, antigen or tumor could in part be related with the set of hormones produced by the immune system. In this way, if the internal homeostasis of the organism is being altered, the nervous system is notified by chemical communication via cytokines, which stimulate the immunological system to respond. Once the malfunction has been controlled, the neuroendocrine system responds producing hormones and neurohormones that regulate the immune response, and prevent it from becoming aggressive towards the organism (Figure 1).

Cytokines are soluble polypeptides released by immune system cells, mainly by macrophages and activated T cells, which may be liberated during the inflammatory process or as a response to antigenic stimuli, acting as local response coordinators and endocrinologically affecting a large number of tissues [2]. Cytokines have traditionally been divided into various specific factors produced by a lymphocyte type or by other immune cells and based on their interleukin action. They are numbered from 1 to 29, which corresponds to the order in which they were discovered.

Thus, the immunologic system not only regulates the magnitude of the response to an antigenic stimulus by means of intrinsic signals from its own cells –cytokine secretion and the idiotype-anti-idiotype network– but receives extrinsic signals from the neuroendocrine system that regulate the magnitude of the response [5, 6]. Analogous to this, the substances of the immunological system such as TNF-α, IL-1, IL-2, IL-6 and interferons (especially IFN-α and IFN-γ), and thymic hormones, regulate the secretion of diverse neuroendocrine gland products, such as hypothalamic releasing factors (CRF, TRH, GnRH), hypophysial peptide hormones (prolactin, melatonin, ACTH, gonadotropins), adrenal and gonadal steroids (glucocorticoids, estradiol, progesterone and testosterone), among others [1-5]. The cells of the neuroendocrine system are also able to produce cytokines (the hypophysis produces IL-6, IL-1, migration inhibitory factor and interferon) [6], and immune cells have similar capacities to endocrine cells (macrophages can metabolize testosterone to DHT). On the other hand, sex hormones play a regulatory role in the humoral and cellular immunologic responses, which can in turn affect hormone levels. The suggestion that gonadal steroids play an important role in the immune response is based on several observations: differences between males and females in immune response level, changes in the immune response during pregnancy, after gonadectomy or sex hormone replacement, and the presence of receptors for certain gonadal hormones in lymphoid organs and circulating immune cells Figure 2) [3-5].

Animals should maintain their internal milieu under tight control for surviving. This formidable task is accomplished by coordinating functions of the nervous, endocrine and immune systems [7]. Feedback/feedforward communication loops among these systems are put in place by short distance cell-cell contacts and/or short, intermediate and long distance interactions mediated by secreted soluble messengers [1] (Figure 1).

An important aspect of cell communication that has emerged as a result of studying neuro-endocrine-immune interactions is the redundancy in the use of some chemical messengers that communicate these systems. Thus, neurotrophins are chemical messengers first identified and characterized in the central nervous system (CNS), but they are also expressed and secreted by immune and endocrine cells, and have immune and endocrine functions [8, 9].

The lack of exclusivity in the use of some cellular messengers by specific systems might be a rule, rather than an exception (Figure 2).

Although strong evidence supports that neurons and immune cells produce hormones, and endocrine and immune cells synthesize and secrete typical neurotransmitters, it remains controversial whether cytokines, the classic immunological messengers, can indeed be produced by neurons and modulate neural function. In this review we discuss evidence supporting the role of cytokines in the regulation of both excitatory and inhibitory neurotransmission in the CNS of mammals and its impact in neurological and psychiatric diseases.

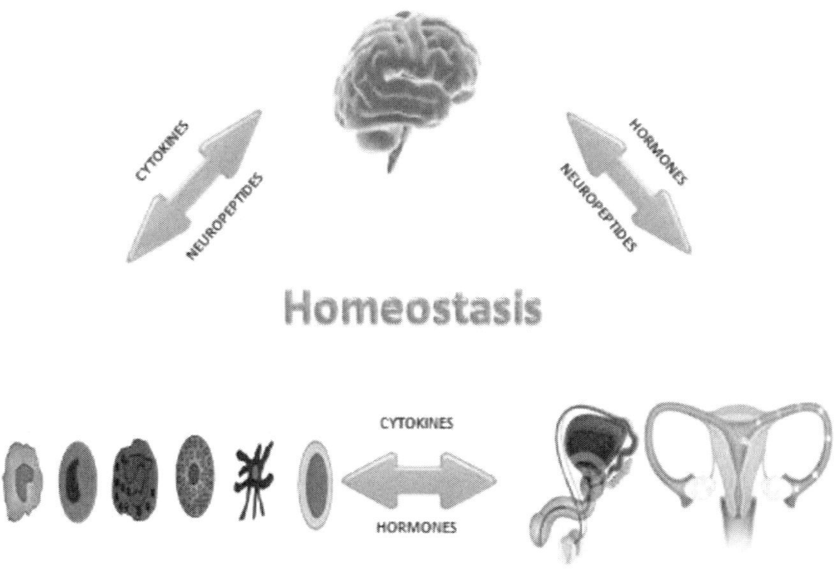

Figure 1. Proposed neuroimmunoendocrinological interactions that occur in higher vertebrates. In physiological conditions there is a crosstalk between the brain, the endocrine (gonads) and the immune systems. External stimuli, such as infections, results in a TH1/TH2 systemic cytokine production of the immune response. Also, the barin is able to actively induce the expression of cytokines, which may affect the brain and the gonadal function.

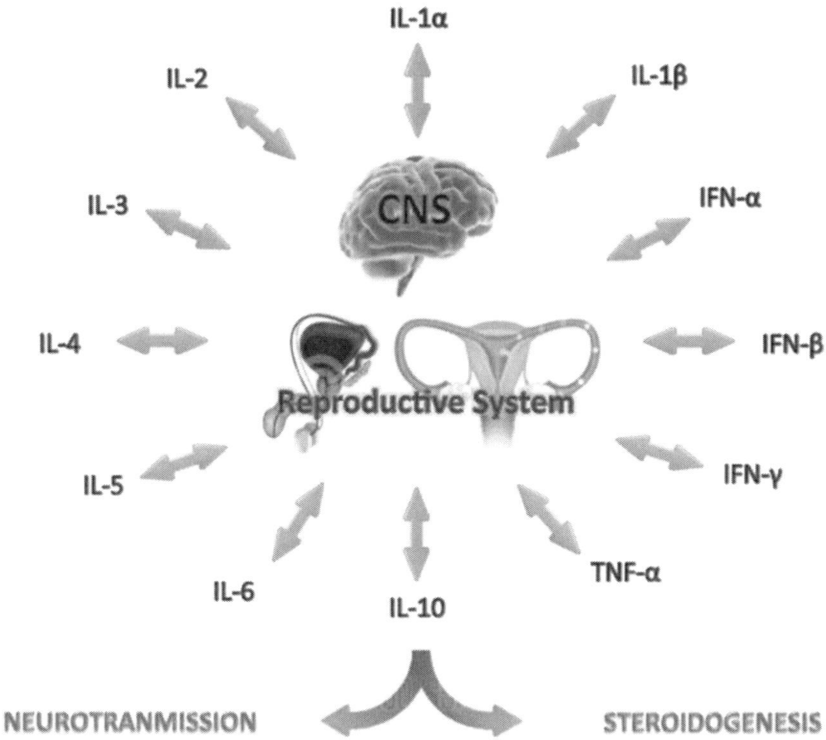

Figure 2. Cytokine effects and production on brain and reproductive system. Besides their effects on immune function, cytokines can influence brain and gonadal function by affecting differently many of the functions of virtually all their cells types. For example, cytokines regulate neurotransmission and gonadal sterooidogenesis. On the other hand, cytokine affect the production of sex steroids, which in turn can have effects on the innate immune response, and may affect subsequent adaptive immunity. In addition, sex steroids also influence the functions of the adaptive immune response cells mainly T and B lymphocytes. These molecules thus are one of the main communicators between brain, endocrine and immune system.

The Neuroimmunoendocrine Network

The immune and neuroendocrine systems are integrated through a complex network of hormones, neurohormones, cytokines, chemokines, neurotransmitters and neuropeptides, which serve to maintain homeostasis [7]. Two of the main components of this network are the hypothalamic-pituitary-adrenocortical (HPA) axis and the hypothalamic-pituitary-gonadal axis (HPG).

The relationship between the HPA and HPG axes and the immune system during acute and chronic inflammatory responses due to stress, infection and autoimmune responses has been well established [10, 11]. An important aspect of cellular communication that has emerged from studies of the neuroendocrine and immune system is the redundancy in the chemical messengers responsible for communication. The identification of a relatively high number of cellular messengers responsible for coordinating interactions between these homeostatic systems may herald a fundamental shift in our understanding of such important phisiologycal process such as neurotransmission, neuromodulation or the host immune response. Thus, there is an extremely complex Neuroimmunoendocrine (NIE) network involving many molecules, including cytokines, neurotransmitters, hormones, and neurohormones, that foresees potent interactions in events generally attributed to the exclusive operation of single systems in response to simple precepts (neurotransmission, reproduction and defense). So much plasticity and multi-functionality in a network are not without a risk. Loss of control in the NIE network could be involved in the physiopathology of some neuropathologies in which inflammation is a prominent effector of pathology, or could lead to the loss of tolerance and autoimmunity, and/or to be involved in the immune compromise of aging. A complex picture of interneuronal communications with multiple synaptic, presynaptic, and parasynaptic interactions is further complicated by the intimate participation of cytokines in these processes, which result in a very complicated network that has to be in a very delicated balance during all ontogenic states of an organism. The mutual regulatory influences between neurotransmitters, neurotrophic, and neuroimmune systems show that in normal conditions they are all working in concert. The increase in the number of factors that determine the final result of interactions between neurons adds new elements to the understanding of the brain function (Figure 1).

LOCAL AVAILABILITY OF CYTOKINES IN THE CENTRAL NERVOUS AND IN REPRODUCTIVE SYSTEMS

Although cytokines have been reported as modulators of brain development, regeneration, and synapses, the origin of these proteins had been controversial since astrocytes produce cytokines and chemokines (Table 1) that attract different types of immunological cells that promote/facilitate their access to the brain through the blood-brain barrier during inflammatory responses [12-16]. Interestingly, astrocytes have the ability to constitutively produce and secrete cytokines, suggesting that these messengers should modulate CNS functioning. Accordingly, primary astrocyte cultures obtained from adult mice synthesize interleukin-6 (IL-6) when exposed to tumor necrosis factor alpha (TNF-α) interleukin-1beta (IL-1β), and interferon-gamma (IFN-γ) [17].

Table 1. Central Nervous System (CNS) and Reproductive System (RS) type cells and its Citokines and interferons secretion

CYTOKINES	TYPE CELL		REFERENCES
	CNS	R. S.	
IL-1 and IL-1β	Astrocytes, neurons of peripheral nervous system.	Leydig cells, follicular theca granulose cells and ovarian cells.	De Simone et al., 1998, Fontana et al., 1984, Schobitz et al., 1993, Breard et al., 1998.
IL-2	Astrocytes.	Leydig cells and ovarian cells.	Ronica et al., 2005, Benveniste et al., 1998, Fontana et al., 1984
IL-3	CNS neurons.	Steroids cells and ovarian cells.	Gorospe et al., 1998, Miller et al., 1991, Yu et al., 1994.
IL-4	Microglia and Glioblastome.	Ovarian, mammary and prostatic epithelial cells.	Ponomarev et al., 2007. Burke et al., 1996
IL-5	Atrocytes and microglial.	Mammary gland, uterus, and ovary cells.	Sferruzzi-Perri et al., 2003, Robertson et al., 2000, Broughton et al., 2012.
IL-6	Astrocytes, neurons from sympathetic and sensory ganglia.	Leydig cells and ovarian cells.	Ronica et al., 2005, Benveniste et al., 1998, Schobitz et al., 1993, Gadient et al., 1994
IL-10	Glial cells, brain endothelial cells, astrocytes.	Female and male reproductive tract epithelial cells.	Cochery-Nouvellon et al., 2009, Robertson et al., 2007.
IFN α, β and γ	Root ganglion neurons, astrocytes, glioblastoma cells.	Female and male reproductive tract cells.	Neumann et al., 1997, Klassen et al., 2003, Vikman et al., 2001, Mendoza-Fernandez et al., 2000, Okada et al., 2005.
TNF-α	Neurons of different brain areas, such as hippocampus, olfactory bulb, cerebellum. Glial cells.	Ovarian, Leydig and theca cells	Friedman et al., 2001, Neumann et al., 2002, Basini et al., 2002, Gonzalez-Navarrete et al., 2007.

It has also been shown that IL-6 and IL-1β regulate their own expression in cultured astrocytes [18, 19]. IL-1β and IL-2 have been detected in astrocyte-conditioned culture media [18-20]. Furthermore, cultured glioblastoma cells produce a variety of interleukins, transforming growth factors and interferons [21]. IL-4 production in the CNS is essential for controlling autoimmune inflammation by inducing a microglial cell phenotype [22]. Also in the CNS, microglial cells produce IL-12 family cytokines, such as IL-12, IL-23, and IL-27, which play critical roles in T cell differentiation, and are important modulators of multiple sclerosis and experimental autoimmune encephalomyelitis (EAE), an animal model of multiple sclerosis [23].

The idea that neurons produce cytokines has been recently accepted [24]. For instance, studies conducted *in vitro,* have documented that fetal rat dorsal root ganglion neurons produce IFN-γ and express its receptor [25, 26]. The presence of astrocytes up-regulates IL-17 and IFN-γ gene expression and protein synthesis in T cells, which is on line with astrocytes' ability to express IL-23 subunit p19 and common IL-12/IL-23 subunit p40, but not IL-12 subunit p35 in co-cultures [27]. These results suggest that astrocytes should contribute to the complex interactions during CNS inflammation by different mechanisms [27]. Moreover, cultured neurons from sympathetic and sensory ganglia express IL-6 mRNA and the protein [28, 29]. Neuronal production of IL-6 is increased following N-Methyl-D-aspartate (NMDA)-mediated depolarization [30]. IL-1β immunoreactive fibers have also been detected in hypothalamic areas [31].

IL-1 and IL-6 receptors have been reported in various neuronal populations along the peripheral nervous system and the CNS [28, 32-35]. TNF-α receptors, p55 and p75, are expressed in oligodendrocytes and mediate apoptotic and trophic signaling in these cells, respectively [36, 37].

Transgenic mice that have a construct of glial fibrillary acidic protein (GFAP) and IL-6 show an enhanced sensitivity to glutamatergic but not cholinergic-induced seizures. However, transgenic mice showing GFAP coupled to TNF-α instead of IL-6 do not present the same sensitivity [38]. Therefore, pre-existing IL-6 production in the CNS not only causes spontaneous neurodegeneration, but also synergizes with other neurotoxic insults to induce a more severe functional neurological impairment [38].

In the next paragraphs, there is a compelling evidence of the role of each known cytokine in both, central nervous system and reproductive system (Figure 2).

Macrophage Migration Inhibitory Factor (MIF)

In addition to their role as immunomodulator, it is known that macrophage migration inhibition factor (MIF) can act upon the anterior pituitary gland as autocrine or paracrine regulators of its functions, including possibly those relative to infections [39]. MIF is produced by many endocrine tissues, such as the anterior pituitary itself, the medial basal hypothalamus [40] and reproductive tissues [41]. It has been shown that MIF stimulates the secretion of luteinizing hormone (LH) and follicle stimulating hormone (FSH) in cultured pituitary cells, to enhance the secretion of adrenocorticotropic hormone (ACTH) through the stimulation of the production of hypothalamic corticotropin-releasing hormone (CRH) [42], and to stimulate the release of prolactin from the anterior pituitary gland. The major endocrine role for MIF is as the most potent known counter-regulator of glucocorticoid action within the immune system [40], although recent evidences suggest also a role in regulating macrophage subsets within the testis of the adult rat [43]. Macrophages, as antigen processing and presenting cells, play key roles in the immune response and are thought to be responsible for the sex hormone-related dimorphism by being targets for sex steroids, while their function is modulated by MIF [44].

Interleukin-1 Beta (IL-1β) and Interleukin-1 Alpha (IL-1α)

Neurotransmission mediated by glutamate and γ-aminobutyric (GABA), key excitatory and inhibitory neurotransmitters, respectively, is modulated by cytokines. *In vitro*, IL-1β increases $GABA\text{-}_A$ mediated inward chloride currents in synaptosomes and cultured neurons of the amygdala and cerebral cortex of the rat [45, 46]. Moreover, *in vivo*, IL-1β systemically injected, increases *c-fos* expression in GABAergic, enkephalinergic, neurotensinergic and CRHergic neurons of the amygdaline complex. This effect is prevented by systemic injection of bicuculline (a $GABA\text{-}_A$ antagonist), and anti-IL-1β antibodies [46-49].

Hypothalamic (preoptic and mediobasal areas) explants, cultured *in vitro* and superfused with IL-1β present an increase in GABA and glycine release without changes in that of glutamate [50]. Furthermore, IL-1β decreases the release of GnRH induced by glutamatergic stimulation through increasing GABA, glycine and/or taurine release [51]. Interestingly, when IL-1β was applied in other areas of the brain, but using concentrations found during inflammatory conditions, it has the opposite effects on GABA-mediated chloride inward currents. Interestingly, this opposite effect is mediated by kinase activity [52]. Moreover, *in vitro* cultured chick cortical neurons, IL-1β decreases excitatory transmission by reducing NMDA-induced calcium inward currents [47, 48].

Experiments *in vitro*, by affinity cross-linking of ^{125}I-Hu-IL-1α to hippocampal membranes, revealed the existence of two types of IL-1 receptor proteins, consistent with the sizes of the type I (85 kD) and type II (60 kD) IL-1 receptors. *In vivo*, mouse brain expresses both type I and II IL-1 receptor mRNA and proteins, supporting the idea that both IL-1 receptors are synthesized and expressed by neurons [53]. Granulocyte-macrophage colony-stimulating factor reduces hypothalamic, but not hippocampal, concentrations of glutamate, GABA, aspartate, norepinephrine and serotonin. Because the specific antagonist for IL-1β blocked this effect, it is likely that IL-1β mediates the effects of granulocyte-macrophage colony-stimulating factor on hypothalamic neurotransmitter concentrations [54, 55]. The effects of IL-1β or its putative second messenger lysophosphatidylcholine on IL-6 release from glioma cells are effectively antagonized by somatostatin and GABA [56].

IL-1 can also regulate neurotransmission mediated by amines such as noradrenaline, dopamine and serotonin. The activity of the locus coeruleus (LC), which is the most important source of noradrenaline inside the brain, was increased after *in vivo* IL-1b microinjection in this area; this effect was blocked by IL-1β receptor antagonist (IL-1 RA) [57, 58]. Furthermore, microinjection of IL-1 RA alone was found to decrease LC activity, raising the possibility that LC neurons are under the influence of tonic excitation by IL-1β [57]

In vivo experiments, in which there was partial chemical lesions of *substantia nigra pars compacta* following 6-hydroxy-dopamine administration as well as the chronic haloperidol treatment, a dopamine type 2 receptor antagonist, led to a sprouting of fibers from the remaining dopaminergic neurons of the *substantia nigra*. Both responses (to 6-hydroxy-dopamine and to haloperidol) were greatly attenuated in animals that were microinjected with IL-1β and IL-6, thus suggesting that both cytokines participate in the normal arborisation and possible regeneration of the nigro-striatal pathway [25, 59], which is damaged in Parkinson's disease [60].

IL-1β decreases open field activity, and increases susceptibility to epileptic seizures induced by pentylenetetrazol [46]. In slices of preoptic area and magnocellular basal forebrain neurons superfused i*n vitro* with IL-1β they decreased their discharge rate during sleep/waking cycle. On the contrary, a subset of sleep-related neurons in the basal forebrain increases their firing rate in the presence of IL-1β, suggesting that the same cytokine can have opposite effects depending of the area of the brain studied [61]. IL-1β has also been reported as a neurotrophic agent for somatostatinergic neurons, modulating in this manner the neuroendocrine response to infection [62]. IL-1β also modulates synaptic plasticity in the hippocampus [63, 64], and it is capable of driving persistent cellular infiltration of the brain parenchyma without engendering explicit neuropathology [65].

In regard to reproduction, IL-1 production increases during the acute phase of infection in response to antigens, bacterial toxins, or tissue damage. IL-1 mediates many responses during disease, including fever, sleep, neutrophilic leukocytosis, acute phase protein synthesis as well as endocrine changes, such as increased release of insulin, glucagons, growth hormone, prolactin, ACTH, TSH, vasopressin and PTH [66, 67]. At testicular level, IL-1α upregulates StAR protein expression and phosphorilation [68], this protein (particularly its phosphorilated form) regulates the translocation of cholesterol from the outer to the inner mitochondrial membrane where steroidogenesis rate limiting step occurs [69]. Both isoforms IL-1α and Il-1β stimulate basal progesterone [70] as well as testosterone [70, 71], DHT [71] and androstenedione [70] secretion by Leydig cells in vitro. In contrast, when stimulated by gonadotropins, particularly by LH/hCG, IL-1α inhibits testosterone secretion [72-77] in Leydig cells. The mechanism by which IL-1 inhibits LH/hCG stimulated steroidogenesis in Leydig cells is dependent on cAMP levels [72, 73]. IL-1 inhibits the steroid production by direct effect on the enzyme, P450 cholesterol side chain cleavage (P450scc), which stimulates the transformation of cholesterol into pregnenolone, the step of entry of cholesterol into steroidogenesis as well as at the level of 17α-hydroxylase/C17-20 lyase (P450c17) that converts progestins into androgens. This effect of IL-1 is due to the decrease in the mRNA that transcribes this enzyme and its protein levels [72, 73, 75] and P450c17 [70, 72, 73]. This regulation seems to be located downstream of cAMP, since Leydig cells cultured in the presence of cAMP analogs (8-Br-cAMP, db-cAMP) still show a dose-dependent decrease in testosterone production [73]. Studies at different ages suggest a similar behavior, administration of IL-1 to immature Leydig cells stimulates testosterone while adult Leydig cells do not show response [78]. In immature hemicastrated rats, local injection of IL-1β induced a significant rise in testosterone secretion [79]. IL-1 effect on Leydig cells seems to be dependent on the presence of IL-1R. In male mice lacking a functional type I IL-1R, IL-1 has not shown steroidogenic effect [80].

Similar IL-1 effects have been observed at ovarian level. IL-1β stimulates basal progesterone secretion by human granulosa and theca cells [81] and small and large follicles [82] in vitro. When stimulated by gonadotropins, IL-1β inhibits both LH/hCG and FSH stimulated progesterone [81, 83-88] and estradiol [81, 88, 89] secretion by follicular theca and granulosa cells [84], affecting cAMP production [84] suggesting an follicle-stage dependent regulatory role of IL-1 on ovarian follicles [82]. In the same fashion, progesterone and estradiol are stimulated by IL-1 in small follicles while in antral gonadotropin-dependent follicles their secretion is inhibited [82]. Similarly to the Leydig cells, granulosa cells cultured in the presence of cAMP analogs show an IL-1 induced decrease in estrogen production suggesting an interleukin steroidogenic downstream regulation [89].

Interleukin-2 (IL-2)

IL-2 is a factor produced by activated T lymphocytes which acts as an autocrine factor on the growth and differentiation of T cells, and stimulates macrophages. *In vitro*, it increases the tumoricidal activity of blood peripheral mononuclear cells and induces the formation of T-cytotoxic cells (NK) and lymphocyte eliminating cells (LAK). *In vitro*, IL-2 administration reduces GABA-induced chloride currents in *aplysia* neurons [90]. Electrophysiological evidence also suggests that IL-2 increases GABA release in hippocampal slices [91]. Glutamate-dependent, dopamine release from mesencephalic neurons is potentiated by low concentrations of IL-2 through the modulation of the NMDA receptor [92, 93]. In neonatal rats, high doses (in the order of □g) of IL-2 significantly potentiated NMDA effects in hippocampal neural excitability. In contrast, low doses of IL-2 markedly decreased the voltage-dependent NMDA response.

The regulation of NMDA receptors activation by IL-2 may contribute to synaptic plasticity in the mesolimbic system and to pathological outcomes associated with this system such as Parkinson disease [93]. IL-2 has been shown to produce a variety of effects in the CNS, and it has recently been proposed as an endogenous brain neurokine; IL-2R beta is an essential subunit for signal transduction by peripheral immune cells and it is expressed in murine forebrain [94]. When administered to rats for long periods, it increases ACTH levels. IL-2 is a potent inhibitor both of hCG-stimulated steroidogenesis and of cAMP formation in Leydig cells. Since it blocks forskoline and 8-bromo cAMP-induced testosterone production, as well as pregnelonone, progesterone, 17α-hydroxypregnelonone and 17α-hydroxyprogesterone, and has no effect on dehydroepiandrosterone and androstendione production, the enzyme it specifically inhibits is P450c17 [95]. The addition of cholesterol does not revert the effect, meaning that P450scc may also be affected. This suggests that the effect of IL-2 is specifically on the steroidogenic enzyme system, and is not due to a toxic effect of the molecule on the cells [96]. The mentioned effect on the steroidogenic enzyme system could be achieved by hindering the steric enzyme-substrate recognition, since IL-2 can modify the binding site in a non-competitive irreversible way. On the other hand, in macrophages, IL-2 can stimulate the conversion of testosterone to dihydrotestosterone, by increasing the enzymatic activity of 5α-reductase [97]. In the ovary, IL-2 has no effect on LH/hCG induced steroid secretion, while it increases FSH induced progesterone synthesis and has no effect on estradiol [98].

Interleukin-3 (IL-3)

This lymphokine is secreted by T helper cells (Th1) and participates in cellular immunity. It promotes the generation of neutrophils, monocytes and macrophages at a microbial infection site, and also stimulates the mechanisms of respiratory discharge and phagocytosis in these cells. In the CNS, IL-3 has been shown to exert a trophic action on septal cholinergic rat neurons *in vitro* and *in vivo*. The presence of IL-3 receptor (IL-3R) ß subunits in septal cholinergic neurons and its role in neuroprotection has been demonstrated. In an ischemic model in gerbils, IL-3 prevents delayed neuronal death in the hippocampal CA1 field through a receptor-mediated expression of Bcl-xL protein, which is known to facilitate neuron survival [46, 47]. On the side of reproduction, it is also knownthat IL-3 to act on T lymphocytes directly, causing an enzymatic activity exclusive of steroid cells: an increase in the activity of 20α-hydroxysteroid dehydrogenase. In ovary cells in culture, it provokes an increase in progesterone production by stimulating the 3β-hydroxysteroid dehydrogenase activity [97].

Interleukin-4 (IL-4)

In general terms, the Interlukin 4 (IL-4) is principally secreted by activated lymphocytes T, NK1, basophils and mast cells. Like wise, IL-4 is capable to induce the differentiation of naïve T cells and the Th2 response. IL-4 is considerate another anti-inflammatory cytokine that play a crucial role in the intrinsic autoimmune response and in contrast to IL-10 its production is limited. In several studies in the brain, indicated that the microglia can respond to IL-4 with increase proliferation and activation, yet a corresponding suppression of MHC class II expression and TNF- α, IL-10, and IL-1β production that could be a critical regulation pathway during CNS inflammation [99]. The IL-4 has also been reported to have mitogenic activity for endothelial cells. In the CNS the IL-4 do not express in Glioma cells, however, some research have found IL-4 mRNA expressed nearly 10% of the primary brain tumors, this expression its probably for the lymphocytic infiltration [100]; should be noted that the local expression of IL-4 can also prevent the brain metastasis [101]. In addition, *in vitro* cultures of encephalitogenic Th1 cells treated with IL-4, decreases IFN-γ production and reduces their pathogenic potential, yet attempts to ameliorate disease induction or progression by co-transfer of Th2 populations has produced mixed results [102]. Recent reports propose the IL-4 use such stimulate the antitumor immune response [37]. In brain tumors the IL-4 production through the stem cells has shown potent antitumor effects in experimental rodent models [37]. Overall, the role of the IL-4 such one of the most potent antitumoral cytokines was demonstrated in these studies and its very significant induction of long-term survival when used in subcutaneous vaccine protocols.

In reproductive system, IL-4 action is mediated through its coupling to the IL-4 receptor (IL-4R) which is expressed in several immune cell types as well as in epithelial cells, including the ovarian cell surface [103]. Likewise, the IL-4 has a role in the alleviation of inflammation and restoration of postovulatory stigma with potential therapeutic advantage in malignancy [104]. IL-4 is a T-lymphocyte-associated cytokine that is involved in several cell immune responses with a principal role in ameliorating inflammation-associated diseases such as cancer through inhibition of Th-1 responses [105, 106]. The pregnancy is associated with a relative increase in Th2-associated immunity, characterized by increased production of the cytokines IL-4. Transactivation of IL-4R commonly results in activation of phosphatidylinositol 3-kinase (PI3K), ERK1/2 MAPK or signal transducers and activators of transcription protein 6 (STAT6) signalling pathways [107]. In this regard, some studies shown that 3 beta-HSD type 1 gene expression is specifically induced by interleukin (IL)-4 in several human cancer cell lines and in normal human mammary and prostatic epithelial cells in primary culture. There is evidence that IL-4 stimulates bifurcating signaling pathways in which the Stat6-signal pathway is involved in differentiation and gene regulation, whereas insulin receptor substrate (IRS) proteins mediate the mitogenic action of IL-4.

Interleukin-5 (IL-5)

The interlukine 5 (IL-5) is member of a discrete family of cytokines that regulates the growth, differentiation, migration and effector function activities of many hematopoietic cells and immunocytes [108]. This cytokine is involved in normal responses to infectious agents, bridging innate and adaptive immunity, is a cytokine that exhibits line age restriction. It stimulates the proliferation, maturation, and functional activation of eosinophils and basophils [108]. The major cellular source of IL-5 is T cells, although mast cells and some extent eosinophils also produce IL-5. The relationship between IL-5 activity and eosinophil function has been strongly linked to the eosinophilic inflammation observed in asthma [108]. Stimulation of eosinophil numbers and function has also been causally linked to the actions of IL-5 in hypereosinophilic syndrome as well as in severe, corticosteroid-resistant occurrences of asthma [108].

In reproductive system Interleukin 5 (IL-5) is expressed in type 2 T lymphocytes and has a key role in driving the differentiation, recruitment and activation of eosinophils. Mice with a null mutation in the interleukin-5 gene ($IL\text{-}5^{-/-}$ mice) have altered type 2 immune responses and severely depleted eosinophil populations [109]. The murine models shown, that in the female reproductive tract, the effect of the IL-5 deficiency, results in the reduction of endometrial eosinophils during the oestrous cycle and in early pregnancy, such as, eosinophils present in the cervix and decidual tissues at the time of parturition are similarly diminished. However, the temporal fluctuations in eosinophil recruitment and localization within these tissues are otherwise unchanged; indicating that interleukin 5 is not a necessary chemotactic agent in the female reproductive tract [110]. Likewise, the birth weights and growth of pups are significantly influenced by interleukin 5 status. All data showed are consistent with the view that eosinophils have a role in endometrial tissue remodelling associated with the oestrous cycle, but indicate that the events of pregnancy and parturition proceed quite normally in the absence of maternal and fetal interleukin 5 [110]. However, the interleukin 5 deficiency on placental growth and function and subsequent weight gain in the newborn indicate that this cytokine may act through the maternal or fetal immune axis to exert subtle influences on reproductive outcome. On the other hand, the administration of estradiol (E2) to ovariectomized mice results in a dramatic increase in uterine growth and an influx of eosinophilic leukocytes [111]. This influx is mediated by stimulation of an E2-dependent eosinophilic chemotactic factor in the uterus (ECF-U). At the present, the role of the eosinophil infiltration in uterus still remains, but some studies shown that this role could involve early growth and/or remodeling processes [109]. In this regard, the ovariectomized mice severely depleted of circulating eosinophils by administration of a purified rat IgG monoclonal antibody against interleukin-5 (IL-5), and after the seven days treated with estradiol, no significant changes show it in the uterine wet weight. In addition, IL-5 antibody administration significantly reduced E2-induced increase in peroxidase activity [111]. However, the possible IL-5 role in other events such as remodeling remains to be elucidated.

Interleukin-6 (IL-6)

IL-6 acts as a differentiation factor in B-cells and it is produced by T-cells. In addition, it is also known to be produced by a large variety of cells such as fibroblasts, endothelial cells, monocytes, hypophysial, and hypothalamic cells. Its levels increase during the acute phase response; it is a growth factor of hematopoyetic cells and increases T cell proliferation (Th2). It is synergistic with IL-1 and can indirectly mediate some of its actions. Receptors to IL-6 are known to be present in neuroendocrine tissue; the binding of the molecule to its receptors modifies the response of these cells.

Another interleukin involved in neurochemical communication is IL-6, which potentiates evoked GABA release from mediobasal hypothalamic explants and posterior pituitary cells in culture [112]. IL-6 also inhibits nociceptive responses to heat, since intraplantar IL-6 injection leads to thermal hypoalgesia in rats [113]. Similarly, IL-6 systemically administered to anesthetized rats, with or without neuropathic pain, inhibits naturally evoked neuronal responses [114].

Long-term exposure of the brain to IL-6, as it has been observed in certain degenerative disorders and infections, reduced adult hippocampal neurogenesis [115]. For instance, the mean firing rate of spontaneously active Purkinje neurons from cerebellar slices *in vitro*, is significantly reduced in IL-6 transgenic mice (they produce higher IL-6 concentrations than parental strain) compared to wild type animals. In addition, a significantly higher proportion of Purkinje neurons from transgenic IL-6 mice slices exhibited an oscillatory pattern of spontaneous firing than in control slices. Purkinje neurons also express high levels of both the IL-6 receptor and its intracellular signaling subunit, indicating that this cytokine directly acts on Purkinje neurons [116-118]. Short-term effects of several cytokines on synaptic transmission are mediated by the activation of intracellular protein kinases. The effects of IL-6 on the expression of paired pulse facilitation, post-tetanic potentiation, and LTP in the CA1 region of the hippocampus are mediated via the activation of the signal transducer and activator of transcription-3 (STAT3), the mitogen-activated protein kinase ERK (MAPK/ERK 1), and the stress-activated protein kinase/c-Jun NH (2)-terminal kinase (SAPK/JNK) [119].

In the CNS, astrocytes are a major inducible source of IL-6. Although this cytokine has beneficial effects in the CNS because of its neurotrophic properties, its overexpression is generally detrimental. Many factors have been shown to induce IL-6 expression by astrocytes, such as TNF-α, IL-1β, IL-6, and oncostatin [120].

In *in vivo* experiments, it has been reported that microinjection of low doses of kainic acid (an agonist of one of glutamate subtypes receptors) induced severe tonic-clonic seizures and death in IL-6 transgenic mice. Moreover, these animals were more sensitive to NMDA-induced seizures. It has been shown that IL-6 is chronically expressed at elevated levels within the CNS in many neurological disorders and may contribute to the pathological and cognitive deficits associated with such disorders [121, 122], while IL-2 is associated with pathological outcomes that are mediated, at least in part, by aberrations in mesolimbic neurotransmission [123]. Also, it has been demonstrated that IL-6 administration reduced scopolamine-induced amnesia as monitored by passive avoidance [54].

Regarding steroidogenesis, in healthy male patient, it has been observed that subcutaneous administration of IL-6 increases its circulating levels, and consequently produce a suppression in testosterone levels without affecting LH [124]. In FSH-stimulated granulosa cells, increasing amounts of IL-6 produce a significant suppression of progesterone biosynthesis. However, basal progesterone production is not influenced by this cytokine [125], but it does not seem to affect LH-induced estradiol or progesterone levels by the ovary although it increases progesterone basal synthesis [126].

IL-6 has a stimulatory effect on estradiol production since it can stimulate aromatization of testosterone to estradiol, increasing the enzymatic activity of P450 aromatase in cultured mammary cancer cells. Moreover, in cultured granulosa cells, the addition of IL-6 and testosterone cause the appearance in few hours of high levels of estradiol, which are not produced with the sole direct addition of testosterone in the same period. Thus, the possible enzymatic targets of IL-6 are the following enzymes: stimulating P450scc and 3β-hydroxysteroid dehydrogenase stimulated by FSH, increasing the capacity of P450 aromatase. The mechanisms of action remain to be determined.

Interleukin 10 (IL-10)

Interleukin 10 (IL-10) is a polypeptide that has been shown to be secreted by multiple cell types, including T and B cells, monocytes, is a Th2 cytokine with a marked anti-inflammatory profile and is a potent immune-regulating cytokine and inhibitor of inflammatory cytokine synthesis [127]. The classical cytokine interleukine 10 (IL-10) is antagonist of IFN-γ by inhibiting its production by Th1 cells. The IL-10 is secreted by Th2 lymphocytes, macrophages, and other cells of the immune system and has various effects on different cell types *in vitro* [123]. Its primary functions include the inhibition of the T-cell proliferation, suppresses pro-inflammatory cytokines, prevents the expression of co-stimulation and adhesion molecules in antigen presenting cells (APC) and leads to a long-lasting antigen-specific anergy in CD4-T cells [123]. On the other hand, the IL-10 is capable of stimulates the B-cell growth and the antibody production, and when the Th2 response is up regulated, it is suggested a central role in the regulation of both Th1 and Th2 cells [128].

In the central nervous system (CNS) normal, cytokines are involved in the regulation of a wide range of processes such as sleep, appetite, memory and learning, and the interactions between the nervous, endocrine and immune system [128]. Interestingly, in vitro studies suggest that cytokines also modulate various phenomena inherent to the development of the CNS such as neuronal maturation, differentiation and astroglial, oligodendroglial. In this sense, IL-10 is capable of inducing survival in neural progenitors as well as promotes growth axodendritico, which takes place during the final stages of neuronal differentiation [128]. However, in vivo expression pattern is unknown space and IL-10 cell during the stages corresponding to the normal development of the brain, which would be of great importance to clarify their possible role throughout this period [128].

In reproductive system, some reports suggest that IL-10 modulates resistance to inflammatory stimuli by downregulating expression of proinflammatory cytokines TNF-α, IL-6, IL-1A, and IL-12, acting to protect against inflammation-induced pathology in the implantation site [127].

Likewise, IL-10 is associated with maternal immunotolerance. IL-10 also down-regulates decidual cell tissue factor expression, the main molecule triggering coagulation activation: this antithrombotic effect may protect the umbilicoplacental vasculature from the 10th week of gestation onward. IL-10 down-regulation may thus dispose to early pregnancy loss (PL) due to maternal immunotolerance defect or late pregnancy failure due to placental vascular insufficiency. In the CNS, the IL-10 is capable to induce the neural progenitor survival as well as promotes the axodendritic growth in the last phases of neuronal differentiation [129]. However, *in vivo* the cellular expression pattern of IL-10 during the stages corresponding to the normal development of the brain is unknown, which would be of great importance to clarify their possible role throughout this period. At the present, some reports propose that IL-10 is present in the normal brain, from birth to maturity, indicating the involvement of this interleukin in normal condition. The brain pattern of temporal and cell expression of IL-10, under physiological conditions, is regulated during the first two postnatal weeks, suggesting its participation in the various processes that characterize the brain development during this stage. After the citotoxic damage in the postnatal brain, both IL-10 and its receptor expression is increased, primarily in glial cells, indicating his involvement in the processes that characterize the inflammatory response associated with immature CNS damage. The IL-10 over-expression in the postnatal citotoxic injured brain carries a deleterious effect on the development of the damaging process. The IL-10 over-expression after the citotoxic damage in the postnatal brain is capable of modulating the main cellular responses that characterize the inflammatory response associated with CNS damage, without inducing changes in the production of cytokines of pro-inflamatory character.

Interferons (IFN-α, IFN-β and IFN-γ)

In recent years, it has been established that interferons are not only important host defense molecules against viral infections and resistance to tumors, but also regulate some normal physiological processes. In fact, the 3 known types of IFN share many biological actions. IFNs have been detected in human amniotic fluid and murine placenta in absence of viral or any other type of infection. These molecules have been suggested to participate in the regulation of fetal development, or in the immunoregulation of the mother's acceptance of the product. They are also known to have a large variety of effects on the endocrine system.

Interferons appear to have various neuromodulatory actions during neurological and infectious diseases in the CNS. For instance, extended release of IFN-γ in the CNS during immunological and infectious conditions may trigger demyelinating disorders and cause disturbances in brain function [130]. Interferons also regulates neural transmission. The application of IFN-α during the peak of synaptogenesis reduces the frequency of spontaneous excitatory activity, but increases that of spontaneous inhibitory postsynaptic currents, thus changing the balance between excitatory and inhibitory neurotransmission [131]. This cytokine increases the frequency and amplitude of excitatory postsynaptic currents and decreases GABAergic neuron activation in the hippocampusof the rat, by reducing AMPA receptor clustering [132].

Superfusion of IFN-α in hippocampal slices inhibits CA1 pyramidal neuron excitatory potentials and reverses or prevents long-term potentiation (LTP), which has been proposed as a cellular mechanism involved in learning and memory. This effect is mediated through non-NMDA receptors [133]. Cultured dorsal horn neurons showed reduced nitric oxide-dependent clustering of AMPA receptor subunit I when exposed to IFN for two weeks [134]. In cultured rat astrocytes, IFN-β regulates IL-6 production. Thus, this pleiotropic cytokine may induce different biological activities in the CNS [134]. Chronic peripheral administration of IFN-α reduces serotonin levels in various brain areas of the rat but the mechanisms involved in this effect are not known [135].

In vivo, structural changes in the brain have been shown in IFN-α (highly producers) transgenic mice, including neurodegeneration with loss of cholinergic neurons, gliosis, angiopathy with mononuclear cell cuffing, progressive calcification affecting basal ganglia and cerebellum, as well as a modest impairment in discrimination learning throughout development. At a functional level, *in vivo* and *in vitro* electrophysiological studies revealed impaired neuronal function and disturbed synaptic plasticity with pronounced hippocampal hyperexcitability in IFN-α transgenic mice [136, 137].

In regards to endocrine and reproductive activities, IFNs have direct action on gonadal steroidogenesis. It has been established that treatment with IFN-α reduces serum progesterone and estradiol concentrations, with no apparent change in LH/hCG and FSH levels. IFN-α inhibits the FSH-stimulated conversion of testosterone to estradiol by cultured Sertoli cells In contrast, in the ovary IFN-α has no effect on progesterone or estradiol production by luteal cells [138]. Pre-treatment of Leydig cells with α or IFN-γ diminishes steroidogenesis and, if the treatment is combined, the effect is summatory. In these systems it has been shown that gonadal inhibition is caused by the capacity of IFN-γ to inhibit the accumulation of basal and LH/hCG stimulated mRNA molecules that code for StAR protein and enzymes P450scc [139] and P450c17 [140] and testosterone production in Leydig cells [141-143]. They also interfere with the enzyme fixation of the substrate (cholesterol) without modifying its structure. In ovaries disaggregated in bioassay, IFN-α inhibits both the basal and the hCG-stimulated production of testosterone and estradiol in a dose-dependent and temporary way. The effect of IFN-α inhibition is caused by interference with substrate (cholesterol) fixation by the enzyme 17β-hydroxysteroid dehydrogenase, and with the accumulation of the P450 aromatase 1 and 2 mRNA.

It has also been shown that IFN-γ can stimulate steroidogenesis in the testicle, increasing the activity of both, 17β-hydroxysteroid dehydrogenase and 5α-reductase [140-143]. In granulosa and theca cells, IFN-γ reduces LH/hCG stimulated progesterone secretion [138, 144, 145] and FSH stimulated estradiol secretion as well as gonadotropin dependent cAMP levels [144, 146]. It also reduces progesterone secretion in response to (Bu)2cAMP [144]. At follicular cells, addition of IFN-γ inhibits the formation of the LH/hCG receptor [146].

Tumor Necrosis Factor Alpha (TNF-α)

TNF-α is produced by macrophages in response to a tumorigenic transformation within the organism. In many of its effects, TNF-α resembles IL-1, however, they are not homologous, since TNF-α has its own receptor and does not directly activate lymphocytes. The injection of this cytokine causes fever, hypotension, response to acute phase proteins, lipase inhibition and release of stress hormones. Macrophage-derived cytokines or growth factors may directly or indirectly promote oligodendroglial proliferation and differentiation, contributing to myelin repair in inflammatory demyelinating diseases [147].

TNF-α is a cytokine rapidly produced in the brain in response to vigorous neuronal activity and tissue injury. TNF-α may protect neurons against excytotoxic and oxidative insults by a mechanism involving activation of the transcription factor NF-κB [148]. It has also been shown that a traumatic lesion to the hippocampus of adult mice induces a transitory expression of TNF-α and IL-1α in neurons of different brain areas, such as hippocampus, olfactory bulb, cerebellum, as well in glial cells in the site of injury [149, 150].

Whole-cell perforated patch clamp recordings in cultured rat hippocampal neurons showed that long-term treatment with TNF-α increases Ca^{2+} current density through L-type voltage-dependent channels, but it decreases currents induced by glutamate, NMDA, AMPA, and kainate. Neurons pre-treated with TNF-α exhibited increased intracellular Ca^{2+} concentrations following membrane depolarization, but reduced intracellular Ca^{2+} concentration in response to excitatory amino acids [151, 152]. Inflammatory mediators such as nitric oxide (NO) and TNF-α are released from glia-enriched mix culture in response to hypoxia/reoxygenation [153, 154]. TNF-α also modulates synaptic maturation and neuronal branching in the hippocampus by controlling the expression of synaptic vesicle-associated proteins [155]. Moreover, TNF-α changes the electrophysiological properties of myenteric neurons via cyclooxygenase metabolites and protein tyrosine phosphorylation [99].

In the ovary, it has been found to induce complex dose-dependent alterations in progesterone and androsterone synthesis, but not in estrogen synthesis. It is interesting to note that TNF-α inhibits gonadotropin-dependent differentiation in isolated murine granulosa cells increasing its proliferation in a dose dependent manner. This effect is mediated by its type 1 receptor (TNFR1), in the TNFR1 knockout TNF administration did not induced granulosa cell proliferation [156]. At steroidogenic level, TNF inhibits basal progesterone production in granulosa and theca cells and stimulates estradiol from small follicles but not cAMP levels [157] It also reduces intracellular levels of StAR protein in granulosa cells [158] and gonadotropin stimulated progesterone and estradiol secretion [159, 160] It lowers the LH/hCG-induced androstendione production by thecal cells from large follicles [161-163] and basal and FSH stimulated progesterone production in preovulatory follicles [164]. In the theca cells, it enhances the conversion of cholesterol to pregnenolone [164], but does not show any effect on cAMP [159]. The data suggest a cAMP downstream downregulation by inhibiting PKA [162]. The TNF receptor does not seem to be implicated in the regulation of these effects since in the TNFR1 knockout mice, administration of TNF does not affect LH/hCG-stimulated accumulation of progesterone, estradiol or cAMP [159]. In follicular fluid the estradiol and progesterone levels are lower when TNF is detectable [165].

TNF-α has been demonstrated to inhibit steroidogenesis in Leydig cells. In vitro, it does not affect the expression of StAR protein on the synthesis of progesterone [166], while intratesticular administration induces a reduction on StAR protein expression and testosterone byosinthesis [167]. TNF is known to suppress gonadotropin (LH/hCG) and cAMP (8-Br-cAMP) induced steroid secretion by Leydig cells [168]. Downstream it suppresses CRE activity but this is not mediated by the NF-κB pathway and the levels of CREB or P-CREB are not affected [168]. At the transcriptional level, TNF-α induces the recruitment of NFκB to the promoter of P450c17 causing the repression of this gen [169].

In a similar behavior to IL-1, TNFα inhibits cAMP stimulated testosterone production [72, 170, 171], as well as mRNA and protein of P450scc [72, 139, 171] and P450c17 [72, 170, 171] and 3β-HSD [72] an basal expression of 3β-HSD [72] but not P450scc basal expression [171]. It reduces in a dose dependent manner LH/hCG induces StAR levels of mRNA and protein [139, 172]. It also promotes the conversion of testosterone to dihydrotestosterone. Therefore, the enzymatic targets of this molecule are inhibition of P450scc and P450c17 in the ovary, and the increase of 5-α reductase activity in the testicle.

Conclusion

The aforementioned data suggest that different cytokines in fact play an important role in the regulation of the function of the gonads, both testes and ovaries. Most of the reviewed molecules have been shown to be produced by steroidogenic cells. Paracrine and autocrine roles have also been demonstrated for them. Here, we paid particular attention on steroidogenesis but other reproductive functions heve been shown to be altered by cytokines such as ovulation and spermatogenesis. Most of the experimental data show basal stimulation and gonadotropin-stimulated downregulation of the synthesis of sex steroids. Local or systemic up regulation of these cytokines, as it happens when an infection occurs, could modify gonadal functions. And it explains the lack or the loss of reproductive capacities when the immune system is highly activated (Table 1 and 2).

In summary, regulation of the ovarian and testicular steroid production depends not only on the complex normal endocrine regulation by the hypothalamus- hypophysial-gonadal axis, but on certain cell-types: lymphocytes (B and T), monocytes, macrophages, and on several representatives of the leukocyte strain, which are normal residents of the ovary and testicle, and regulate gonadal steroidogenesis by secretion of interleukins (Figure 2). New data in neurosciences rapidly accumulating in the past years suggest a revision of many long-established and widely accepted paradigms.

Table 2. Citokines an interferones effects to Central Nervous System (CNS) and Reproductive System (RS)

Cytokines	Effects		References
	CNS	R. S.	
IL-1	Regulate the secretion of diverse neuroendocrine, such as hypothalamic releasing factors. IL-1 also regulates neurotransmission mediated by amines such as noradrenaline, dopamine and serotonin. Likewise, mediates many responses during disease, including fever, sleep, neutrophilic leukocytosis, acute phase protein synthesis as well as endocrine changes, such as increased release of insulin, glucagons, growth hormone, prolactin ACTH, TSH, vasopressin and PTH.	Inhibits LH/hCG stimulated steroidogenesis in Leydig cells is dependent on cAMP levels. Inhibits the steroid production by direct effect on the enzyme, P450 cholesterol side chain cleavage (P450scc)	Blalock et al., 1989, Kennedy et al., 1991, Borsody 2002, Pitzel et al., 1993, Tsai et al., 2000, Xiong et al., 1993, Hales et al., 1992, Lin et al., 1991.
IL-1β	Increases GABA-A mediated inward chloride currents in synaptosomes. Increases c-fos expression in GABAergic, enkephalinergic, neurotensinergic and CRHergic neurons of the amygdaline complex.	Stimulates the basal progesterone, testosterone and androstenedione secretion in Leyding cells.	Hu et al., 2000, Miller et al., 1991 and 1994, Yu et al., 1994, Mazzoni 1997,
IL-1α	Upregulates StAR protein expression and phosphorilation [68], this protein (particularly its phosphorilated form) regulates the translocation of cholesterol from the outer to the inner mitochondrial membrane where steroidogenesis rate limiting step occurs	Stimulates the basal progesterone, testosterone and androstenedione secretion in Leyding cells.	Stocco et al., 1996

Table 2. (Continued)

Cytokines	Effects		References
	CNS	R. S.	
IL-2	Increases GABA release in hippocampal slices and reduces GABA-induced chloride currents in aplysia neurons	Is a potent inhibitor both of hCG-stimulated steroidogenesis and of cAMP formation in Leydig cells. In the ovary, IL-2 has no effect on LH/hCG induced steroid secretion, while it increases FSH induced progesterone synthesis and has no effect on estradiol. The regulation of NMDA receptors activation by IL-2 may contribute to synaptic plasticity in the mesolimbic system and to pathological outcomes	Sawada et al., 1992, Seto et al., 1997, Mikuni et al., 1995, McCann et al., 2000,
IL-3	IL-3 has been shown to exert a trophic action on septal cholinergic rat neurons. In the presence of IL-3 receptor (IL-3R) ß subunits in septal cholinergic neurons and its role in neuroprotection has been demonstrated. Likewise its capable to prevents delayed neuronal death in the hippocampal CA1 field through a receptor-mediated expression of Bcl-xL protein.	In the reproductive system Il-3 act on T lymphocytes directly, causing an enzymatic activity exclusive of steroid cells: an increase in the activity of 20a-hydroxysteroid dehydrogenase. In ovary cells in culture, it provokes an increase in progesterone production by stimulating the 3b-hydroxysteroid dehydrogenase activity.	Gorospe et al., 1998, Miller et al., 1991, Yu et al., 1994.
IL-4	The microglia respond to IL-4 with increase proliferation and activation, yet a corresponding suppression of MHC class II expression and TNF- α, IL-10, and IL-1β production that could be a critical regulation pathway during CNS	IL-4 has a role in the alleviation of inflammation and restoration of postovulatory stigma with potential therapeutic advantage in malignancy. In the pregnancy is associated with a relative increase in Th2-associated immunity,	Rehn et al., 2004, Weilemann et al., 2003, Benedetti et al., 1999, Papacleovoulou et al., 2009, Reichel et al., 2000.

Cytokines	Effects		References
	CNS	R. S.	
	inflammation. IL-4 production through the stem cells has shown potent antitumor effects in experimental rodent models, such as prevent the brain metastasis.	characterized by increased production of the cytokines IL-4.	
IL-5	Stimulates the proliferation, maturation, and functional activation of eosinophils and basophils associated to inflammation. Regulates the growth, differentiation, migration and effector function activities of many hematopoietic cells and immunocytes.	Is expressed in type 2 T lymphocytes and has a key role in driving the differentiation, recruitment and activation of eosinophils that have a role in endometrial tissue remodelling associated with the oestrous cycle. Deficiency on placental growth and function and subsequent weight gain in the newborn indicate that this cytokine may act through the maternal or fetal immune axis to exert subtle influences on reproductive outcome.	Broughton et al., 2012, Robertson et al., 2000, Perez et al., 1996.
IL-6	Another interleukin involved in neurochemical communication is IL-6, which potentiates evoked GABA release from mediobasal hypothalamic explants and posterior pituitary cells in culture. Systemically administered, inhibits naturally evoked neuronal responses. Long-term exposure of the brain to IL-6, as it has been observed in certain degenerative disorders and infections, reduced adult hippocampal neurogenesis. Although this cytokine has beneficial effects in the CNS because of its neurotrophic properties, its overexpression is generally detrimental.	Subcutaneous administration of IL-6 produce a suppression in testosterone levels without affecting LH. In FSH-stimulated granulosa cells, increasing amounts of IL-6 produce a significant suppression of progesterone biosynthesis. IL-6 has a stimulatory effect on estradiol production since it can stimulate aromatization of testosterone to estradiol, increasing the enzymatic activity of P450 aromatase.	De Laurentiis et al., 2000, Brenn et al., 2007, Vallieres et al., 2002, Van Wagoner et al., 1999, Tsigos et al., 1999, Gorospe et al., 1992.

Table 2. (Continued)

Cytokines	Effects		References
	CNS	R. S.	
IL-10	Inhibitor of inflammatory cytokine synthesis. Is capable of inducing survival in neural progenitors as well as promotes growth axodendritico, which takes place during the final stages of neuronal differentiation. Some reports propose that IL-10 is present in the normal brain, from birth to maturity, indicating the involvement of this interleukin in normal condition.	Modulates resistance to inflammatory stimuli by downregulating expression of proinflammatory cytokines TNF-α, IL-6, IL-1A, and IL-12, acting to protect against inflammation-induced pathology in the implantation site. Also, down-regulates decidual cell tissue factor expression, the main molecule triggering coagulation activation: this antithrombotic effect may protect the umbilicoplacental vasculature. Likewise, IL-10 is associated with maternal immunotolerance.	Robertson et al., 2007. Ransohoff et al., 2006. Cochery-Nouvellon et al., 2009.
IFN α, β and γ	Interferons appear to have various neuromodulatory actions during neurological and infectious diseases in the CNS and extended release of IFN-□ in during immunological and infectious conditions may trigger demyelinating disorders and cause disturbances in brain function. The application of IFN-α during the peak of synaptogenesis reduces the frequency of spontaneous excitatory activity, but increases that of spontaneous inhibitory postsynaptic currents, thus changing the balance between excitatory and inhibitory neurotransmission and	Interferons have a direct action on gonadal steroidogenesis. It has been established that treatment with IFN-α reduces serum progesterone and estradiol concentrations, with no apparent change in LH/hCG and FSH levels. IFN-α inhibits the FSH stimulated conversion of testosterone to estradiol by cultured Sertoli cells In contrast, in the ovary IFN-α has no effect on progesterone or estradiol production by luteal cells. In the testicle, IFN-γ can stimulate steroidogenesis, increasing the activity of both, 17b-hydroxysteroid dehydrogenase and 5a-reductase. In	Miljkovic et al., 2007, Yang et al., 2004, Brask et al., 2004, Vikman et al., 2001, Wang et al., and Fukuoka et al., 1992, Fairchild et al., 1991, Gorospe et al., 1988.

Cytokines	Effects		References
	CNS	R. S.	
	increases the frequency and amplitude of excitatory postsynaptic currents and decreases GABAergic neuron activation in the hippocampusof by reducing AMPA receptor clustering. Likewise, Induce the astrocytes to express IL-23 subunit p19 and common IL-12/IL-23 subunit p40.	granulose and theca cells, IFN-γ reduces LH/hCG stimulated progesterone secretion and 13 FSH stimulated estradiol secretion as well as gonadotropin dependent cAMP levels.	
TNF-α	Cytokine rapidly produced in the brain in response to vigorous neuronal activity and tissue injury. TNF-α may protect neurons against excytotoxic and oxidative insults by a mechanism involving activation of the transcription factor NF-κB Regulate the secretion of diverse neuroendocrine products hypophysial peptide hormones. TNF-α□also modulates synaptic maturation and neuronal branching in the hippocampus by controlling the expression of synaptic vesicle-associated proteins.	In the ovary, TNF-a inhibits gonadotropin-dependent differentiation in isolated murine granulosa cells increasing its proliferation in a dose dependent manner. At steroidogenic level, TNF inhibits basal progesterone production in granulosa and theca cells and stimulates estradiol from small follicles but not cAMP levels. It also reduces intracellular levels of StAR protein in granulosa cells [158] and gonadotropin stimulated progesterone and estradiol secretion. It lowers the LH/hCG-induced androstendione production by thecal cells from large follicles and basal and FSH stimulated progesterone production in preovulatory follicles. In the theca cells, it enhances the conversion of cholesterol to pregnenolone, but does not show any effect on cAMP. TNF-α has been demonstrated to inhibit steroidogenesis in Leydig cells.	Filipov et al., 2005, Son 2004, Basini et al., 2002, Roby et al., 1999, Hales 1994, Spicer et al., 1998, Zachow et al., 1993, Golan et al., 2004.

This paper reviewed some data leading to new concepts of the life and functions of neurons. Other molecules, the cyokines, which originally were believed exclusive of the immune system, regulate all neurotransmitters. These findings open a whole new theorethical concept of bi-directional communication between the nervous and the immune system under normal circumstances, not necessarily during disease or infection. Finally, the development of drugs specifically targeted against cytokines may be useful in the treatment of neuropathologies in which immune inflammation has a protagonic role. For instance, the specific targeting of IL-6/sIL-6R pathway will be a promising new approach for the treatment of neurodegenerative diseases.

Acknowledgments

Financial support: Grant # IN-214011 from Programa de Apoyo a Proyectos de Investigación e Innovación Tecnológica (PAPIIT) from the Dirección General de Asuntos del Personal Académico (DGAPA) from Universidad Nacional Autónoma de México (UNAM), and Grant number 176803, from Programa de Fondos Sectoriales CB-SEP, Consejo Nacional de Ciencia y Tecnología (CONACyT), both of them to Jorge Morales Montor. Karen E Nava Castro has a Posdoctoral Fellowship from Consejo Nacional de Ciencia y Tecnología (CONACyT), Hugo Aguilar Díaz has a Posdoctoral Fellowship from DGAPA,UNAM.

References

[1] Blalock, JE. A molecular basis for bidirectional communication between the immune and neuroendocrine systems. *Physiol Rev.*, 1989, 69(1), 1-32.

[2] Kennedy, RL; Jones, TH. Cytokines in endocrinology: their roles in health and in disease. *J Endocrinol.*, 1991, 129(2), 167-78.

[3] Ansar Ahmed, S; Penhale, WJ; Talal, N. Sex hormones, immune responses, and autoimmune diseases. Mechanisms of sex hormone action. *Am J Pathol.*, 1985, 121(3), 531-51.

[4] Grossman, CJ; Roselle, GA; Mendenhall, CL. Sex steroid regulation of autoimmunity. *J Steroid Biochem Mol Biol.*, 1991, 40(4-6), 649-59.

[5] Schuurs, AH; Verheul, HA. Effects of gender and sex steroids on the immune response. *J Steroid Biochem.*, 1990, 35(2), 157-72.

[6] Buzzetti, R; McLoughlin, L; Scavo, D; Rees, LH. A critical assessment of the interactions between the immune system and the hypothalamo-pituitary-adrenal axis. *J Endocrinol.*, 1989, 120(2), 183-7.

[7] Besedovsky, HO; del Rey, A. Immune-neuro-endocrine interactions: facts and hypotheses. *Endocr Rev.*, 1996, 17(1), 64-102. Epub 1996/02/01.

[8] Peck, R. Neuropeptides modulating macrophage function. *Ann N Y Acad Sci.*, 1987, 496264-70. Epub 1987/01/01.

[9] Webster, JI; Tonelli, L; Sternberg, EM. Neuroendocrine regulation of immunity. *Annu Rev Immunol.*, 2002, 20125-63. Epub 2002/02/28.

[10] Cutolo, M; Villaggio, B; Foppiani, L; Briata, M; Sulli, A; Pizzorni, C; Faelli, F; Prete, C; Felli, L; Seriolo, B; Giusti, M. The hypothalamic-pituitary-adrenal and gonadal axes in rheumatoid arthritis. *Ann N Y Acad Sci.*, 2000, 917835-43. Epub 2001/03/28.

[11] Grossman, CJ; Roselle, GA. The interrelationship of the HPG-thymic axis and immune system regulation. *J Steroid Biochem.*, 1983, 19(1B), 461-7. Epub 1983/07/01.

[12] Yoshida, K; Kakihana, M; Chen, LS; Ong, M; Baird, A; Gage, FH. Cytokine regulation of nerve growth factor-mediated cholinergic neurotrophic activity synthesized by astrocytes and fibroblasts. *Journal of neurochemistry*, 1992, 59(3), 919-31.

[13] Benveniste, EN; Kwon, J; Chung, WJ; Sampson, J; Pandya, K; Tang, LP. Differential modulation of astrocyte cytokine gene expression by TGF-beta. *Journal of immunology*, 1994, 153(11), 5210-21.

[14] Hu, S; Martella, A; Anderson, WR; Chao, CC. Role of cytokines in lipopolysaccharide-induced functional and structural abnormalities of astrocytes. *Glia*, 1994, 10(3), 227-34.

[15] Feldhaus, B; Dietzel, ID; Heumann, R; Berger, R. Effects of interferon-gamma and tumor necrosis factor-alpha on survival and differentiation of oligodendrocyte progenitors. *J Soc Gynecol Investig.*, 2004, 11(2), 89-96.

[16] Croitoru-Lamoury, J; Guillemin, GJ; Boussin, FD; Mognetti, B; Gigout, LI; Cheret, A; Vaslin, B; Le Grand, R; Brew, BJ; Dormont, D. Expression of chemokines and their receptors in human and simian astrocytes: evidence for a central role of TNF alpha and IFN gamma in CXCR4 and CCR5 modulation. *Glia*, 2003, 41(4), 354-70.

[17] De Simone, R; Levi, G; Aloisi, F. Interferon gamma gene expression in rat central nervous system glial cells. *Cytokine*, 1998, 10(6), 418-22.

[18] Aronica, E; Gorter, JA; Rozemuller, AJ; Yankaya, B; Troost, D. Activation of metabotropic glutamate receptor 3 enhances interleukin (IL)-1beta-stimulated release of IL-6 in cultured human astrocytes. *Neuroscience*, 2005, 130(4), 927-33.

[19] Benveniste, EN. Cytokine actions in the central nervous system. *Cytokine & growth factor reviews*, 1998, 9(3-4), 259-75.

[20] Fontana, A; Grob, PJ. Astrocyte-derived interleukin-1-like factors. *Lymphokine research*, 1984, 3(1), 11-6.

[21] Fontana, A; Hengartner, H; de Tribolet, N; Weber, E. Glioblastoma cells release interleukin 1 and factors inhibiting interleukin 2-mediated effects. *Journal of immunology*, 1984, 132(4), 1837-44.

[22] Ponomarev, ED; Maresz, K; Tan, Y; Dittel, BN. CNS-derived interleukin-4 is essential for the regulation of autoimmune inflammation and induces a state of alternative activation in microglial cells. The Journal of neuroscience: the official journal of the Society for *Neuroscience*, 2007, 27(40), 10714-21.

[23] Xu, J; Drew, PD. Peroxisome proliferator-activated receptor-gamma agonists suppress the production of IL-12 family cytokines by activated glia. *Journal of immunology*, 2007, 178(3), 1904-13.

[24] Tsakiri, N; Kimber, I; Rothwell, NJ; Pinteaux, E. Interleukin-1-induced interleukin-6 synthesis is mediated by the neutral sphingomyelinase/Src kinase pathway in neurones. *British journal of pharmacology*, 2008, 153(4), 775-83.

[25] Neumann, H; Schmidt, H; Wilharm, E; Behrens, L; Wekerle, H. Interferon gamma gene expression in sensory neurons: evidence for autocrine gene regulation. *The Journal of experimental medicine*, 1997, 186(12), 2023-31.

[26] Klassen, HJ; Imfeld, KL; Kirov, II; Tai, L; Gage, FH; Young, MJ; Berman, MA. Expression of cytokines by multipotent neural progenitor cells. *Cytokine*, 2003, 22(3-4), 101-6.

[27] Miljkovic, D; Momcilovic, M; Stojanovic, I; Stosic-Grujicic, S; Ramic, Z; Mostarica-Stojkovic, M. Astrocytes stimulate interleukin-17 and interferon-gamma production in vitro. *Journal of neuroscience research*, 2007, 85(16), 3598-606.

[28] Schobitz, B; de Kloet, ER; Sutanto, W; Holsboer, F. Cellular localization of interleukin 6 mRNA and interleukin 6 receptor mRNA in rat brain. *The European journal of neuroscience*, 1993, 5(11), 1426-35.

[29] Gadient, RA; Otten, U. Identification of interleukin-6 (IL-6)-expressing neurons in the cerebellum and hippocampus of normal adult rats. *Neuroscience letters*, 1994, 182(2), 243-6.

[30] Sallmann, S; Juttler, E; Prinz, S; Petersen, N; Knopf, U; Weiser, T; Schwaninger, M. Induction of interleukin-6 by depolarization of neurons. *The Journal of neuroscience : the official journal of the Society for Neuroscience*, 2000, 20(23), 8637-42.

[31] Breder, CD; Dinarello, CA; Saper, CB. Interleukin-1 immunoreactive innervation of the human hypothalamus. *Science*, 1988, 240(4850), 321-4.

[32] Gadient, RA; Otten, U. Differential expression of interleukin-6 (IL-6) and interleukin-6 receptor (IL-6R) mRNAs in rat hypothalamus. *Neuroscience letters*, 1993, 153(1), 13-6.

[33] Gadient, RA; Otten, U. Postnatal expression of interleukin-6 (IL-6) and IL-6 receptor (IL-6R) mRNAs in rat sympathetic and sensory ganglia. *Brain research*, 1996, 724(1), 41-6.

[34] Pfeffer, K. Biological functions of tumor necrosis factor cytokines and their receptors. *Cytokine & growth factor reviews*, 2003, 14(3-4), 185-91.

[35] Pejovic, V; Soskic, V; Pan, W; Kastin, AJ. Brain proteome of mice lacking the receptors for tumor necrosis factor alpha. *Proteomics*, 2004, 4(5), 1461-4.

[36] Akassoglou, K; Bauer, J; Kassiotis, G; Pasparakis, M; Lassmann, H; Kollias, G; Probert, L. Oligodendrocyte apoptosis and primary demyelination induced by local TNF/p55TNF receptor signaling in the central nervous system of transgenic mice: models for multiple sclerosis with primary oligodendrogliopathy. *Am J Pathol.*, 1998, 153(3), 801-13.

[37] Benedetti, S; Bruzzone, MG; Pollo, B; DiMeco, F; Magrassi, L; Pirola, B; Cirenei, N; Colombo, MP; Finocchiaro, G. Eradication of rat malignant gliomas by retroviral-mediated, in vivo delivery of the interleukin 4 gene. *Cancer research*, 1999, 59(3), 645-52.

[38] Samland, H; Huitron-Resendiz, S; Masliah, E; Criado, J; Henriksen, SJ; Campbell, IL. Profound increase in sensitivity to glutamatergic- but not cholinergic agonist-induced seizures in transgenic mice with astrocyte production of IL-6. *Journal of neuroscience research*, 2003, 73(2), 176-87.

[39] Bacher, M; Meinhardt, A; Lan, HY; Dhabhar, FS; Mu, W; Metz, CN; Chesney, JA; Gemsa, D; Donnelly, T; Atkins, RC; Bucala, R. MIF

expression in the rat brain: implications for neuronal function. *Molecular medicine*, 1998, 4(4), 217-30.

[40] Bucala, R. Neuroimmunomodulation by macrophage migration inhibitory factor (MIF). *Ann N Y Acad Sci.*, 1998, 84074-82.

[41] Meinhardt, A; Bacher, M; McFarlane, JR; Metz, CN; Seitz, J; Hedger, MP; de Kretser, DM; Bucala, R. Macrophage migration inhibitory factor production by Leydig cells: evidence for a role in the regulation of testicular function. *Endocrinology*, 1996, 137(11), 5090-5.

[42] Angeli, A; Masera, RG; Sartori, ML; Fortunati, N; Racca, S; Dovio, A; Staurenghi, A; Frairia, R. Modulation by Cytokines of Glucocorticoid Action. *Annals of the New York Academy of Sciences*, 1999, 876(1), 210-20.

[43] Meinhardt, A; Bacher, M; Metz, C; Bucala, R; Wreford, N; Lan, H; Atkins, R; Hedger, M. Local regulation of macrophage subsets in the adult rat testis: examination of the roles of the seminiferous tubules, testosterone, and macrophage-migration inhibitory factor. *Biol Reprod.*, 1998, 59(2), 371-8.

[44] Unanue, ER; Allen, PM. The basis for the immunoregulatory role of macrophages and other accessory cells. *Science*, 1987, 236(4801), 551-7.

[45] Hu, S; Sheng, WS; Ehrlich, LC; Peterson, PK; Chao, CC. Cytokine effects on glutamate uptake by human astrocytes. *Neuroimmunomodulation*, 2000, 7(3), 153-9.

[46] Miller, LG; Galpern, WR; Dunlap, K; Dinarello, CA; Turner, TJ. Interleukin-1 augments gamma-aminobutyric acidA receptor function in brain. *Molecular pharmacology*, 1991, 39(2), 105-8.

[47] Yu, B; Shinnick-Gallagher, P. Interleukin-1 beta inhibits synaptic transmission and induces membrane hyperpolarization in amygdala neurons. *The Journal of pharmacology and experimental therapeutics*, 1994, 271(2), 590-600.

[48] Miller, LG; Fahey, JM. Interleukin-1 modulates GABAergic and glutamatergic function in brain. *Ann N Y Acad Sci.*, 1994, 739292-8.

[49] Mazzoni, IE; Kenigsberg, RL. Microglia from the developing rat medial septal area can affect cholinergic and GABAergic neuronal differentiation in vitro. *Neuroscience*, 1997, 76(1), 147-57.

[50] Feleder, C; Refojo, D; Nacht, S; Moguilevsky, JA. Interleukin-1 stimulates hypothalamic inhibitory amino acid neurotransmitter release. *Neuroimmunomodulation*, 1998, 5(1-2), 1-4.

[51] Feleder, C; Arias, P; Refojo, D; Nacht, S; Moguilevsky, J. Interleukin-1 inhibits NMDA-stimulated GnRH secretion: associated effects on the release of hypothalamic inhibitory amino acid neurotransmitters. *Neuroimmunomodulation*, 2000, 7(1), 46-50.

[52] Wang, S; Cheng, Q; Malik, S; Yang, J. Interleukin-1beta inhibits gamma-aminobutyric acid type A (GABA(A)) receptor current in cultured hippocampal neurons. *The Journal of pharmacology and experimental therapeutics*, 2000, 292(2), 497-504.

[53] Parnet, P; Amindari, S; Wu, C; Brunke-Reese, D; Goujon, E; Weyhenmeyer, JA; Dantzer, R; Kelley, KW. Expression of type I and type II interleukin-1 receptors in mouse brain. *Brain research Molecular brain research*, 1994, 27(1), 63-70.

[54] Bianchi, M; Clavenna, A; Bondiolotti, GP; Ferrario, P; Panerai, AE. GM-CSF affects hypothalamic neurotransmitter levels in mice: involvement of interleukin-1. *Neuroreport*, 1997, 8(16), 3587-90.

[55] McCann, SM; Kimura, M; Karanth, S; Yu, WH; Rettori, V. Role of nitric oxide in the neuroendocrine responses to cytokines. *Ann N Y Acad Sci.*, 1998, 840174-84.

[56] Spangelo, BL; Horrell, S; Goodwin, AL; Shroff, S; Jarvis, WD. Somatostatin and gamma-aminobutyric acid inhibit interleukin-1 beta-stimulated release of interleukin-6 from rat C6 glioma cells. *Neuroimmunomodulation*, 2004, 11(5), 332-40.

[57] Borsody, MK; Weiss, JM. Alteration of locus coeruleus neuronal activity by interleukin-1 and the involvement of endogenous corticotropin-releasing hormone. *Neuroimmunomodulation*, 2002, 10(2), 101-21.

[58] Ho, A; Blum, M. Induction of interleukin-1 associated with compensatory dopaminergic sprouting in the denervated striatum of young mice: model of aging and neurodegenerative disease. *The Journal of neuroscience : the official journal of the Society for Neuroscience*, 1998, 18(15), 5614-29.

[59] Parish, CL; Finkelstein, DI; Tripanichkul, W; Satoskar, AR; Drago, J; Horne, MK. The role of interleukin-1, interleukin-6, and glia in inducing growth of neuronal terminal arbors in mice. *The Journal of neuroscience: the official journal of the Society for Neuroscience*, 2002, 22(18), 8034-41.

[60] Parati, EA; Bez, A; Ponti, D; Sala, S; Pozzi, S; Pagano, SF. Neural stem cells. Biological features and therapeutic potential in Parkinson's disease. *Journal of neurosurgical sciences*, 2003, 47(1), 8-17.

[61] Alam, MN; McGinty, D; Bashir, T; Kumar, S; Imeri, L; Opp, MR; Szymusiak, R. Interleukin-1beta modulates state-dependent discharge activity of preoptic area and basal forebrain neurons: role in sleep regulation. *The European journal of neuroscience*, 2004, 20(1), 207-16.
[62] Scarborough, DE; Lee, SL; Dinarello, CA; Reichlin, S. Interleukin-1 beta stimulates somatostatin biosynthesis in primary cultures of fetal rat brain. *Endocrinology*, 1989, 124(1), 549-51.
[63] Schneider, H; Pitossi, F; Balschun, D; Wagner, A; del Rey, A; Besedovsky, HO. A neuromodulatory role of interleukin-1beta in the hippocampus. *Proceedings of the National Academy of Sciences of the United States of America*, 1998, 95(13), 7778-83.
[64] Ikegaya, Y; Delcroix, I; Iwakura, Y; Matsuki, N; Nishiyama, N. Interleukin-1beta abrogates long-term depression of hippocampal CA1 synaptic transmission. *Synapse*, 2003, 47(1), 54-7.
[65] Shaftel, SS; Carlson, TJ; Olschowka, JA; Kyrkanides, S; Matousek, SB; O'Banion, MK. Chronic interleukin-1beta expression in mouse brain leads to leukocyte infiltration and neutrophil-independent blood brain barrier permeability without overt neurodegeneration. The Journal of neuroscience : *the official journal of the Society for Neuroscience*, 2007, 27(35), 9301-9.
[66] Pitzel, L; Jarry, H; Wuttke, W. Effects and interactions of prostaglandin F2 alpha, oxytocin, and cytokines on steroidogenesis of porcine luteal cells. *Endocrinology*, 1993, 132(2), 751-6.
[67] Tsai, JA; Rong, H; Torring, O; Matsushita, H; Bucht, E. Interleukin-1beta upregulates PTHrP-mRNA expression and protein production and decreases TGF-beta in normal human osteoblast-like cells. *Calcif Tissue Int.*, 2000, 66(5), 363-9.
[68] Renlund, N; Jo, Y; Svechnikova, I; Holst, M; Stocco, DM; Soder, O; Svechnikov, K. Induction of steroidogenesis in immature rat Leydig cells by interleukin-1alpha is dependent on extracellular signal-regulated kinases. *J Mol Endocrinol*, 2006, 36(2), 327-36.
[69] Stocco, DM; Clark, BJ. Role of the steroidogenic acute regulatory protein (StAR) in steroidogenesis. *Biochem Pharmacol*, 1996, 51(3), 197-205.
[70] Verhoeven, G; Cailleau, J; Van Damme, J; Billiau, A. Interleukin-1 stimulates steroidogenesis in cultured rat Leydig cells. *Mol Cell Endocrinol*, 1988, 57(1-2), 51-60.
[71] Colon, E; Svechnikov, KV; Carlsson-Skwirut, C; Bang, P; Soder, O. Stimulation of steroidogenesis in immature rat Leydig cells evoked by

interleukin-1alpha is potentiated by growth hormone and insulin-like growth factors. *Endocrinology*, 2005, 146(1), 221-30.

[72] Xiong, Y; Hales, DB. Differential effects of tumor necrosis factor-alpha and interleukin-1 on 3 beta-hydroxysteroid dehydrogenase/delta 5-->delta 4 isomerase expression in mouse Leydig cells. *Endocrine*, 1997, 7(3), 295-301.

[73] Hales, DB. Interleukin-1 inhibits Leydig cell steroidogenesis primarily by decreasing 17 alpha-hydroxylase/C17-20 lyase cytochrome P450 expression. *Endocrinology*, 1992, 131(5), 2165-72.

[74] Mauduit, C; Chauvin, MA; Hartmann, DJ; Revol, A; Morera, AM; Benahmed, M. Interleukin-1 alpha as a potent inhibitor of gonadotropin action in porcine Leydig cells: site(s) of action. *Biol Reprod*, 1992, 46(6), 1119-26.

[75] Lin, T; Guo, H; Calkins, JH; Wang, D; Chi, R. Recombinant monocyte-derived interleukin-1 receptor antagonist reverses inhibitory effects of interleukin-1 on Leydig cell steroidogenesis. *Mol Cell Endocrinol*, 1991, 78(3), 205-9.

[76] Calkins, JH; Sigel, MM; Nankin, HR; Lin, T. Interleukin-1 inhibits Leydig cell steroidogenesis in primary culture. *Endocrinology*, 1988, 123(3), 1605-10.

[77] Gerendai, I; Banczerowski, P; Csernus, V. Interleukin 1-beta injected into the testis acutely stimulates and later attenuates testicular steroidogenesis of the immature rat. *Endocrine*, 2005, 28(2), 165-70.

[78] Svechnikov, KV; Sultana, T; Soder, O. Age-dependent stimulation of Leydig cell steroidogenesis by interleukin-1 isoforms. *Mol Cell Endocrinol*, 2001, 182(2), 193-201.

[79] Gerendai, I; Banczerowski, P; Csernus, V; Halasz, B. Innervation and serotoninergic receptors of the testis interact with local action of interleukin-1beta on steroidogenesis. *Auton Neurosci.*, 2007, 131(1-2), 21-7.

[80] Cohen, PE; Pollard, JW. Normal sexual function in male mice lacking a functional type I interleukin-1 (IL-1) receptor. *Endocrinology*, 1998, 139(2), 815-8.

[81] Chen, HF; Shew, JY; Chao, KH; Chang, LJ; Ho, HN; Yang, YS. Luteinizing hormone up-regulates the expression of interleukin-1 beta mRNA in human granulosa-luteal cells. *Am J Reprod Immunol*, 2000, 43(3), 125-33.

[82] Baratta, M; Basini, G; Bussolati, S; Tamanini, C. Effects of interleukin-1 beta fragment (163-171) on progesterone and estradiol-17 beta release

by bovine granulosa cells from different size follicles. *Regul Pept.*, 1996, 67(3), 187-94.

[83] Kohen, P; Castro, A; Caballero-Campo, P; Castro, O; Vega, M; Makrigiannakis, A; Simon, C; Carvallo, P; Devoto, L. Interleukin-1beta (IL-1beta) is a modulator of human luteal cell steroidogenesis: localization of the IL type I system in the corpus luteum. *J Clin Endocrinol Metab.*, 1999, 84(11), 4239-45.

[84] Breard, E; Delarue, B; Benhaim, A; Feral, C; Leymarie, P. Inhibition by gonadotropins of interleukin-1 production by rabbit granulosa and theca cells: effects on gonadotropin-induced progesterone production. *Eur J Endocrinol*, 1998, 138(3), 328-36.

[85] Dawood, MY; Chellaram, R; Khan-Dawood, FS. Interleukin-1 beta inhibits in vitro pulsatile progesterone secretion and stimulates prostaglandin F2 alpha secretion by micro-retrodialyzed baboon corpus luteum. *Horm Metab Res.*, 1997, 29(10), 483-90.

[86] Terranova, PF; Rice, VM. Review: cytokine involvement in ovarian processes. *Am J Reprod Immunol.*, 1997, 37(1), 50-63.

[87] Donesky, BW; Dias de Moura, M; Tedeschi, C; Hurwitz, A; Adashi, EY; Payne, DW. Interleukin-1beta inhibits steroidogenic bioactivity in cultured rat ovarian granulosa cells by stimulation of progesterone degradation and inhibition of estrogen formation. *Biol Reprod.*, 1998, 58(5), 1108-16.

[88] Kasson, BG; Gorospe, WC. Effects of interleukins 1, 2 and 3 on follicle-stimulating hormone-induced differentiation of rat granulosa cells. *Mol Cell Endocrinol*, 1989, 62(1), 103-11.

[89] Zhou, MH; Galway, AB. [Inhibitory effect of interleukin-1 beta on follicle stimulating hormone (FSH) induced estrogen production by cultured rat granulosa cells]. *Sheng Li Xue Bao.*, 1991, 43(1), 67-72.

[90] Sawada, M; Hara, N; Ichinose, M. Interleukin-2 inhibits the GABA-induced Cl- current in identified Aplysia neurons. *Journal of neuroscience research*, 1992, 33(3), 461-5.

[91] Seto, D; Kar, S; Quirion, R. Evidence for direct and indirect mechanisms in the potent modulatory action of interleukin-2 on the release of acetylcholine in rat hippocampal slices. *British journal of pharmacology*, 1997, 120(6), 1151-7.

[92] Alonso, R; Chaudieu, I; Diorio, J; Krishnamurthy, A; Quirion, R; Boksa, P. Interleukin-2 modulates evoked release of [3H]dopamine in rat cultured mesencephalic cells. *Journal of neurochemistry*, 1993, 61(4), 1284-90.

[93] McCann, SM; Kimura, M; Karanth, S; Yu, WH; Mastronardi, CA; Rettori, V. The mechanism of action of cytokines to control the release of hypothalamic and pituitary hormones in infection. *Ann N Y Acad Sci.*, 2000, 9174-18.

[94] Petitto, JM; Huang, Z. Molecular cloning of a partial cDNA of the interleukin-2 receptor-beta in normal mouse brain: in situ localization in the hippocampus and expression by neuroblastoma cells. *Brain research*, 1994, 650(1), 140-5.

[95] Guo, H; Calkins, JH; Sigel, MM; Lin, T. Interleukin-2 is a potent inhibitor of Leydig cell steroidogenesis. *Endocrinology*, 1990, 127(3), 1234-9.

[96] Meikle, AW; Cardoso de Sousa, JC; Dacosta, N; Bishop, DK; Samlowski, WE. Direct and indirect effects of murine interleukin-2, gamma interferon, and tumor necrosis factor on testosterone synthesis in mouse Leydig cells. *J Androl.*, 1992, 13(5), 437-43.

[97] Gorospe, WC; Kasson, BG. Lymphokines from concanavalin-A-stimulated lymphocytes regulate rat granulosa cell steroidogenesis in vitro. *Endocrinology*, 1988, 123(5), 2462-71.

[98] Mikuni, M. [Effect of interleukin-2 and interleukin-6 on ovary in the ovulatory period--establishment of the new ovarian perfusion system and influence of interleukins on ovulation rate and steroid secretion]. *Hokkaido Igaku Zasshi*, 1995, 70(4), 561-72.

[99] Rehn, M; Hubschle, T; Diener, M. TNF-alpha hyperpolarizes membrane potential and potentiates the response to nicotinic receptor stimulation in cultured rat myenteric neurones. *Acta physiologica Scandinavica*, 2004, 181(1), 13-22.

[100] Joshi, BH; Leland, P; Asher, A; Prayson, RA; Varricchio, F; Puri, RK. In situ expression of interleukin-4 (IL-4) receptors in human brain tumors and cytotoxicity of a recombinant IL-4 cytotoxin in primary glioblastoma cell cultures. *Cancer research*, 2001, 61(22), 8058-61.

[101] Weilemann, F; Steinmetz, A; Kirsch, M; Buttler, A; Kunze, S; Kuhlisch, E; Schackert, HK; Schackert, G. Prevention of brain metastasis formation by local expression of interleukin-4 or hemagglutinin antigen. *Zentralblatt fur Neurochirurgie*, 2003, 64(2), 65-70.

[102] Racke, MK; Bonomo, A; Scott, DE; Cannella, B; Levine, A; Raine, CS; Shevach, EM; Rocken, M. Cytokine-induced immune deviation as a therapy for inflammatory autoimmune disease. *The Journal of experimental medicine*, 1994, 180(5), 1961-6.

[103] Burke, F; Relf, M; Negus, R; Balkwill, F. A cytokine profile of normal and malignant ovary. *Cytokine*, 1996, 8(7), 578-85.
[104] Papacleovoulou, G; Hogg, K; Fegan, KS; Critchley, HO; Hillier, SG; Mason, JI. Regulation of 3beta-hydroxysteroid dehydrogenase type 1 and type 2 gene expression and function in the human ovarian surface epithelium by cytokines. *Molecular human reproduction*, 2009, 15(6), 379-92.
[105] Nelms, K; Keegan, AD; Zamorano, J; Ryan, JJ; Paul, WE. The IL-4 receptor: signaling mechanisms and biologic functions. *Annu Rev Immunol*, 1999, 17701-38.
[106] Nagai, S; Toi, M. Interleukin-4 and breast cancer. *Breast cancer*, 2000, 7(3), 181-6.
[107] Reichel, M; Nelson, BH; Greenberg, PD; Rothman, PB. The IL-4 receptor alpha-chain cytoplasmic domain is sufficient for activation of JAK-1 and STAT6 and the induction of IL-4-specific gene expression. *Journal of immunology*, 1997, 158(12), 5860-7.
[108] Broughton, SE; Dhagat, U; Hercus, TR; Nero, TL; Grimbaldeston, MA; Bonder, CS; Lopez, AF; Parker, MW. The GM-CSF/IL-3/IL-5 cytokine receptor family: from ligand recognition to initiation of signaling. *Immunological reviews*, 2012, 250(1), 277-302.
[109] Sferruzzi-Perri, AN; Robertson, SA; Dent, LA. Interleukin-5 transgene expression and eosinophilia are associated with retarded mammary gland development in mice. *Biol Reprod*, 2003, 69(1), 224-33.
[110] Robertson, SA; Mau, VJ; Young, IG; Matthaei, KI. Uterine eosinophils and reproductive performance in interleukin 5-deficient mice. *Journal of reproduction and fertility*, 2000, 120(2), 423-32.
[111] Perez, MC; Furth, EE; Matzumura, PD; Lyttle, CR. Role of eosinophils in uterine responses to estrogen. *Biol Reprod.*, 1996, 54(1), 249-54.
[112] De Laurentiis, A; Pisera, D; Lasaga, M; Diaz, M; Theas, S; Duvilanski, B; Seilicovich, A. Effect of interleukin-6 and tumor necrosis factor-alpha on GABA release from mediobasal hypothalamus and posterior pituitary. *Neuroimmunomodulation*, 2000, 7(2), 77-83.
[113] Flatters, SJ; Fox, AJ; Dickenson, AH. Nerve injury alters the effects of interleukin-6 on nociceptive transmission in peripheral afferents. *European journal of pharmacology*, 2004, 484(2-3), 183-91.
[114] Brenn, D; Richter, F; Schaible, HG. Sensitization of unmyelinated sensory fibers of the joint nerve to mechanical stimuli by interleukin-6 in the rat: an inflammatory mechanism of joint pain. *Arthritis and rheumatism*, 2007, 56(1), 351-9.

[115] Vallieres, L; Campbell, IL; Gage, FH; Sawchenko, PE. Reduced hippocampal neurogenesis in adult transgenic mice with chronic astrocytic production of interleukin-6. The Journal of neuroscience : *the official journal of the Society for Neuroscience*, 2002, 22(2), 486-92.
[116] Nelson, TE; Campbell, IL; Gruol, DL. Altered physiology of Purkinje neurons in cerebellar slices from transgenic mice with chronic central nervous system expression of interleukin-6. *Neuroscience*, 1999, 89(1), 127-36.
[117] Nelson, TE; Netzeband, JG; Gruol, DL. Chronic interleukin-6 exposure alters metabotropic glutamate receptor-activated calcium signalling in cerebellar Purkinje neurons. *The European journal of neuroscience*, 2004, 20(9), 2387-400.
[118] Nelson, TE; Ur, CL; Gruol, DL. Chronic interleukin-6 exposure alters electrophysiological properties and calcium signaling in developing cerebellar purkinje neurons in culture. *Journal of neurophysiology*, 2002, 88(1), 475-86.
[119] Tancredi, V; D'Antuono, M; Café, C; Giovedi, S; Bue, MC; D'Arcangelo, G; Onofri, F; Benfenati, F. The inhibitory effects of interleukin-6 on synaptic plasticity in the rat hippocampus are associated with an inhibition of mitogen-activated protein kinase ERK. *Journal of neurochemistry*, 2000, 75(2), 634-43.
[120] Van Wagoner, NJ; Oh, JW; Repovic, P; Benveniste, EN. Interleukin-6 (IL-6) production by astrocytes: autocrine regulation by IL-6 and the soluble IL-6 receptor. *The Journal of neuroscience : the official journal of the Society for Neuroscience*, 1999, 19(13), 5236-44.
[121] Gruol, DL; Nelson, TE. Physiological and pathological roles of interleukin-6 in the central nervous system. *Molecular neurobiology*, 1997, 15(3), 307-39.
[122] Kushima, Y; Hama, T; Hatanaka, H. Interleukin-6 as a neurotrophic factor for promoting the survival of cultured catecholaminergic neurons in a chemically defined medium from fetal and postnatal rat midbrains. *Neuroscience research*, 1992, 13(4), 267-80.
[123] Moore, KW; de Waal Malefyt, R; Coffman, RL; O'Garra, A. Interleukin-10 and the interleukin-10 receptor. *Annu Rev Immunol*, 2001, 19683-765.
[124] Tsigos, C; Papanicolaou, DA; Kyrou, I; Raptis, SA; Chrousos, GP. Dose-dependent effects of recombinant human interleukin-6 on the pituitary-testicular axis. *J Interferon Cytokine Res.*, 1999, 19(11), 1271-6.

[125] Gorospe, WC; Hughes, FM Jr.; Spangelo, BL. Interleukin-6: effects on and production by rat granulosa cells in vitro. *Endocrinology*, 1992, 130(3), 1750-2.

[126] Van der Hoek, KH; Woodhouse, CM; Brannstrom, M; Norman, RJ. Effects of interleukin (IL)-6 on luteinizing hormone- and IL-1beta-induced ovulation and steroidogenesis in the rat ovary. *Biol Reprod*, 1998, 58(5), 1266-71.

[127] Robertson, SA; Care, AS; Skinner, RJ. Interleukin 10 regulates inflammatory cytokine synthesis to protect against lipopolysaccharide-induced abortion and fetal growth restriction in mice. *Biol Reprod.*, 2007, 76(5), 738-48.

[128] Ransohoff, RM. A mighty mouse: building a better model of multiple sclerosis. *The Journal of clinical investigation*, 2006, 116(9), 2313-6.

[129] Cochery-Nouvellon, E; Nguyen, P; Attaoua, R; Cornillet-Lefebvre, P; Mercier, E; Vitry, F; Gris, JC. Interleukin 10 gene promoter polymorphisms in women with pregnancy loss: preferential association with embryonic wastage. *Biol Reprod.*, 2009, 80(6), 1115-20.

[130] Yang, L; Blumbergs, PC; Jones, NR; Manavis, J; Sarvestani, GT; Ghabriel, MN. Early expression and cellular localization of proinflammatory cytokines interleukin-1beta, interleukin-6, and tumor necrosis factor-alpha in human traumatic spinal cord injury. *Spine*, 2004, 29(9), 966-71.

[131] Brask, J; Kristensson, K; Hill, RH. Exposure to interferon-gamma during synaptogenesis increases inhibitory activity after a latent period in cultured rat hippocampal neurons. *The European journal of neuroscience*, 2004, 19(12), 3193-201.

[132] Vikman, KS; Owe-Larsson, B; Brask, J; Kristensson, KS; Hill, RH. Interferon-gamma-induced changes in synaptic activity and AMPA receptor clustering in hippocampal cultures. *Brain research*, 2001, 896(1-2), 18-29.

[133] Mendoza-Fernandez, V; Andrew, RD; Barajas-Lopez, C. Interferon-alpha inhibits long-term potentiation and unmasks a long-term depression in the rat hippocampus. *Brain research*, 2000, 885(1), 14-24.

[134] Okada, K; Kuroda, E; Yoshida, Y; Yamashita, U; Suzumura, A; Tsuji, S. Effects of interferon-beta on the cytokine production of astrocytes. *Journal of neuroimmunology*, 2005, 159(1-2), 48-54.

[135] Sato, T; Suzuki, E; Yokoyama, M; Semba, J; Watanabe, S; Miyaoka, H. Chronic intraperitoneal injection of interferon-alpha reduces serotonin levels in various regions of rat brain, but does not change levels of

serotonin transporter mRNA, nitrite or nitrate. *Psychiatry and clinical neurosciences*, 2006, 60(4), 499-506.
[136] Campbell, IL; Krucker, T; Steffensen, S; Akwa, Y; Powell, HC; Lane, T; Carr, DJ; Gold, LH; Henriksen, SJ; Siggins, GR. Structural and functional neuropathology in transgenic mice with CNS expression of IFN-alpha. *Brain research*, 1999, 835(1), 46-61.
[137] Gu, C; Casaccia-Bonnefil, P; Srinivasan, A; Chao, MV. Oligodendrocyte apoptosis mediated by caspase activation. *The Journal of neuroscience : the official journal of the Society for Neuroscience*, 1999, 19(8), 3043-9.
[138] Wang, HZ; Lu, SH; Han, XJ; Zhou, W; Sheng, WX; Sun, ZD; Gong, YT. Inhibitory effect of interferon and tumor necrosis factor on human luteal function in vitro. *Fertil Steril.*, 1992, 58(5), 941-5.
[139] Lin, T; Hu, J; Wang, D; Stocco, DM. Interferon-gamma inhibits the steroidogenic acute regulatory protein messenger ribonucleic acid expression and protein levels in primary cultures of rat Leydig cells. *Endocrinology*, 1998, 139(5), 2217-22.
[140] Orava, M; Voutilainen, R; Vihko, R. Interferon-gamma inhibits steroidogenesis and accumulation of mRNA of the steroidogenic enzymes P450scc and P450c17 in cultured porcine Leydig cells. *Mol Endocrinol.*, 1989, 3(6), 887-94.
[141] Orava, M; Cantell, K; Vihko, R. Human leukocyte interferon inhibits human chorionic gonadotropin stimulated testosterone production by porcine Leydig cells in culture. *Biochem Biophys Res Commun.*, 1985, 127(3), 809-15.
[142] Orava, M; Cantell, K; Vihko, R. Treatment with preparations of human leukocyte interferon decreases serum testosterone concentrations in men. *Int J Cancer*, 1986, 38(2), 295-6.
[143] Orava, M. Comparison of the inhibitory effects of interferons-alpha and -gamma on testosterone production in porcine Leydig cell culture. *J Interferon Res.*, 1989, 9(1), 135-41.
[144] Fukuoka, M; Yasuda, K; Emi, N; Fujiwara, H; Iwai, M; Takakura, K; Kanzaki, H; Mori, T. Cytokine modulation of progesterone and estradiol secretion in cultures of luteinized human granulosa cells. *J Clin Endocrinol Metab*, 1992, 75(1), 254-8.
[145] Fairchild, DL; Pate, JL. Modulation of bovine luteal cell synthetic capacity by interferon-gamma. *Biol Reprod.*, 1991, 44(2), 357-63.

[146] Gorospe, WC; Tuchel, T; Kasson, BG. Gamma-interferon inhibits rat granulosa cell differentiation in culture. *Biochem Biophys Res Commun.*, 1988, 157(3), 891-7.
[147] Diemel, LT; Copelman, CA; Cuzner, ML. Macrophages in CNS remyelination: friend or foe? *Neurochemical research*, 1998, 23(3), 341-7.
[148] Filipov, NM; Seegal, RF; Lawrence, DA. Manganese potentiates in vitro production of proinflammatory cytokines and nitric oxide by microglia through a nuclear factor kappa B-dependent mechanism. *Toxicological sciences : an official journal of the Society of Toxicology*, 2005, 84(1), 139-48.
[149] Friedman, WJ. Cytokines regulate expression of the type 1 interleukin-1 receptor in rat hippocampal neurons and glia. *Experimental neurology*, 2001, 168(1), 23-31.
[150] Neumann, H; Schweigreiter, R; Yamashita, T; Rosenkranz, K; Wekerle, H; Barde, YA. Tumor necrosis factor inhibits neurite outgrowth and branching of hippocampal neurons by a rho-dependent mechanism. *The Journal of neuroscience : the official journal of the Society for Neuroscience*, 2002, 22(3), 854-62.
[151] Furukawa, K; Mattson, MP. The transcription factor NF-kappaB mediates increases in calcium currents and decreases in NMDA- and AMPA/kainate-induced currents induced by tumor necrosis factor-alpha in hippocampal neurons. *Journal of neurochemistry*, 1998, 70(5), 1876-86.
[152] Liu, B; Li, H; Brull, SJ; Zhang, JM. Increased sensitivity of sensory neurons to tumor necrosis factor alpha in rats with chronic compression of the lumbar ganglia. *Journal of neurophysiology*, 2002, 88(3), 1393-9.
[153] Wang, JY; Wang, JY. Hypoxia/Reoxygenation induces nitric oxide and TNF-alpha release from cultured microglia but not astrocytes of the rat. *The Chinese journal of physiology*, 2007, 50(3), 127-34.
[154] Di Santo, E; Foddi, MC; Ricciardi-Castagnoli, P; Mennini, T; Ghezzi, P. DHEAS inhibits TNF production in monocytes, astrocytes and microglial cells. *Neuroimmunomodulation*, 1996, 3(5), 285-8.
[155] Golan, H; Levav, T; Mendelsohn, A; Huleihel, M. Involvement of tumor necrosis factor alpha in hippocampal development and function. *Cerebral cortex*, 2004, 14(1), 97-105.
[156] Son, DS; Arai, KY; Roby, KF; Terranova, PF. Tumor necrosis factor alpha (TNF) increases granulosa cell proliferation: dependence on c-Jun and TNF receptor type 1. *Endocrinology*, 2004, 145(3), 1218-26.

[157] Basini, G; Mainardi, GL; Bussolati, S; Tamanini, C. Steroidogenesis, proliferation and apoptosis in bovine granulosa cells: role of tumour necrosis factor-alpha and its possible signalling mechanisms. *Reprod Fertil Dev.*, 2002, 14(3-4), 141-50.

[158] Sasson, R; Winder, N; Kees, S; Amsterdam, A. Induction of apoptosis in granulosa cells by TNF alpha and its attenuation by glucocorticoids involve modulation of Bcl-2. *Biochem Biophys Res Commun.*, 2002, 294(1), 51-9.

[159] Roby, KF; Son, DS; Terranova, PF. Alterations of events related to ovarian function in tumor necrosis factor receptor type I knockout mice. *Biol Reprod.*, 1999, 61(6), 1616-21.

[160] Hales, HA; Peterson, CM; Mitchell, MD; Jones, KP; Hatasaka, HH; Poulson, AM. Tumor necrosis factor-alpha inhibits ovulation and steroidogenesis, but not prostaglandin production in the perfused rat ovary. *J Soc Gynecol Investig.*, 1994, 1(1), 59-64.

[161] Spicer, LJ. Tumor necrosis factor-alpha (TNF-alpha) inhibits steroidogenesis of bovine ovarian granulosa and thecal cells in vitro. Involvement of TNF-alpha receptors. *Endocrine*, 1998, 8(2), 109-15.

[162] Zachow, RJ; Tash, JS; Terranova, PF. Tumor necrosis factor-alpha attenuation of luteinizing hormone-stimulated androstenedione production by ovarian theca-interstitial cells: inhibition at loci within the adenosine 3',5'-monophosphate-dependent signaling pathway. *Endocrinology*, 1993, 133(5), 2269-76.

[163] Roby, KF; Terranova, PF. Tumor necrosis factor alpha alters follicular steroidogenesis in vitro. *Endocrinology*, 1988, 123(6), 2952-4.

[164] Roby, KF; Terranova, PF. Effects of tumor necrosis factor-alpha in vitro on steroidogenesis of healthy and atretic follicles of the rat: theca as a target. *Endocrinology*, 1990, 126(5), 2711-8.

[165] Punnonen, J; Heinonen, PK; Teisala, K; Kujansuu, E; Jansen, CT; Punnonen, R. Demonstration of tumor necrosis factor-alpha in preovulatory follicular fluid: its association with serum 17 beta-estradiol and progesterone. *Gynecol Obstet Invest.*, 1992, 33(2), 80-4.

[166] Gonzalez-Navarrete, F; Eisner, V; Morales, P; Castro, O; Pommer, R; Quiroga, C; Lavandero, S; Devoto, L. Tumor necrosis factor-alpha activates nuclear factor-kappaB but does not regulate progesterone production in cultured human granulosa luteal cells. *Gynecol Endocrinol*, 2007, 23(7), 377-84.

[167] Morales, V; Santana, P; Diaz, R; Tabraue, C; Gallardo, G; Lopez Blanco, F; Hernandez, I; Fanjul, LF; Ruiz de Galarreta, CM.

Intratesticular delivery of tumor necrosis factor-alpha and ceramide directly abrogates steroidogenic acute regulatory protein expression and Leydig cell steroidogenesis in adult rats. *Endocrinology*, 2003, 144(11), 4763-72.

[168] Arai, KY; Roby, KF; Terranova, PF. Tumor necrosis factor alpha (TNF) suppresses cAMP response element (CRE) activity and nuclear CRE binding protein in MA-10 mouse Leydig tumor cells. *Endocrine*, 2005, 27(1), 17-24.

[169] Hong, CY; Park, JH; Ahn, RS; Im, SY; Choi, HS; Soh, J; Mellon, SH; Lee, K. Molecular mechanism of suppression of testicular steroidogenesis by proinflammatory cytokine tumor necrosis factor alpha. *Mol Cell Biol.*, 2004, 24(7), 2593-604.

[170] Li, X; Youngblood, GL; Payne, AH; Hales, DB. Tumor necrosis factor-alpha inhibition of 17 alpha-hydroxylase/C17-20 lyase gene (Cyp17) expression. *Endocrinology*, 1995, 136(8), 3519-26.

[171] Xiong, Y; Hales, DB. The role of tumor necrosis factor-alpha in the regulation of mouse Leydig cell steroidogenesis. *Endocrinology*, 1993, 132(6), 2438-44.

[172] Mauduit, C; Gasnier, F; Rey, C; Chauvin, MA; Stocco, DM; Louisot, P; Benahmed, M. Tumor necrosis factor-alpha inhibits leydig cell steroidogenesis through a decrease in steroidogenic acute regulatory protein expression. *Endocrinology*, 1998, 139(6), 2863-8.

In: Neuro-Immune Interactions ... ISBN: 978-1-62948-646-8
Editor: Oscar González-Pérez

Chapter 7

NEUROIMMUNE CROSSTALK IN OBESITY

Norma A. Moy-Lopez*[*]*, Jorge Guzman-Muñiz, Jorge Collas-Aguilar, Roberto Montes-Delgado and Oscar Gonzalez-Perez

Laboratory of Neuroscience, School of Psychology, University of Colima, Colima, Mexico

ABSTRACT

The central nervous system (CNS) plays an important role in the regulation of food intake and energy expenditure in response to different signals (hormones, neuronal or nutrient stimulus). In the brain, lipid metabolism and transport system differ from that of peripheral tissues. These lipids are involved in important metabolic pathways, which are regularly related to the energy homeostasis of cells. Imbalances in the metabolism of lipids are closely associated with the development of several diseases such as: eating disorders, metabolic syndrome, Alzheimer's disease, Huntington's disease and Niemann–Pick type C disease. These metabolic defects modify cholesterol biosynthesis, lipid transport and lipoprotein assembly, receptors that mediate the cellular uptake of lipids and signaling molecules. Specifically in the CNS, there are several studies demonstrating that hypothalamic lipid metabolism is a crucial process to regulate energy homeostasis. In particular, the arcuate

[*] Corresponding author: Norma A. Moy-Lopez, Facultad de Psicologia, Universidad de Colima, Av. Universidad 333, Colima, COL 28040, Mexico, Tel: +52(312)316-1091, Email: moynor@ucol.mx.

nucleus is a critical structure in appetite regulation and the mechanism of obesity. Thus, high energy intake leads to a state of chronic nutrient excess that promotes systemic and neural inflammation. Moreover, neurons and glia express receptors for metabolic hormones, such as leptin and insulin, and can be stimulated in response to increased weight gain. This interaction generates an activation of inflammatory pathways in hypothalamus and other brain areas that may lead to leptin resistance and defective regulation of energy homeostasis. This chapter is focused on the neurological and immune response in obesity. Herein, we describe the obesity regulation by CNS and the role of neurons and glial cells in the inflammatory process.

Acronyms

CNS)	Central nervous system
BBB	blood–brain barrier
ApoE	Apolipoprotein E
Apos	Apolipoproteins
LDL-R	low density lipoprotein receptor
AD	Alzheimer's disease
PPARγ	peroxisome proliferator-activated receptor gamma
VMH	ventromedial nuclei of the hypothalamus
ARC	arcuate nucleus
PVN	paraventricular nucleus
LHA	lateral hypothalamic area
NPY	neuropeptide Y
AgRP	agouti-related peptide
POMC	pro-opiomelanocortin
CART	cocaine- and amphetamine-regulated transcripts
GHSR	growth hormone secretagogue receptor
DHA	docosahexaenoic acid
AA	arachidonic acid
IL-1	interleukin-1
IL-6	interleukin-6
TNF-α	tumor necrosis factor-alpha
JNK	c-Jun N-terminal kinase
TLR	toll-like receptor
PAMPs	pathogen-associated molecular pattern
ObR or LepR	leptin receptor

1. Lipid Metabolism in the CNS

Lipids represent 50–60% of cellular components. The different glycerophospholipid species, together with sphingolipids, cholesterol, acylglycerols and fatty acids are the principal components of cell membranes (Table 1), and determine the structure and plasticity of somatic, dendritic and axonal membranes of neurons (Adibhatla and Hatcher, 2008, Jordan et al., 2010, Veloso et al., 2011).

Table 1. Principal lipids present in the neurons and glia membranes

Lipid Type	Subtypes
Glycerophospholipids	• Phosphatidylcholine • Phosphatidylethanolamine • Phosphatidylserine • Phosphatidylinositol
Sphingolipids	• Sphingomyelin • Ceramide • Glycosphingolipids (Gangliosides)
Sterol lipids	• Cholesterol • Cholesterol esters
Glycerolipids	• Acylglycerol
Fatty acyls	• Free fatty acids and conjugates

The lipid metabolism in the CNS (Figure 1) is different from that of peripheral tissues because the CNS is partially segregated from systemic circulation by the blood–brain barrier (BBB) (Dietschy, 2009, Hayashi, 2011). This BBB formed by tight junctions between capillary endothelial cells prevents lipoproteins exchanges, which are responsible for intercellular transport of sterols and other lipids (Pfrieger and Ungerer, 2011, Orth and Bellosta, 2012, Segatto et al., 2012). Consequently, lipoproteins do not cross the BBB of mouse, rat and human brain; hence, labeled cholesterol peripherally administrated is not found in the CNS (Hayashi, 2011). Unlike other organs, brain cholesterol is primarily derived by *de novo* synthesis. Therefore, brain cells have implemented their specific way to handle cholesterol metabolism (Veloso et al., 2011, Chen et al., 2013).

Cholesterol *de novo* synthesis is different within brain regions. This metabolic process depends on the expression of cholesterol-synthesizing enzymes, sterol-sensing factors, intracellular transporters, cholesterol shuttle proteins, and lipoprotein receptors (Orth and Bellosta, 2012). Astrocytes and neurons synthesize cholesterol and lipoproteins in the brain. Cholesterol is associated with lipoproteins, which are produced by astrocytes only. Astrocytes and microglia, but not neurons, express apolipoprotein E (ApoE) (Chen et al., 2013). Apolipoproteins (Apos) are the protein component of lipoproteins responsible for lipid transport. Lipoproteins are formed by linking apoproteins to free cholesterol, cholesterol esters, phospholipids or triacylglycerols (Woods et al., 2012). ApoE is highly expressed in the CNS and mediates the transport of cholesterol by interacting with cell surface receptors of the low density lipoprotein (LDL-R) and low-density lipoprotein receptor-related protein 1 (LRP1). After ApoE-receptor interaction, the lipid transport is completed by endocytosis (Rebeck et al., 2006). ApoE is produced within the CNS and interacts with Aβ (a cleavage product of amyloid precursor protein: Amyloid β), promoting the formation of amyloid fibrils from soluble Aβ in the CNS (Orth and Bellosta, 2012). Overproduction of Aβ is one of the most important characteristics in Alzheimer's disease (AD) that promotes the formation of amyloid plaques. This evidence suggests that cholesterol is importance in AD development and progression (Adibhatla and Hatcher, 2008, Matsuzaki, 2010).

On the other hand, ApoE is involved in other functions including: immunomodulation, oxidative stress, stabilization of neuronal microtubules, synaptic plasticity and apoptosis (Elliott et al., 2010, Hayashi, 2011). In the hypothalamus, ApoE also acts as a homeostatic factor that partially mediates the inhibitory effects of leptin. Moreover, glial cells express receptors for metabolic hormones, such as leptin and insulin. These receptors may be activated in response to increased weight gain and dietary challenges. Another relevant biological sensor of lipid concentrations in the brain is the peroxisome proliferator-activated receptor gamma (PPARγ), which is expressed in astrocytes and neurons. PPARγ is involved in central regulation of energy metabolism in states of leptin resistance (Garcia-Caceres et al., 2012). Therefore, the control center for the systemic energy balance is the hypothalamus. This cerebral structure not only regulates food intake and energy expenditure, but also the utilization and partitioning of nutrients, glucose homoeostasis and lipid metabolism.

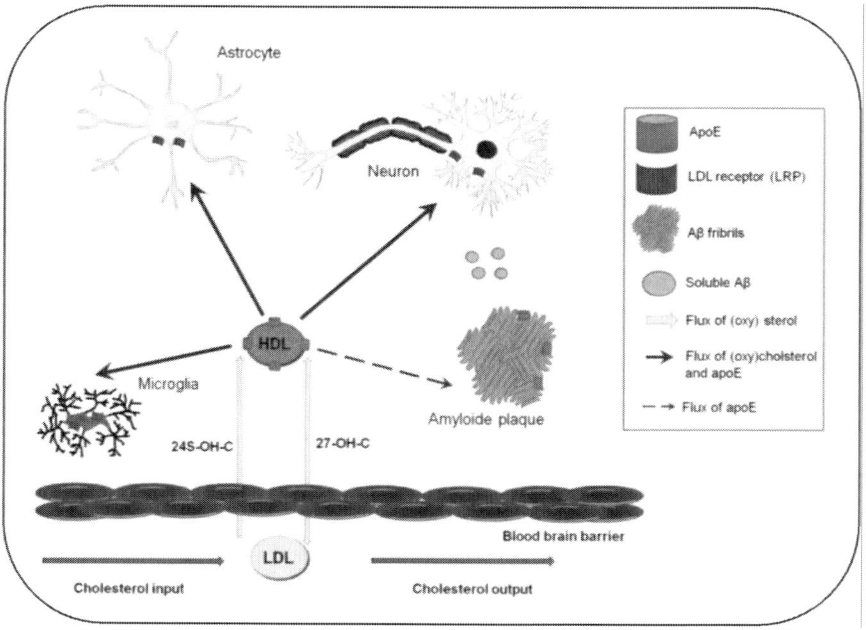

Figure 1. Cholesterol *de novo* synthesis in the brain. Cholesterol can be converted to 24S-hydroxycholesterol (24S-OH-C) and 27-hydroxycholesterol (27-OH-C) in the CNS. These sterols can cross the BBB because of the hydroxylated side chains. 24S-OH-C is produced only in the CNS. Astrocytes and microglia cells secrete HDL-like lipoproteins composed of cholesterol and phospholipids and ApoE. Cholesterol synthesis in neural cells can be regulated by the ApoE-mediated uptake of lipoproteins via the LDL receptor family. The availability of cholesterol and ApoE have been involved in the formation of amyloid fibrils from soluble Aβ in the CNS.

2. Hypothalamic Signals in Obesity

CNS controls energy balance by involving a complex network between several brain regions and the rest of the body. There are two mechanisms of this balance: energy intake (food intake) and energy expenditure (physical activity, metabolism, and body temperature regulation) (Faulconbridge and Hayes, 2011, Velloso and Schwartz, 2011). The brain needs to obtain information about the energy status of the periphery to promote appropriate responses and metabolic changes to maintain energy balance (Morton et al., 2006, Sanchez-Lasheras et al., 2010).

The control of food intake may suffer various alterations that can promote an increase in energy intake. These factors include the preference for high energy dense foods, weak post-prandial inhibitory signaling, strong hunger traits (associated with low leptin levels followed by weight loss) and consumption of fatty foods (Blundell et al., 2008). The chronic imbalance between the energy intake and energy expenditure could be an epigenetic factor that produces different metabolic syndromes. The obesity is an example of this imbalance, because it is a state in where the energy intake exceeds energy expenditure. In fact, a subtle mismatch (less than 0.5%) in caloric intake over the energy expenditure is sufficient to cause weight gain (Suzuki et al., 2012).

Energy homeostasis involves a complex network of hypothalamic and extra-hypothalamic neurons that transduce hormonal and nutrient signals that regulate the caloric intake and energy expenditure to stabilize body fat storage (Figure 2). Clearly, the hypothalamus is crucial in the control of food intake and energy balance. Hypothalamic lesion studies offered the first evidence of the role of brain in body weight control and the pathogenesis of obesity and diabetes (Velloso and Schwartz, 2011). In this experiments, the ventromedial nuclei of the hypothalamus (VMH), including the arcuate nucleus (ARC), paraventricular nucleus (PVN) and dorsal hypothalamus were identified as important brain regions in the development of hyperphagia and obesity. Besides, lesions in lateral hypothalamic area (LHA) resulted in hypophagia and anorexia (Gao and Horvath, 2007). In the ARC, there are two neuronal populations: neurons that stimulate food intake and co-express neuropeptide Y (NPY) and agouti-related peptide (AgRP) and, neurons that co-express pro-opiomelanocortin (POMC) and cocaine- and amphetamine-regulated transcripts (CART), which suppress food intake (Suzuki et al., 2012). NPY and AgRP neuronal groups are regulated by insulin, leptin, and ghrelin (Jordan et al., 2010). Insulin and leptin levels secretion is directly proportional to body fat, which indicates that these hormones provide information about the total amount of body fat and help regulate long- term energy stores (Arble and Sandoval, 2013). Thus, the hypothalamus is the primary integrative region for nutrient-related signals, which include central and peripheral neuronal inputs as well as hormonal signals.

Insulin secretion from pancreas is regulated by feeding (after meal consumption) and its blood levels vary directly proportional to body adiposity. Insulin crosses the blood-brain barrier and its receptors are in the ARC nucleus in the hypothalamus, an area implicated in energy balance regulation. Direct administration of insulin into hypothalamus or adjacent third ventricle inhibits food intake and decreases body weight (Woods et al., 1979, Dietschy, 2009, Konner et al., 2009, Hayashi, 2011).

Leptin is an adipocyte-derived hormone that increases in proportion to body fat mass and can be used as biomarker of adiposity. Activation of hypothalamic leptin signaling increases activity of POMC/CART neurons and decreases NPY/AgRP neuronal activity (Sahu, 2003), resulting in reduced food intake and enhanced energy expenditure (Yu and Kim, 2012). Leptin levels are associated with immune response in malnourished infants, which have low plasma leptin and impaired immune response. Moreover, leptin signaling deficiency impairs humoral and cellular immune response (Fernandez-Riejos et al., 2010). In the last section, we analyze the relationship between leptin and immune/inflammatory responses in the obesity.

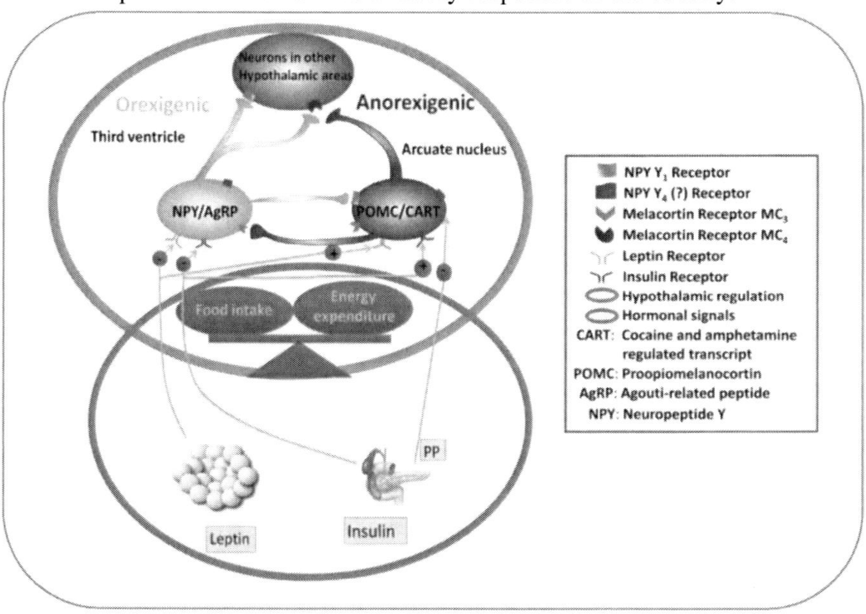

Figure 2. Regulation of energy homeostasis. Food intake is regulated by a complex system of peripheral and central signals. Peripheral regulation involves "satiety signals" and "adiposity signals" triggered by insulin and leptin. In the ARC, leptin activate POMC/CART neurons (orexigenic effect) and inhibit NYP/AgRP neurons (anorexigenic effect).

Ghrelin is another hormone involved in the regulation of lipid metabolism. This hormone is secreted from the upper tract of intestine and some hypothalamic neurons. Ghrelin stimulates the release of growth hormone from the pituitary gland, and regulates feeding and energy homoeostasis via GHSR (growth hormone secretagogue receptor) in the hypothalamus (Pang and Han, 2012), where NPY and AgRP neurons are the primary targets (Nakazato et al., 2001).

Taking together, this evidence indicates that leptin, ghrelin, and other hormones that control energy metabolism may be affected by other immune response, synaptic plasticity and the structural connections of neurons/glia in the hypothalamus as well as other brain regions. Some of these processes are related to hypothalamic inflammation, which is important in obesity development mediated by glial cells (Streit et al., 2004).

3. From Immune System to Brain Signaling: Obesity Implications

Reciprocal interactions between the brain and the immune system have been implicated in the pathogenesis of metabolic syndromes, a group of metabolic disorders that include abdominal obesity, insulin resistance (glucose intolerance), atherogenic dyslipidemia and overexpression of prothrombotic and proinflammatory markers (Olufadi and Byrne, 2008, Bruce-Keller et al., 2009, Capuron and Miller, 2011, Tahergorabi and Khazaei, 2013). Cerebral and immunological interaction are also implied in cognitive decline and mood disorders (Bruce-Keller et al., 2009, Taha et al., 2012).

Dysregulation of lipid metabolism is particularly important in the brain, because this organ is highly enriched with polyunsaturated fatty acids, docosahexaenoic acid (DHA) and arachidonic acid (AA). DHA and AA are essential for mediating neuroreceptor signaling. Likewise, in neuroinflammation and excitotoxicity process, there is excessive releasing of AA. Unesterified AA is a precursor of prostaglandins, thromboxanes, leukotrienes, which have important roles in regulating the neuroinflammatory response (Uauy et al., 2001, Green et al., 2008, Burke and Dennis, 2009, Taha et al., 2012). In the brain, the BBB partially restricts the access of immune cells and mediators from the blood. This anatomical condition limits the immune response. However, the brain has an innate immune activation to respond local and systemic inflammatory signal through a complex communication between neurons and glial cells (Laflamme and Rivest, 2001, Thaler et al., 2010). In response to injury, infection or disease, neural cells generate inflammatory mediators, including proinflammatory cytokines, such as interleukin-1(IL-1), interleukin-6 (IL-6), and tumor necrosis factor-alpha (TNF-α), prostaglandins, free radicals and complement, which produce adhesion molecules, recruit immune cells, and activate microglia (Lucas et al., 2006, Emanuela et al., 2012). In obesity, other factors are associated with the response of the glia cells, because adipose tissue is an important source of proinflammatory cytokines and other proteins with similar effects, such as: IL-1, leptin and adiponectin (Figure 3).

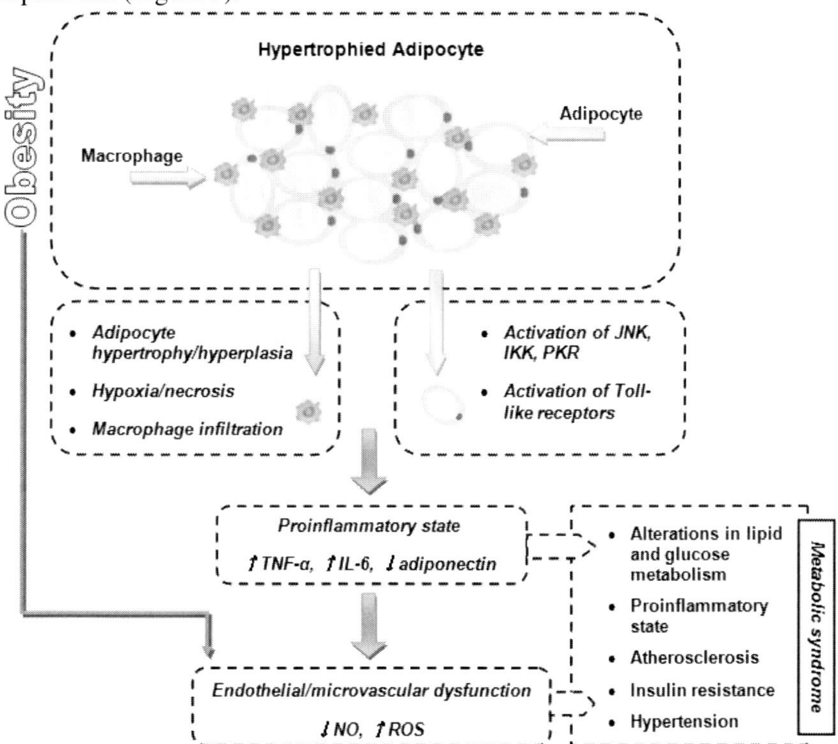

Figure 3. Overview of the effect of both lipids and cytokines in inflammation process (Metabolic syndrome and Obesity). TNF-*α:* tumor necrosis factor alpha; IL-6: interleukin 6; NO: nitric oxide; ROS: reactive oxygen species; JNK: c-jun N-terminal kinase; IKK: Inhibitor of k kinase; PKR: protein kinase R.

In obese mice, adipose hypoxia is associated with increased expression of inflammatory genes and decreased expression of adiponectin (Ye et al., 2007). In parallel, hypoxia induces a strong activation of the c-Jun N-terminal kinase (JNK) (Kunz et al., 2001). This signaling pathway contributes to inflammation, macrophage recruitment and mediates metabolic response to obesity, including insulin resistance (Han et al., 2013). Furthermore, JNK regulates brain development, repair, and memory formation as well as it is a potent effector of neuroinflammation and neuronal death (Haeusgen et al., 2009).

Adipose tissue participates in the physiological regulation of immune responses via toll-like receptor (TLR) signaling cascades, TLRs play central roles in the innate immune response by recognizing structural patterns in diverse microbial molecules (Lowther et al., 1970). In the brain, microglia and astrocytes express a number of TLRs, which allow the recognition of pathogen-associated molecular pattern (PAMPs) and endogenous TLR agonists (Kielian, 2006). Hypothalamic TLR2 is related to obesity control (Shechter et al., 2013).

4. Obesity, Inflammation and Leptin

Adipose tissue comprises not only adipocytes, but also blood vessels, nerve terminals, adipocyte precursors and leukocytes. These cellular components are collectively known as "stromal vascular compartment" (SVC) (Patel et al., 2013). Adipose tissue was primarily considered as a passive reservoir for energy deposition and storage. The discovery of leptin and other adipose tissue-derived humoral mediators (e.g., adiponectin and resistin), collectively referred to as "adipokines", changes the traditional view of adipocytes as passive reservoirs. To date, adipose tissue is considered as a complex, essential and highly active metabolic organ (Bluher, 2005, Kadowaki et al., 2006, Nishimura et al., 2009). Adipokines are important determinants of both insulin resistance and obesity, either through a traditional hormonal effect, or local effects on adipocytes. The effects of obesity include an increase in circulating cytokines and a decrease in protective factors, being the communication between inflammatory and metabolic cells an important aspect of this process. Obesity induces a chronic low-grade inflammation in diverse tissues, including the hypothalamus, which triggers alterations in insulin and leptin sensitivity (Wang et al., 2012). The cerebral inflammatory responses are primarily promoted by microglia cells and astrocytes (Garcia-Caceres et al., 2012).

The endocrine hormone leptin is a 167-amino-acid protein that is mainly produced by adipocytes and plasmatic levels are closely correlated to body fat (Harvey, 2013). Circulating leptin provides a negative feedback control on feeding behavior and energy balance (Thaler et al., 2010). This biochemical system can be regulated by physiological or pathological factors (Table 2) including brain injury, diet-induced obesity, leptin treatment, triglycerides, glucose and insulin (Pan et al., 2008b, Hsuchou et al., 2010).

The biological actions of leptin are mediated by the leptin receptor (ObR or LepR), a member of the interleukin-6 receptor family that lacks endogenous kinase activity (Tartaglia et al., 1995, Williams et al., 2009, Pan et al., 2012, Harvey, 2013). The areas with the highest level of LepR expression are the arcuate nucleus and median eminence of the hypothalamus followed by dentate gyrus and CA1 region of the hippocampus. Most of the mRNA leptin signals appear to be in hypothalamic NPY neurons (Pan et al., 2012). In the ARC nucleus, there are two populations of leptin-responsive neurons that play a significant role in body weight control by communicating the status of energy storages. A regulatory pathway consists of neurons co-expressing NPY and AgRP, which mediate food intake, whereas an adjacent set of ARC neurons co-expressing POMC and CART suppress food intake (Dieguez et al., 2011, Mainardi et al., 2013). The lack of leptin signaling in ob/ob and db/db mice results in a reduction in the brain weight and the expression of glial fibrillary acidic protein in the hypothalamus (Ahima et al., 1999), as well as in the ApoE levels that inhibits the effects of leptin in food intake (Figure 4). During the period of fasting or high-fat diet intake, astrocytes transport higher concentrations of fatty acids and ketone bodies from the peripheral circulation to the brain. The monocarboxylate transporter (MCT)-1 is the main transporter of ketone bodies in the CNS. This transporter is expressed by astrocytes, neurons and endothelial cells. Interestingly, long-term HFD intake increases the number and size of glial cells (gliosis) in the hypothalamus. Indeed, it seems that neuronal inflammation is constrained by glial signals that, in turn, limit weight gain. Thus, these recent studies suggest the role of hypothalamic inflammation and leptin in obesity pathogenesis during high-fat diet (Morris and Rui, 2009, Thaler et al., 2010, Garcia-Caceres et al., 2012).

Table 2. Mediators of leptin transport across the BBB

State or substance	Effect on transport	Description	Reference

Fasting ↑	↓	Food deprivation can decrease the blood-to-brain transport of leptin	(Kastin and Akerstrom, 2000)
Glucose/ Insulin ↑	↑	Glucose and Insulin can increase leptin transport, but they probably are not the principal factors responsible for the regulatory effect of the BBB on leptin entry into the brain.	(Kastin and Akerstrom, 2001)
Obesity ↑	↓	The impaired transport of leptin across the brain develops in tandem with obesity and is reversible with even modest weight reduction.	(Banks and Farrell, 2003)
Triglycerides ↓	↑	Decreasing triglycerides may potentiate the anorectic effect of leptin by enhancing leptin transport across the BBB.	(Banks et al., 2004)
Alcohol ↑	↑	Increased leptin permeation across the brain occurred concomitantly with brain disruption after 2 weeks of forced alcohol ingestion.	(Pan et al., 2008a)
C-reactive protein ↑	↓	It is thought that CRP contributes to leptin resistance by preventing leptin from crossing the BBB.	(Hsuchou et al., 2012)

In addition to the effect of leptin in regulating energy balance, this protein plays also a key role in brain development. In this regard, it is well-known that leptin has significant effects on proliferation, maintenance, and differentiation of neuronal and glial cells. During the early postnatal period, there is an increase in circulating leptin concentrations, but despite this elevation, neonates maintain a high level of food intake. Furthermore, feeding behavior and metabolic responses to exogenous leptin administration are absent until near the time of weaning (Vickers and Sloboda, 2012, Cojocaru et al., 2013). Leptin functions in the brain include the modulation of the excitability of hippocampal neurons by activating potassium channels. Since leptin receptor-deficient mice have impaired spatial learning ability, it has been suggested that leptin signaling may also influence synaptic plasticity (Oomura et al., 2006).

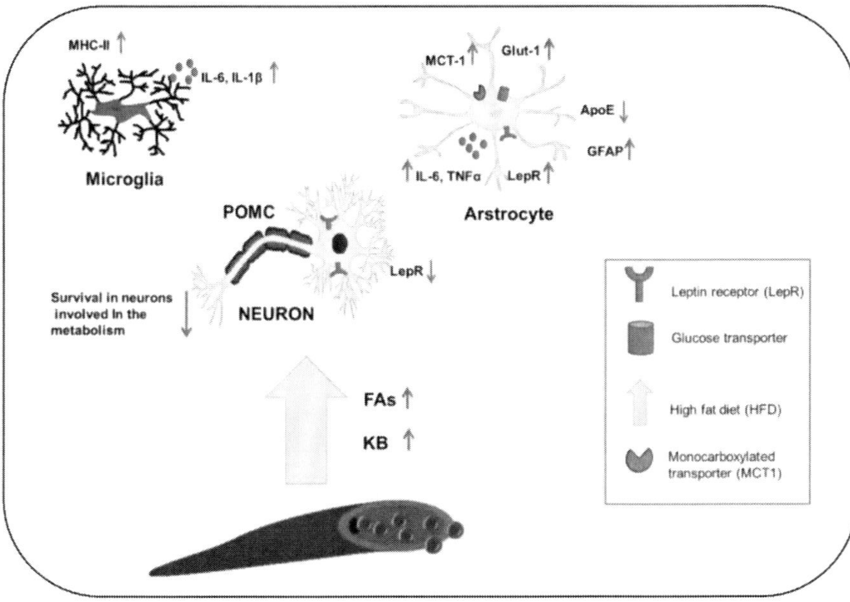

FA: Fatty Acids. KB: Ketone Bodies. GFAP: Glial fibrillary acidic protein. MHC: Major Histocompatibility Complex. MCT: Monocarboxylated transporter. ApoE: Apolipoprotein E.

Figure 4. Schematic representation of glial changes associated with modifications in synaptic protein and hypothalamic cytokine concentrations. HFD intake increases the reactive gliosis, and this affect the cytoarchitecture of the ARC.

CONCLUSION

Inflammatory and innate immune responses in peripheral tissues can be activated by serum lipids, such as cholesterol and fatty acids. In the brain, hypothalamic neurons respond to peripheral lipid signals by modifying the synthesis and releases of both neuropeptides and hormones. Leptin informs the brain about the status of energy availability and lipid metabolism having effects on the activation of POMC/CART neurons and inhibiting NPY/AgRP neurons, which inhibits feeding and increases energy expenditure. Glial cells express several receptors for hormones involved in appetite control and food intake. Thus, astrocytes play a crucial role in modulating the local environment of nutrient sensing neurons in the hypothalamus. Therefore, the hypothalamic regulation of energy balance is severely compromised by over nutrition, particularly in obesity state, which induces neuroinflammation involving an abnormal cytokine production and activation of inflammatory signaling pathways. In addition, increasing evidence indicates that leptin acts as a pro-inflammatory cytokine. Nevertheless, the effect of leptin in the brain is not only restricted to hypothalamic regulation of energy balance, but also regulates of the learning, memory, reward, motivation, neuroprotection, reproduction and growth.

Acknowledgment

This work was supported in part by grants from the PROMEP (103.5/12/4857) and Fondo Ramón Álvarez-Buylla de Aldana (FRABA 846/13).

References

Adibhatla, R. M. & Hatcher, J. F. (2008). Altered lipid metabolism in brain injury and disorders. *Sub-cellular biochemistry*, *49*, 241-268.

Ahima, R. S., Bjorbaek, C., Osei, S. & Flier, J. S. (1999). Regulation of neuronal and glial proteins by leptin: implications for brain development. *Endocrinology*, *140*, 2755-2762.

Arble, D. M. & Sandoval, D. A. (2013). CNS control of glucose metabolism: response to environmental challenges. *Frontiers in neuroscience*, *7*, 20.

Banks, W. A., Coon, A. B., Robinson, S. M., Moinuddin, A., Shultz, J. M., Nakaoke, R. & Morley, J. E. (2004). Triglycerides induce leptin resistance at the blood-brain barrier. *Diabetes*, *53*, 1253-1260.

Banks, W. A. & Farrell, C. L. (2003). Impaired transport of leptin across the blood-brain barrier in obesity is acquired and reversible. *American journal of physiology Endocrinology and metabolism*, *285*, E10-15.

Bluher, M. (2005). Transgenic animal models for the study of adipose tissue biology. *Best practice & research Clinical endocrinology & metabolism*, *19*, 605-623.

Blundell, J. E., Levin, F., King, N. A., Barkeling, B., Gustafsson, T., Hellstrom, P. M., Holst, J. J. & Naslund, E. (2008). Overconsumption and obesity: peptides and susceptibility to weight gain. *Regulatory peptides*, *149*, 32-38.

Bruce-Keller, A. J., Keller, J. N. & Morrison, C. D. (2009). Obesity and vulnerability of the CNS. *Biochimica et biophysica acta*, *1792*, 395-400.

Burke, J. E. & Dennis, E. A. (2009). Phospholipase A2 structure/function, mechanism, and signaling. *Journal of lipid research*, *50*, Suppl, S237-242.

Capuron, L. & Miller, A. H. (2011). Immune system to brain signaling: neuropsychopharmacological implications. *Pharmacology & therapeutics*, *130*, 226-238.

Cojocaru, M., Cojocaru, I. M., Silosi, I. & Rogoz, S. (2013). Role of leptin in autoimmune diseases. *Maedica*, *8*, 68-74.

Chen, J., Zhang, X., Kusumo, H., Costa, L. G. & Guizzetti, M. (2013). Cholesterol efflux is differentially regulated in neurons and astrocytes: implications for brain cholesterol homeostasis. *Biochimica et biophysica acta*, *1831*, 263-275.

Dieguez, C., Vazquez, M. J., Romero, A., Lopez, M. & Nogueiras, R. (2011). Hypothalamic control of lipid metabolism: focus on leptin, ghrelin and melanocortins. *Neuroendocrinology*, *94*, 1-11.

Dietschy, J. M. (2009). Central nervous system: cholesterol turnover, brain development and neurodegeneration. *Biological chemistry*, *390*, 287-293.

Elliott, D. A., Weickert, C. S. & Garner, B. (2010). Apolipoproteins in the brain: implications for neurological and psychiatric disorders. *Clinical lipidology*, *51*, 555-573.

Emanuela, F., Grazia, M., Marco, de R., Maria, Paola, L., Giorgio, F., & Marco, B. (2012). Inflammation as a Link between Obesity and Metabolic Syndrome. *Journal of nutrition and metabolism*, *2012*, 476380.

Faulconbridge, L. F. & Hayes, M. R. (2011). Regulation of energy balance and body weight by the brain: a distributed system prone to disruption. *The Psychiatric clinics of North America*, *34*, 733-745.

Fernandez-Riejos, P., Najib, S., Santos-Alvarez, J., Martin-Romero, C., Perez-Perez, A., Gonzalez-Yanes, C. & Sanchez-Margalet, V. (2010). Role of leptin in the activation of immune cells. *Mediators of inflammation, 2010*, 568343.

Gao, Q. & Horvath, T. L. (2007). Neurobiology of feeding and energy expenditure. *Annual review of neuroscience*, *30*, 367-398.

Garcia-Caceres, C., Fuente-Martin, E., Argente, J. & Chowen, J. A. (2012). Emerging role of glial cells in the control of body weight. *Molecular metabolism*, *1*, 37-46.

Green, J. T., Orr, S. K. & Bazinet, R. P. (2008). The emerging role of group VI calcium-independent phospholipase A2 in releasing docosahexaenoic acid from brain phospholipids. *Journal of lipid research*, *49*, 939-944.

Haeusgen, W., Boehm, R., Zhao, Y., Herdegen, T. & Waetzig, V. (2009). Specific activities of individual c-Jun N-terminal kinases in the brain. *Neuroscience*, *161*, 951-959.

Han, M. S., Jung, D. Y., Morel, C., Lakhani, S. A., Kim, J. K., Flavell, R. A. & Davis, R. J. (2013). JNK expression by macrophages promotes obesity-induced insulin resistance and inflammation. *Science*, *339*, 218-222.

Harvey, J. (2013). Leptin regulation of neuronal morphology and hippocampal synaptic function. *Frontiers in synaptic neuroscience*, *5*, 3.

Hayashi, H. (2011). Lipid metabolism and glial lipoproteins in the central nervous system. *Biological & pharmaceutical bulletin*, *34*, 453-461.

Hsuchou, H., Kastin, A. J., Mishra, P. K. & Pan, W. (2012). C-reactive protein increases BBB permeability: implications for obesity and neuroinflammation. *Cellular physiology and biochemistry: international journal of experimental cellular physiology, biochemistry, and pharmacology*, *30*, 1109-1119.

Hsuchou, H., Kastin, A. J., Tu, H., Joan Abbott, N., Couraud, P. O. & Pan, W. (2010). Role of astrocytic leptin receptor subtypes on leptin permeation across hCMEC/D3 human brain endothelial cells. *Journal of neurochemistry*, *115*, 1288-1298.

Jordan, S. D., Konner, A. C. & Bruning, J. C. (2010). Sensing the fuels: glucose and lipid signaling in the CNS controlling energy homeostasis. *Cellular and molecular life sciences: CMLS*, *67*, 3255-3273.

Kadowaki, T., Yamauchi, T., Kubota, N., Hara, K., Ueki, K. & Tobe, K. (2006). Adiponectin and adiponectin receptors in insulin resistance, diabetes, and the metabolic syndrome. *The Journal of clinical investigation*, *116*, 1784-1792.

Kastin, A. J. & Akerstrom, V. (2000). Fasting, but not adrenalectomy, reduces transport of leptin into the brain. *Peptides*, *21*, 679-682.

Kastin, A. J. & Akerstrom, V. (2001). Glucose and insulin increase the transport of leptin through the blood-brain barrier in normal mice but not in streptozotocin-diabetic mice. *Neuroendocrinology*, *73*, 237-242.

Kielian, T. (2006). Toll-like receptors in central nervous system glial inflammation and homeostasis. *Journal of neuroscience research*, *83*, 711-730.

Konner, A. C., Klockener, T. & Bruning, J. C. (2009). Control of energy homeostasis by insulin and leptin: targeting the arcuate nucleus and beyond. *Physiology & behavior*, *97*, 632-638.

Kunz, M., Ibrahim, S., Koczan, D., Thiesen, H. J., Kohler, H. J., Acker, T., Plate, K. H., Ludwig, S., Rapp, U. R., Brocker, E. B., van Muijen, G. N., Flory, E. & Gross, G. (2001). Activation of c-Jun NH2-terminal kinase/stress-activated protein kinase (JNK/SAPK). is critical for hypoxia-induced apoptosis of human malignant melanoma. *Cell growth & differentiation: the molecular biology journal of the American Association for Cancer Research*, *12*, 137-145.

Laflamme, N. & Rivest, S. (2001). Toll-like receptor 4: the missing link of the cerebral innate immune response triggered by circulating gram-negative bacterial cell wall components. *FASEB journal: official publication of the Federation of American Societies for Experimental Biology*, *15*, 155-163.

Lowther, C. P., MacLeod, R. D. & Williamson, J. (1970). Evaluation of early diagnostic services for the elderly. *British medical journal*, *3*, 275-277.

Lucas, S. M., Rothwell, N. J. & Gibson, R. M. (2006). The role of inflammation in CNS injury and disease. *British journal of pharmacology*, *147* Suppl 1, S232-240.

Mainardi, M., Pizzorusso, T. & Maffei, M. (2013). Environment, leptin sensitivity, and hypothalamic plasticity. *Neural plasticity*, *2013*, 438072.

Matsuzaki, K. (2010). [Ganglioside cluster-mediated aggregation and cytotoxicity of amyloid beta-peptide: molecular mechanism and inhibition]. *Yakugaku zasshi: Journal of the Pharmaceutical Society of Japan*, *130*, 511-515.

Morris, D. L. & Rui, L. (2009). Recent advances in understanding leptin signaling and leptin resistance. *American journal of physiology Endocrinology and metabolism*, *297*, E1247-1259.

Morton, G. J., Cummings, D. E., Baskin, D. G., Barsh, G. S. & Schwartz, M. W. (2006). Central nervous system control of food intake and body weight. *Nature*, *443*, 289-295.

Nakazato, M., Murakami, N., Date, Y., Kojima, M., Matsuo, H., Kangawa, K. & Matsukura, S. (2001). A role for ghrelin in the central regulation of feeding. *Nature*, *409*, 194-198.

Nishimura, S., Manabe, I. & Nagai, R. (2009). Adipose tissue inflammation in obesity and metabolic syndrome. *Discovery medicine*, *8*, 55-60.

Olufadi, R. & Byrne, C. D. (2008). Clinical and laboratory diagnosis of the metabolic syndrome. *Journal of clinical pathology*, *61*, 697-706.

Orth, M. & Bellosta, S. (2012). Cholesterol: its regulation and role in central nervous system disorders. *Cholesterol*, *2012*, 292598.

Pan, W., Barron, M., Hsuchou, H., Tu, H. & Kastin, A. J. (2008a). Increased leptin permeation across the blood-brain barrier after chronic alcohol ingestion. *Neuropsychopharmacology: official publication of the American College of Neuropsychopharmacology*, *33*, 859-866.

Pan, W., Hsuchou, H., He, Y., Sakharkar, A., Cain, C., Yu, C. & Kastin, A. J. (2008b). Astrocyte leptin receptor (ObR). and leptin transport in adult-onset obese mice. *Endocrinology*, *149*, 2798-2806.

Pan, W., Hsuchou, H., Jayaram, B., Khan, R. S., Huang, E. Y., Wu, X., Chen, C. & Kastin, A. J. (2012). Leptin action on nonneuronal cells in the CNS: potential clinical applications. *Annals of the New York Academy of Sciences*, *1264*, 64-71.

Pang, Z. P. & Han, W. (2012). Regulation of synaptic functions in central nervous system by endocrine hormones and the maintenance of energy homoeostasis. *Bioscience reports*, *32*, 423-432.

Patel, P. S., Buras, E. D. & Balasubramanyam, A. (2013). The role of the immune system in obesity and insulin resistance. *Journal of obesity*, *2013*, 616193.

Pfrieger, F. W. & Ungerer, N. (2011). Cholesterol metabolism in neurons and astrocytes. *Progress in lipid research*, *50*, 357-371.

Rebeck, G. W., LaDu, M. J., Estus, S., Bu, G. & Weeber, E. J. (2006). The generation and function of soluble apoE receptors in the CNS. *Molecular neurodegeneration*, *1*, 15.

Sahu, A. (2003). Leptin signaling in the hypothalamus: emphasis on energy homeostasis and leptin resistance. *Frontiers in neuroendocrinology*, *24*, 225-253.

Sanchez-Lasheras, C., Konner, A. C. & Bruning, J. C. (2010). Integrative neurobiology of energy homeostasis-neurocircuits, signals and mediators. *Frontiers in neuroendocrinology*, *31*, 4-15.

Segatto, M., Trapani, L., Lecis, C. & Pallottini, V. (2012). Regulation of cholesterol biosynthetic pathway in different regions of the rat central nervous system. *Acta Physiol (Oxf).*, *206*, 62-71.

Shechter, R., London, A., Kuperman, Y., Ronen, A., Rolls, A., Chen, A. & Schwartz, M. (2013). Hypothalamic neuronal toll-like receptor 2 protects against age-induced obesity. *Scientific reports*, *3*, 1254.

Streit, W. J., Mrak, R. E. & Griffin, W. S. (2004). Microglia and neuroinflammation: a pathological perspective. *Journal of neuroinflammation*, *1*, 14.

Suzuki, K., Jayasena, C. N. & Bloom, S. R. (2012). Obesity and appetite control. *Experimental diabetes research*, *2012*, 824305.

Taha, A. Y., Gao, F., Ramadan, E., Cheon, Y., Rapoport, S. I. & Kim, H. W. (2012). Upregulated expression of brain enzymatic markers of arachidonic and docosahexaenoic acid metabolism in a rat model of the metabolic syndrome. *BMC neuroscience*, *13*, 131.

Tahergorabi, Z. & Khazaei, M. (2013). The relationship between inflammatory markers, angiogenesis, and obesity. *ARYA atherosclerosis*, *9*, 247-253.

Tartaglia, L. A., Dembski, M., Weng, X., Deng, N., Culpepper, J., Devos, R., Richards, G. J., Campfield, L. A., Clark, F. T., Deeds, J., Muir, C., Sanker, S., Moriarty, A., Moore, K. J., Smutko, J. S., Mays, G. G., Wool, E. A., Monroe, C. A. & Tepper, R. I. (1995). Identification and expression cloning of a leptin receptor, OB-R. *Cell*, *83*, 1263-1271.

Thaler, J. P., Choi, S. J., Schwartz, M. W. & Wisse, B. E. (2010). Hypothalamic inflammation and energy homeostasis: resolving the paradox. *Frontiers in neuroendocrinology*, *31*, 79-84.

Uauy, R., Hoffman, D. R., Peirano, P., Birch, D. G. & Birch, E. E. (2001). Essential fatty acids in visual and brain development. *Lipids*, *36*, 885-895.

Veloso, A., Fernandez, R., Astigarraga, E., Barreda-Gomez, G., Manuel, I., Giralt, MT., Ferrer, I., Ochoa, B., Rodriguez-Puertas, R. & Fernandez, J. A. (2011). Distribution of lipids in human brain. *Analytical and bioanalytical chemistry*, *401*, 89-101.

Velloso, L. A. & Schwartz, M. W. (2011). Altered hypothalamic function in diet-induced obesity. *Int J Obes (Lond).*, *35*, 1455-1465.

Vickers, M. H. & Sloboda, D. M. (2012). Leptin as mediator of the effects of developmental programming. Best practice & research *Clinical endocrinology & metabolism*, *26*, 677-687.

Wang, X., Ge, A., Cheng, M., Guo, F., Zhao, M., Zhou, X., Liu, L. & Yang, N. (2012). Increased hypothalamic inflammation associated with the susceptibility to obesity in rats exposed to high-fat diet. *Experimental diabetes research*, *2012*, 847246.

Williams, K. W., Scott, M. M. & Elmquist, J. K. (2009). From observation to experimentation: leptin action in the mediobasal hypothalamus. *The American journal of clinical nutrition*, *89*, 985S-990S.

Woods, A. G., Sokolowska, I., Taurines, R., Gerlach, M., Dudley, E., Thome, J. & Darie, C. C. (2012). Potential biomarkers in psychiatry: focus on the cholesterol system. *Journal of cellular and molecular medicine*, *16*, 1184-1195.

Woods, S. C., Lotter, E. C., McKay, L. D. & Porte, D. Jr. (1979). Chronic intracerebroventricular infusion of insulin reduces food intake and body weight of baboons. *Nature*, *282*, 503-505.

Ye, J., Gao, Z., Yin, J. & He, Q. (2007). Hypoxia is a potential risk factor for chronic inflammation and adiponectin reduction in adipose tissue of ob/ob and dietary obese mice. *American journal of physiology Endocrinology and metabolism*, *293*, E1118-1128.

Yu, J. H. & Kim, M. S. (2012). Molecular mechanisms of appetite regulation. *Diabetes & metabolism journal*, *36*, 391-398.

In: Neuro-Immune Interactions ...
Editor: Oscar González-Pérez
ISBN: 978-1-62948-646-8

Chapter 8

THE ROLE OF GLIA IN STRESS-GLUCOCORTICOID EFFECTS IN THE BRAIN

Fernando Jauregui-Huerta[1], Aidee Uribe Gonzalez[1], Joaquin Garcia-Estrada[2], Yaveth Ruvalcaba-Delgadillo[1], Rodrigo Ramos-Zuñiga[1], Alfredo Feria-Velasco[3] and Sonia Luquin[1]

[1]Departamento de Neurociencias. Centro Universitario de ciencias de la Salud. Universidad de Guadalajara, México

[2]Laboratorio de Neuroendocrinología celular, Centro de Investigación Biomédica de Occidente CIBO, IMSS. Guadalajara, México

[3]Laboratorio de Neurobiología Celular. Centro Universitario de Ciencias Biológico Agropecuarias. Universidad de Guadalajara, México

ABSTRACT

Stress hormones are strong modulators of brain activity. Given the adaptive nature of stress, hormones released during stress response influence a myriad of brain phenomena including development, plasticity, neurogenesis, homeostasis, central immune response and cognition. In addition to the well-known role of neurons in the stress-brain interaction, glial cells have recently become crucial for the knowledge of this topic. Glial cells are viewed now as important as neurons for the normal function of the brain. There is a growing body of knowledge showing that glial cells crucially affect brain development, homeostasis, synaptic activity, immunity and cognition. It is now unthinkable the hormone-brain interaction without glia. The confluent actions of both, stress hormones and glial cells in brain adaptive capability, make allowed us to explore the otherwise underestimated relationship between stress, hormones and glial cells. This chapter summarizes what is known about stress hormones, its main effects on brain, and the mediating role of glial cells. We choose the central immune response and the homeostatic support as the main scenario where this interaction occurs.

INTRODUCTION

Stress response includes a myriad of changes aiming to return the stability of the internal milieu once it becomes compromised. The hypothalamic corticotropin-releasing hormone (CRH) and the locus coeruleus noradrenaline (LC-NA) orchestrate those adaptive responses by regulating the hypothalamic-pituitary-adrenal (HPA) axis and adrenomedullary sympathetic nervous system, respectively. Individual homeostasis is ensured through the action of glucocorticoids (GCs) -the end product of HPA axis- and catecholamines (CAs) -the main effectors of sympathetic nervous system- (de Kloet, 2003). Catecholamines conduce the initial response to threats provoking rapid and short-lived physiological changes through neural innervation of peripheral organs like heart and blood vessels (Fisher & Brown, 1991). These spatial and time limited actions of CAs contrasts with the more delayed and extended pathways through GCs exert their actions. The highly lipophilic nature of GCs confers them the ability to access brain targets and exert enduring actions on central and peripheral cells. GCs regulate metabolism, influence immune/inflammatory processes, affects blood pressure and regulate cell growth. They modulate the activity of about 10% of our genes (Buckingham, 2006). For this reason, cortisol/corticosterone (the main GC hormones) has received the most attention referring to the stress effects on brain.

Actions of GC on brain are restricted (but not reduced) by the expression of two known corticosteroid receptors: the mineralocorticoid receptor (MR) and the glucocorticoid receptor (GR). They are intracellular receptors capable to regulate the transcription of target genes (De Kloet, Vreugdenhil, Oitzl, & Joels, 1998). Differential actions are promoted depending on the union of GC to MR, GR or both. Such phenomenon is possible because of the differing affinity of these receptors. The MR has high affinity for GCs (about 0.5-2nM). In brain, the distribution of MRs is restricted to the hippocampus, septum, amygdala, locus coeruleus, entorhinal cortex and, in lesser amount, to the hypothalamus. MRs are active when circulating levels of GCs are low, so, they regulate the basal tone of the HPA axis. GRs in the other hand have about 10 fold lower affinity for GCs (10-20nM). They are highly active during periods of abundant secretion of GCs as occurs on circadian peak or stressing conditions. GRs are highly expressed in the limbic system and hypothalamic and pituitary cells that exert negative feedback on the HPA axis. GRs are involved in energy metabolism, cellular homeostasis, restriction of stress-induced responses, behavioral adaptation and information storage (de Kloet, 2003; de Kloet, Oitzl, & Joels, 1999; Lopez, Akil, & Watson, 1999; Lupien, et al., 2005; Maschke, Rupp, & Hecht, 2000; Ozawa, 2005). Figure 1 Illustrates HPA axis function and the main GR-MR mechanisms.

The effects of stress hormones on brain have been widely investigated. It is now known that steroid hormones associated to stress responses may produce both, deleterious and beneficial effects on brain function. If so, early studies focused on deleterious effects of glucocorticoid deregulation on hippocampus and other brain regions, there are now a number of studies reporting adaptive actions of these hormones on cognition, development, central immune response, plasticity and other brain functions (McEwen, 2006).

Regarding damaging stress effects on brain, evidence has accumulated. It has been reported suppressive effects of GCs on neurogenesis (Gonzalez-Perez, et al., 2011; Gould & Tanapat, 1999; Jauregui-Huerta, et al., 2011), atrophic effects on dendrites (Magarinos & McEwen, 1995), compromising actions on cell survival (Joels, et al., 2004; Ramos-Remus, Gonzalez-Castaneda, Gonzalez-Perez, Luquin, & Garcia-Estrada, 2002), deregulation in neurotransmitter systems (J. J. Kim & Diamond, 2002; Zschocke, et al., 2005), imbalances in pathways related to cell adhesion molecules and neurotrophic factors (Sandi, et al., 2005), impairing effects on memory (Jauregui-Huerta, Ruvalcaba-Delgadillo, Garcia-Estrada, et al., 2010; Sandi & Pinelo-Nava, 2007; Sandi, et al., 2005) and so on. Stress has also been proposed as a main factor in the origin or progression of pathologies like depression, anxiety, schizophrenia, drug abuse, dementia and sleep disturbances (Korte, Koolhaas, Wingfield, & McEwen, 2005; McEwen, 2006; Pacak & Palkovits, 2001; Rabat, et al., 2004).

Moreover, structural changes have been reported in brain areas involved in the regulation of HPA system, cognition, emotion and motivation of subjects exposed to severe stress conditions. It has been consistently reported smaller hippocampal or temporal lobe volumes in chronically stressed subjects (Gianaros, et al., 2007).

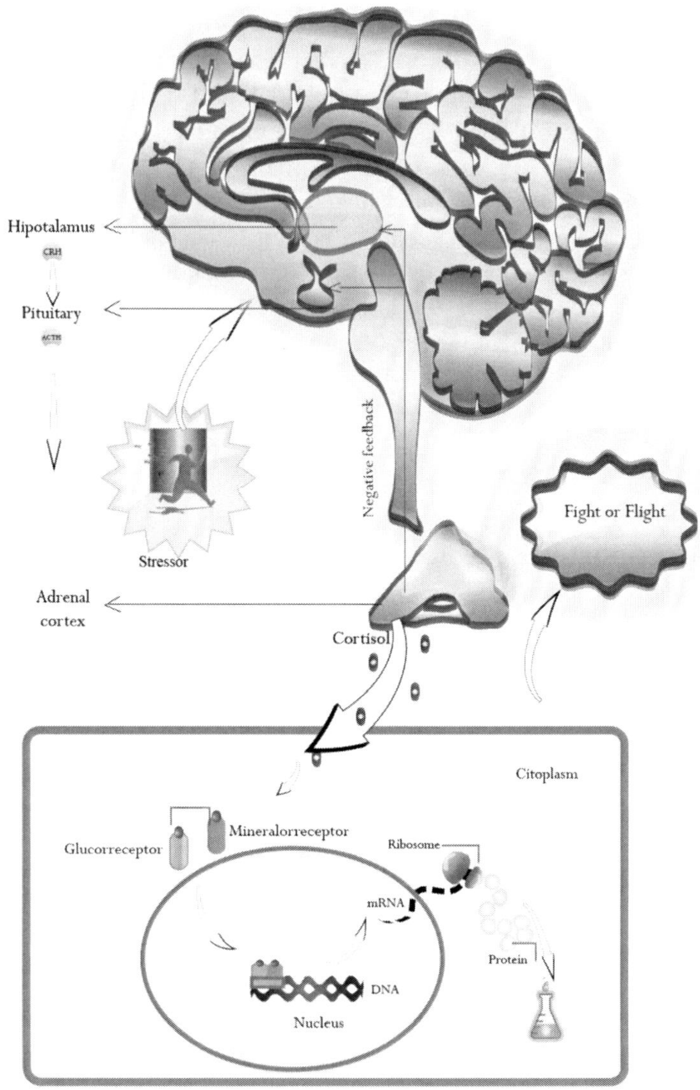

Figure 1. Stress-HPA System. When the brain perceives stress, the hypothalamus releases corticotropin-releasing factor (CRF), which triggers the release of adrenocorticotropic (ACTH) from the pituitary gland. ACTH travels through the bloodstream and stimulates the adrenal glands to release glucocorticoids (i.e., cortisol) (GCs). MR-GR receptors reside predominantly in the cytoplasm. Upon hormone binding, they are translocated into the nucleus where they act as regulators of gene transcription. Within the nucleus, these ligand-activated receptors interact with other transcription factors or bind to specific DNA response elements resulting in the up- or downregulation of the expression of numerous genes.

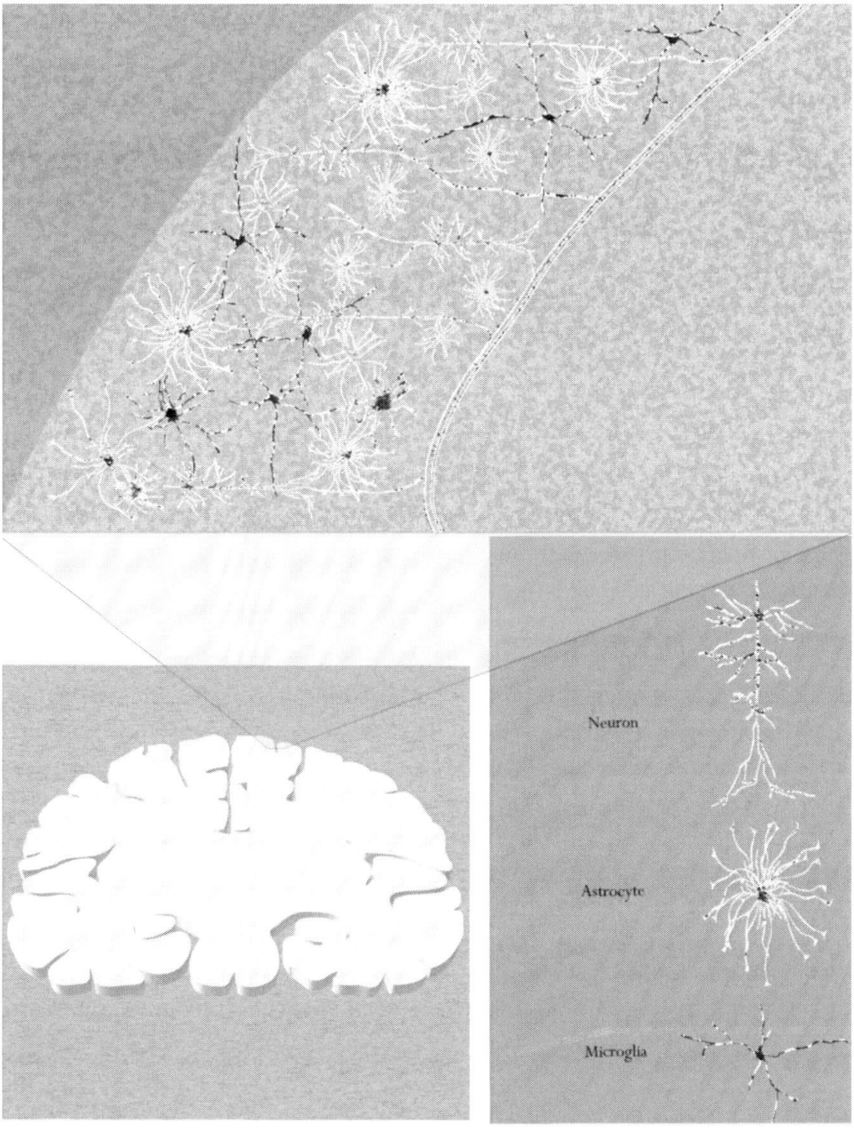

Figure 2. Glial cells. The Central Nervous System consists of neurons and glial cells. Glial cells include microglia, astrocytes and oligodendrocytes (not shown).

The amygdala and the prefrontal cortex are also targets of chronic stress. Studies demonstrating hippocampal shrinkage have also demonstrated amygdala hypertrophy and loss of dendritic spines in prefrontal cortex (McLaughlin, Gomez, Baran, & Conrad, 2007; Vyas, Mitra, Shankaranarayana

Rao, & Chattarji, 2002). Controversy exists however on whether these changes are caused by inhibition of neurogenesis, dendritic shrinkage or other mechanisms (Banasr, et al., 2008; Elder, De Gasperi, & Gama Sosa, 2006; Jauregui-Huerta, Ruvalcaba-Delgadillo, Gonzalez-Castaneda, et al., 2010). Thus far, the consistent finding of glial cell changes into the altered hippocampal and/or prefrontal cortex of stressed subjects placed these extraordinary cells in the eye of stress specialists.

Glial cells include in fact two heterogeneous groups of cells living in the Nervous System: Microglia and Macroglia. Figure 2 illustrates these major cell types.

Microglia encompasses a group of cells that phenotypically and functionally resembles macrophages. Microglia originates from mesodermal macrophages that invade the Nervous System during early development (Napoli & Neumann, 2009). Traditionally they have been exclusively viewed as the immune cells of the brain which best characterized function was the cleaning of cell debris through phagocytosis mechanisms. It has been in recent years however that new discoveries noted that microglial cells supports brain functions not only as surveyors, but also as active modulators of neuronal circuits, cognition and neurogenesis (Ekdahl, 2012; Marin & Kipnis, 2013). Microglial cells posses receptors for neurotransmitters, neuropeptides, hormones, immune signals and growing factors that allows them to scan the brain microenvironment and detect at early stages any disturbing condition (Rivest, 2009). When they detect damage, they become "activated" changing their phenotype, altering their morphology and changing its proliferative pattern to prevent or restore homeostasis in the brain (Hanisch & Kettenmann, 2007; Kreutzberg, 1996; Napoli & Neumann, 2009).

Macroglia represents the most large and diffused cell type in the Nervous System. Unlike microglia, macroglia share its ectodermal origin with nerve cells. This group includes ependymal cells, Schwann-oligodendroglial cells and astroglial cells.

Ependymal cells comprise the "simple ciliated epithelium that lines the ventricular surface of the central nervous system, extending from the lateral ventricles to the filum terminale" (Del Bigio, 2010). Such specialized epithelium is mostly known for its structural role lining the cavities of the nervous system and forming the walls of the ventricles. There is now evidence supporting its role in neurogenesis where they are proposed as crucial trophic and metabolic supporters. They may also be important regulators of water fluxes at the ventricle wall and, its cilia has been postulated a leading helper in neuroblast migration from the lateral ventricle to the olfactory bulb (Sawamoto, et al., 2006).

Oligodendroglial and Schwann cells are mostly known for their role forming the myelin sheath that covers the axon to facilitate nerve conduction in the central and peripheral nervous system respectively. Recent evidence supports a more proactive role of this cells affecting essential brain functions like neuronal transmission, metabolic support, structural integrity, immune response and neural regeneration after damage (Lee, et al., 2012; Peferoen, Kipp, van der Valk, van Noort, & Amor, 2013). It is worth to mention at this point the so called NG2-glia discovered 20 years ago as oligodendrocyte precursor cells (Raff, Miller, & Noble, 1983). They represent for itself the fourth major type of glia and nowadays the only progenitor cell outside of the known mammalian brain niches of neurogenesis. If so, NG2-glia offers more questions than answers and its main function remains to be their oligodendrocyte precursor role, the suggestion exists for their participation in functions like myelination and neural circuits plasticity (Dimou & Gotz, 2012; Etxeberria, Mangin, Aguirre, & Gallo, 2010).

Astroglial cells are the main type of glia in the mammalian brain and include all those cells who do not belong to the lineage of neurons, oligodendrocytes/NG2 or microglia (Parpura & Verkhratsky, 2012). In the past, these cells were defined for their supporting role for neurons, their star-like morphology and the expression of the glial fibrillar acidic protein (GFAP). Nevertheless, we know now that astrocytes include a very versatile group of cells that not necessarily express GFAP or star-like form. The best known function of astroglia remains joined to their homeostatic proficiency although a number of functions were recently added including regulation of the central immune response, modulation of neuroendocrine functions, regulation of synaptogenesis, neurogenesis and gliogenesis, guidance in neuronal migration and regulation of synaptic activity (Araque, Parpura, Sanzgiri, & Haydon, 1999; Caudle, 2006; Fields & Stevens-Graham, 2002; Garcia-Segura & McCarthy, 2004; Parpura & Verkhratsky, 2012).

From data presented in preceding paragraphs, it is easy to note that both, stress hormones and glial cells are key modulators of some of the most important brain functions. Both of them are also common actors in the physiopathology of some of the most prevalent diseases of the brain. Therefore, it is reasonable to suppose that glial cells and stress hormones may interact in different ways to face brain demands. We are coping then with two of the most powerful tools to secure the otherwise principal function of the brain: adaptation. We review in the next section two main facts proposed to sustain this interaction.

The Central Immune Response Interplay

The Central Nervous System (CNS) is an immune "specialized" organ characterized by an anti-inflammatory microenvironment lacking of lymphatic tissue and antigen presenting cells. The CNS remains "separated" from the rest of the body by a complex system named blood-brain-barrier (BBB) which in turn is formed by endothelial cells, astrocytes, pericytes, perivascular macrophages and basal lamina (Daneman, 2012). As pointed above, immune actions in brain are mostly conducted by microglia, astrocytes and in a lesser extent by oligodendrocytes and neurons (Peferoen, et al., 2013). Immune activity in the CNS is mainly directed to protect the nervous system from damage caused by inflammation. As occurs in the rest of the body, whether immune actions are beneficial or detrimental for the nervous system depends on the magnitude and degree of regulation of these responses. Whereas in one hand for example the immune mediators contribute crucially to the perfect early shaping of the brain, it is known in the other hand that the loss of regulation of the immune response is also a crucial step in neurodegeneration (Amor & Woodroofe, 2013). Glial cells are central players in the context of regulation of the immune response versus damage. They change their behavior once the CNS is threatened. The first cells that become activated and migrate to the lesioned site are microglial cells. They initiate much of the following glial reaction. NG2 cells react also in early stages increasing their proliferation. Astrocytes react latter in a complex manner that includes morphological, functional and gene expression pattern changes. These actions are also known as *gliosis* (Robel, Berninger, & Gotz, 2011).

Regarding stress, it has been deeply discussed whether stress hormones exert pro or anti-inflammatory actions on brain (Cutolo, Buttgereit, & Straub, 2011; Sorrells & Sapolsky, 2007). It may be expected that actions of stress hormones on brain follows either the classical anti-inflammatory behavior, or the newest rule described for peripheral organs where basal or low stress hormone levels stimulate immune responses and higher levels suppress immune actions (Munck, Guyre, & Holbrook, 1984). As discussed by Sorrells and Sapolsky, in CNS coexist both anti-inflammatory and pro-inflammatory responses under stress. The direction of this response may depend in opinion of the referred authors on factors like the brain region in question, the use of synthetic versus endogenous GCs or the timing of hormone exposure versus inflammatory challenge (Sorrells & Sapolsky, 2007). We would like to add the cell type on this scenario highlighting the obvious role of glial cells.

Microglia, the primary immune effector cell in brain represents a key element for understanding how stress hormones may affect the CNS. Studies aiming to elucidate microglial responses to stress hormones have revealed multiple and sometimes opposing results (Carrillo-de Sauvage, et al., 2013). Consistent with the immunosuppressive rule, early in vitro studies demonstrated that treatment of microglial cells with GCs might produce strong suppressing actions by decreasing its proliferative rate (Woods, Poulsen, & Gall, 1999), affecting negatively its pro-inflammatory cytokine production, and decreasing its production of free radicals (Drew & Chavis, 2000; Huo, Rangarajan, Ling, & Dheen, 2011; Sierra, Gottfried-Blackmore, Milner, McEwen, & Bulloch, 2008; Tanaka, et al., 1997). These anti-inflammatory actions have been confirmed in vivo by treating spinal cord damaged subjects with the synthetic GC methilprednisolone (Schroter, Lustenberger, Obermair, & Thallmair, 2009). In the other hand, we may also found enhancing effects of GCs over microglia. A detailed review of published data shows that not only the treatment of experimental animals with exogenous GCs but also the exposure to diverse stress models produce pro-inflammatory actions in microglia ranging from morphological activation to enhanced interleukin expression or increased proliferation (Frank, Baratta, Sprunger, Watkins, & Maier, 2007; Minami, et al., 1991; Nair & Bonneau, 2006; Pugh, et al., 1999; Sugama, 2009; Sugama, Fujita, Hashimoto, & Conti, 2007). Even when the direction of the response is still confuse, it is clear now that microglia respond to stress hormones. Such undeniable fact has been addressed for contemporary authors to propose that these hormone-induced microglial activation and the following microglial actions may conduce to maladaptive neuronal networks and consequently contribute to the etiology of some neuropsychiatric disorders (Kato, Hayakawa, Monji, & Kanba, 2013). In this line of evidence, the most widely affecting neuropsychiatric disorder and also stress-related disorder namely depression, has been proposed as an inflammatory illness where microglial deregulation has consistently be found (Frick, Williams, & Pittenger, 2013).

Inflammatory actions of microglia have also gained some status in the understanding of addictive disorders where GCs and stress has been hypothesized to exert sensitizing actions on microglia who maximize inflammatory responses when the CNS is challenged with drugs of abuse (Frank, Watkins, & Maier, 2011).

Astrocytes are also important regulators of immune activity through mediators that include cytokines, chemokines and neurotrophic factors. As pointed above, they react after microglia amplifying the local, initial innate response and modifying the BBB permeability to attract peripheral adaptive immune cells into the brain. Activated astrocytes exhibit some morphological and gene expression changes namely astrogliosis. Astrogliosis may occur not only in inflammatory conditions but also in neurodegenerative or trauma situations. A hallmark of reactive astrocytes is its hypertrophic aspect mostly associated to the glial fibrillary acidic protein (GFAP). This protein is the main intermediate filament component and its changes have been associated to a number of brain pathologies. There are obviously a number of studies trying to elucidate the GFAP response to the otherwise expected anti-inflammatory actions of stress hormones. Accounting for this, it has been reported that the chronic treatment with corticosterone down-regulates GFAP by decreasing mRNA content in the rat brain (Bridges, Slais, & Sykova, 2008; O'Callaghan, Brinton, & McEwen, 1991). This down-regulation of the astrocytic activity may even last in the long term as seen in various limbic regions of adult rats exposed to an early-life chronic stress model (Leventopoulos, et al., 2007). In counterpart, there is also evidence showing that chronic corticosterone or chronic stress actually may up-regulate GFAP in dose and subregion-dependent fashion (Bridges, et al., 2008; Ramos-Remus, et al., 2002). As occurs with microglia, astrocytes are also implicated in the pathogenesis of depression. The use of GFAP as immunohistochemical marker for these cells showed a significant reduction in the number of GFAP+ cells of depressed patients (Muller, et al., 2001). In this line of evidence, postmortem studies of subjects with a history of high-dose steroid treatment have also demonstrated a significant reduction in the number of astrocytes (Rajkowska, 2003; Rajkowska & Miguel-Hidalgo, 2007) suggesting that such phenomena may involve both glia and GCs in the course of depression. Beyond GFAP, anti-inflammatory-like actions of stress and/or its hormones over astrocytes have been also demonstrated experimentally by depleting brain gliogenesis after stress or dexamethasone exposure (Czeh, et al., 2007; Gonzalez-Perez, et al., 2011; Sabolek, Herborg, Schwarz, & Storch, 2006).

Oligodendrocytes have been longer considered immunologically inert cells which role in immune response remained as the victim of some aberrant responses. The recent uncover of a number of receptors for immune-regulatory factors and the complementary fact that oligodendrocytes produce indeed those factors have placed oligodendroglia as a new intriguing immunocompetent cell (Peferoen, et al., 2013). If so, literature regarding direct effects of GCs on oligodendroglia is scarce, the few existing reports points to a marked immunosuppressive action of these hormones on this cell type. From a therapeutic point of view, it is largely known that one major application of GCs is the treatment of Multiple Sclerosis, the most prevalent autoimmune disease of the CNS which hallmark is demyelination and axonal loss. Although immunosuppressive actions of GCs in multiple sclerosis have been mainly associated to their ability to induce apoptosis in infiltrating immune cells (mostly T cells), to reduce inflammatory actions of microglia an to regulate the BBB (Reichardt, Gold, & Luhder, 2006), it is likely to expect direct actions on oligodendroglia. In this line of evidences, it has been reported that GCs may affect oligodendrocytes by suppressing the proliferation rate of the NG2 progenitor cells (Alonso, 2000). Additional reports established that they also regulate key oligodendroglial proteins such as glycerol phosphate dehydrogenase (GPDH), myelin basic protein (MBP) and proteolipid protein (PLP) (Kumar, Cole, Chiappelli, & de Vellis, 1989). Such suppressive actions have recently been proposed as a potential cause for the oligodendrocyte alterations seen in depression and other stress related pathologies (Edgar & Sibille, 2012).

THE METABOLIC SUPPORT INTERPLAY

As stated before, both, glial cells and stress hormones are crucially involved in brain metabolism. Glial cells provide metabolic support for neurons. Supporting actions of glial cells include provision of energy substrates, regulation of cerebral extracellular ion concentrations, driving of water homeostasis, control of the brain microcirculation and regulation of synaptic processes (neurotransmitter systems, synaptogenesis, synaptic pruning and synaptic networks). Through these actions, glial cells play an important role in the regulation of behavior, mood and cognition.

In the other part of the equation, glucocorticoids are mostly known for their metabolic actions. In fact, they were named like this attending their role in the regulation of the metabolism of glucose. As main stress effectors, they are responsible of many of the adaptive actions conducted for the brain during threatening conditions.

Therefore, they modulate not only energy metabolism but also other essential brain functions including synaptic transmission, neurogenesis or development. By affecting these physiological processes, they are also potent modulators of mood, cognition and behavior.

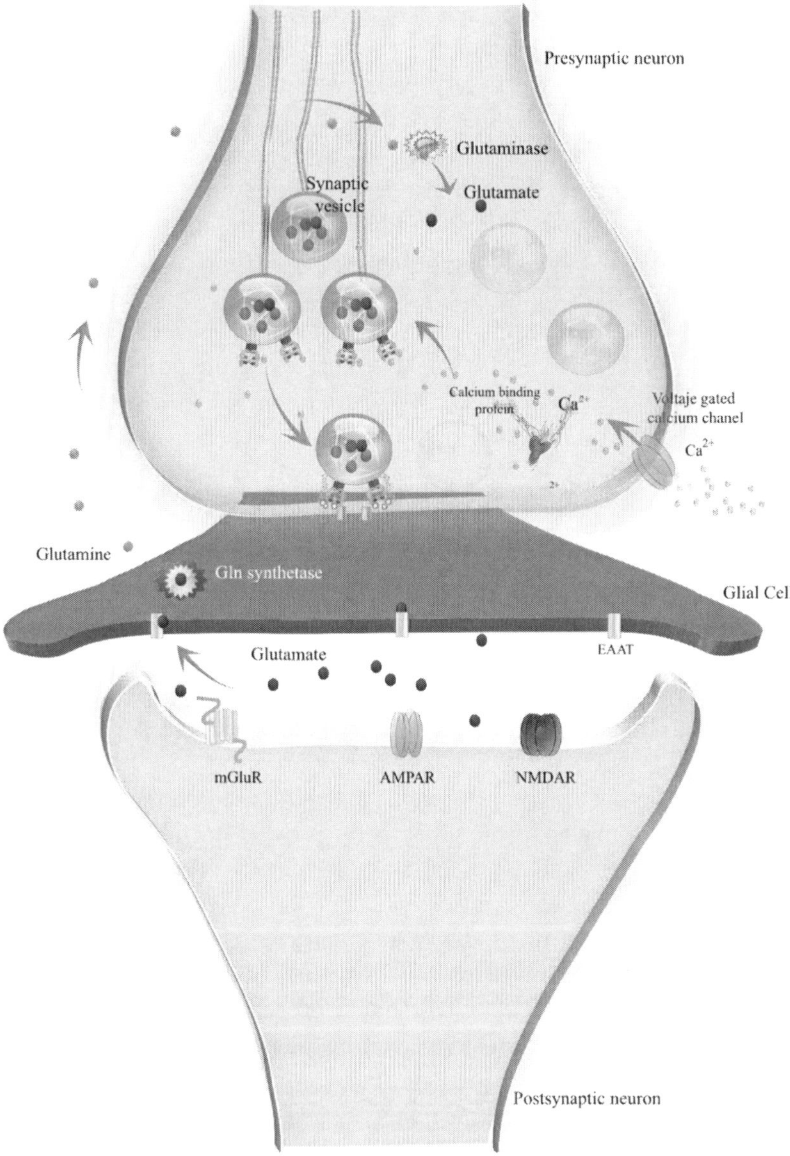

Figure 3. Glutamate tripartite synapse. The tripartite synapse model involves the presynaptic neuron (blue, top), the postsynaptic neuron (blue, down) and the glial cell (pink, middle). After synthesis, glutamate is packaged in synaptic vesicles that release it into the extracellular space. Once released, glutamate binds to its receptor(s) and then is cleared from the synapse by glial cells. Glial cells converts glutamate to glutamine and exports it to neurons where glutamine is again converted to glutamate.

The metabolic interplay between glia and GCs is particularly evident in the case of the excitatory synapse. It is believed that GCs affects the brain following an inverse-U pattern where heightened and prolonged levels of this hormone produces deleterious effects on synaptic plasticity, cognition, dendritic arbors and spine density (McEwen, 2000). The excitatory glutamatergic synapse is a key element to the comprehension of these damaging effects (Timmermans, Xiong, Hoogenraad, & Krugers, 2013). Glutamatergic neurotransmission occurs mainly in the context of the so-called tripartite synapse. Figure 3 illustrates the tripartite glutamate synapse.

Besides its role as excitatory neurotransmitter, glutamate is a key intermediary metabolite with multiple intracellular functions that requires high concentrations within cells. The main source of brain glutamate is glucose provided by blood and glutamine provided by glia. At synaptic level, glutamate exists in presynaptic vesicles that are released into the extracellular space to bind postsynaptic receptors (both, the ionotropics NMDA, AMPA and Kainate, and the metabotropics mGluR1 to mGluR8). Postsynaptic actions include membrane depolarization, activation of intracellular cascades and regulation of protein traffic and synthesis. Glia clears glutamate from the synapse through excitatory amino acid transporters (EAATs). Once in glia, glutamate is converted to glutamine by glutamine synthetase (GS) and subsequently returned to neurons (Kessler, 2013).

A current hypothesis sustains that excessive glutamatergic activity is one of the major causes conducting to deleterious effects of stress in neurons (atrophy of dendrites, impaired synaptic plasticity, reduced neurogenesis and diminished spine density) (Popoli, Yan, McEwen, & Sanacora, 2012). Mechanisms underlying this phenomenon are multiple. GCs for example may inhibit glucose uptake among brain cells. Diminished glucose in turn declines ATP levels and consequently the amount of energy available for neurons and glial cells to face the costly tasks of glutamate clearance is insufficient (Sorrells & Sapolsky, 2007). The problem may become bigger due to the probed fact that the GR, MR activation may also increase glutamate release in the presynaptic side and disturb the traffic of glutamate receptors in the postsynaptic side (Popoli, et al., 2012).

More important for this document is the questionless fact that GCs may directly affect glial cells. It was first discovered the existence of both GR and MR receptors in glial cells (Bohn, Howard, Vielkind, & Krozowski, 1991). Thereafter, a number of glial specific genes and functions have been proposed to be under regulation of stress hormones. Figure 4 enlists some of these genes.

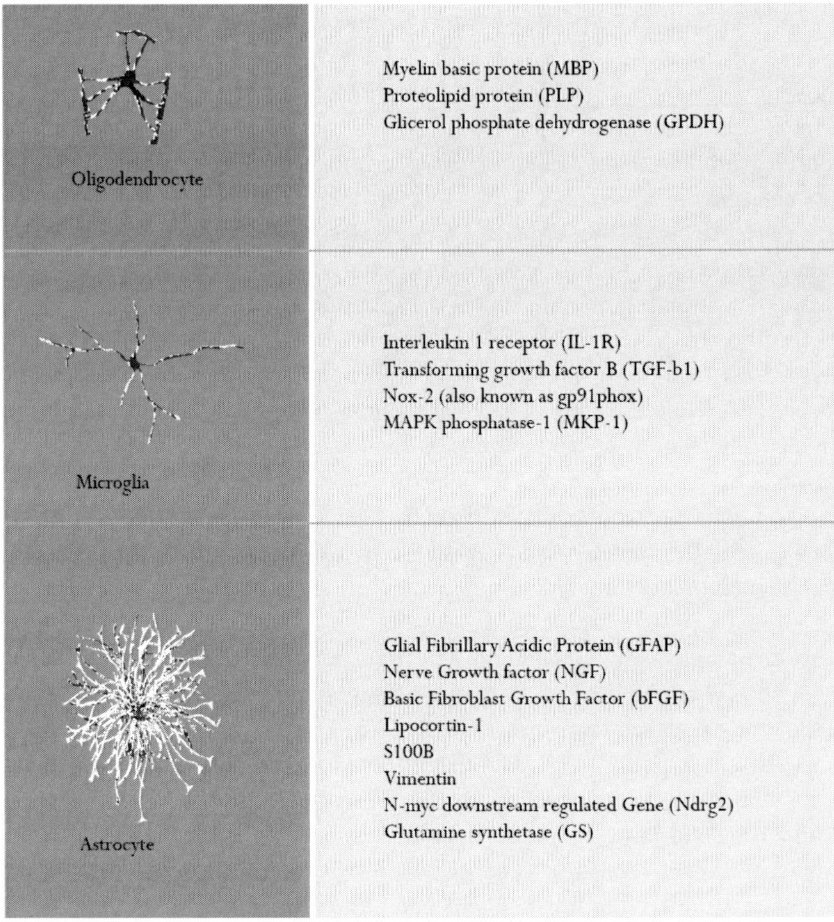

Figure 4. Examples of glucocorticoid-regulated genes in oligodendrocytes (top) (Kumar, et al., 1989), microglia (middle) (Gottschall, Koves, Mizuno, Tatsuno, & Arimura, 1991; Huo, et al., 2011; Nichols, Agolley, Zieba, & Bye, 2005) and astrocytes (Bridges, et al., 2008; McLeod & Bolton, 1995; Nichols, et al., 2005; Niu, Hinkle, & Wise, 1997; Vardimon, et al., 1999) (botton).

Glutamine synthetase (GS) is one of the most important glial proteins involved in the glutamate cycle. This enzyme resides in astrocytes where uses glutamate to synthesize glutamine. Most of the glutamine derived from astroglia is shuttled to neurons where is degraded to glutamate. As pointed above, glutamate is mainly used as excitatory neurotransmitter but serves also as precursor of the inhibitory neurotransmitter gamma-aminobutyric acid (GABA). Another portion of glutamine helps as an energy metabolite and the remaining part leaves the brain to blood in order to avoid overconcentration (Albrecht, Sonnewald, Waagepetersen, & Schousboe, 2007). Accordingly, all these steps may be disrupted by the presence of stress hormones. Particularly, it has been demonstrated that GCs may directly affect the expression of GS (Vardimon, Ben-Dror, Avisar, Oren, & Shiftan, 1999). If so, rat models of chronic stress have failed to find direct effects on GS, they have also demonstrated that the entire cycle suffers unbalances under these conditions (Banasr, et al., 2010).

Excitatory amino acid transporters (EAATs) are other major glial proteins involved in the glutamate-glutamine cycle. EAAT2 is the most important of these transporters and is expressed markedly in glia. This transporter is highly efficient in clearing glutamate from the extracellular space. Regarding this, there is experimental evidence sustaining that stress may affect glutamate transport (Almeida, et al., 2010; Zink, Vollmayr, Gebicke-Haerter, & Henn, 2010). Studies trying to elucidate this effect suggest that GCs have a central role because treatment of rats with this hormone biphasically affects the expression of GLT1, the main isoform of EAAT2 (Autry, et al., 2006; Reagan, et al., 2004; Zschocke, et al., 2005).

Both, the reduced glial ability to process glutamine and the insufficient capacity to clear glutamate from the extracellular space may contribute in a very determinant way to the excitotoxic environment proposed on the basis of the major pathological changes partnering stress related pathologies. If we add to this mechanisms the reported reduction in numbers of astrocytes (we need to take into account that one astrocyte may assist thousands of synapses) seen in stressed or depressed subjects, it becomes clear that glial cells undoubtedly take a protagonic part in the comprehension of stress pathologies. It is not surprising in this context that other glial cells different from astrocytes may be involved. This suggestion has been confirmed by experiments showing that microglial changes in proliferative rate associated to stress, depends directly on the activation of the glutamate NMDA receptor (Nair & Bonneau, 2006).

Additional evidence for the supporting-metabolic interaction between glial cells and stress hormones may be extracted from studies on calcium associated processes. A key molecule in calcium homeostasis is the calcium binding protein S100β. S100β is found primarily in the cytoplasm of astrocytes, although it may be also found in the extracellular space. A variety of cellular actions have been described under the influence of S100β. Those actions include cell growth, energy metabolism, calcium homeostasis and synaptic plasticity (Donato, 2001; Rothermundt, Peters, Prehn, & Arolt, 2003). Its close relationship with these processes has placed S100β in the focus of many investigations trying to establish its use as biomarker in a number of pathological conditions, including cardiomiopathies, neurodegenerative disorders and cancer (Scaccianoce, Del Bianco, Pannitteri, & Passarelli, 2004). Stress-related pathologies include also changes in S100β protein. Even controversial, those changes seem to adjust to a biphasic pattern. It has been reported for example that maternal administration of the synthetic glucocorticoid betamethasone correlates with reduced serum and brain levels of S100β in the neonate (Bruschettini, et al., 2005). In the other hand, acute stress exposure may produce increases in the concentration of cerebrospinal fluid S100β of adult rats (Margis, et al., 2004). Depression, a clinical condition characterized by a stress-like activation of the endocrine system, have been frequently associated to changes in S100β levels specially when depressive symptoms come along with renal disease, myocardial infarction or neurological disorders (J. K. Kim, Kim, Kim, & Song, 2012; Tulner, et al., 2009; Uher & Bob, 2012). So, it is clear that S100β respond actively to the presence of stress hormones in a way that may depend on time of exposure, developmental stage or associated conditions. Apart from S100β, GCs may also affect calcium dynamics by modifying calcium signals. A revealing study aiming to elucidate the mechanisms behind the edemolytic effect of glucocorticoids in brain, found that GC treatment increased both, resting cytosolic calcium levels and the extent and amplitude of calcium waves in astrocytes (Simard, et al., 1999). Therefore, a myriad of calcium-dependent processes controlled by glia may fall under control of GCs.

The blood brain barrier (BBB) represents another point where the supporting role of glia may interact with GCs. Endothelial cells interconnected by tight junctions interact with astrocytes, pericytes and neurons to form the neurovascular unit that selectively controls the homeostasis of the CNS. Astrocytes endfeet envelops the vessels and play an important role in the induction and maintenance of the BBB by secreting soluble factors that regulate endothelial tight junctions. They also control water flux trough a specific water channel namely aquaporin-4 (Nico & Ribatti, 2012). Besides the well documented effects of GCs on BBB barrier which include regulation of P-glycoprotein, angiopoietin-1, vascular endothelial growth factor (VEGF), multidrug resistance transporters and matrix metalloproteinases (MMPs) and their endogenous inhibitors (TIMPs) (Hartmann, et al., 2009; Iqbal, Gibb, & Matthews, 2011; H. Kim, et al., 2008; Narang, et al., 2008), it now must be added regulatory activities of GCs over BBB linking astrocytes. These astrocyte-dependent activities may involve regulation of the tight junction proteins occludin, claudin-5 and ZO-1 (Kroll, et al., 2009). Finally, vasoactive actions of GCs may depend on astrocytes as pointed by a recent report confirming that adrenomedullin (a novel vasodilatory peptide expressed and secreted by astrocytes) is also target of glucocorticoids (Liverani & Paul, 2013).

CONCLUSION

The central immune response and the metabolic support of glial cells represents an amazing meeting point that offers new unexplored opportunities to fully understand the complex relationship between stress hormones and the central nervous system. These elements are also an enormous opportunity to gain comprehension of the complex mechanisms underlying pathologies characterized by stress-like activation of hormonal systems and to found new targets for therapeutic interventions. Much remains to be explored about it in the coming years.

REFERENCES

Albrecht, J., Sonnewald, U., Waagepetersen, H. S., & Schousboe, A. (2007). Glutamine in the central nervous system: function and dysfunction. *Front Biosci.,* 12, 332-343.

Almeida, R. F., Thomazi, A. P., Godinho, G. F., Saute, J. A., Wofchuk, S. T., Souza, D. O., et al., (2010). Effects of depressive-like behavior of rats on brain glutamate uptake. *Neurochem. Res.,* 35(8), 1164-1171.

Alonso, G. (2000). Prolonged corticosterone treatment of adult rats inhibits the proliferation of oligodendrocyte progenitors present throughout white and gray matter regions of the brain. *Glia,* 31(3), 219-231.

Amor, S., & Woodroofe, N. (2013). Review series on immune responses in neurodegenerative diseases: innate and adaptive immune responses in neurodegeneration and repair. *Immunology*.

Araque, A., Parpura, V., Sanzgiri, R. P., & Haydon, P. G. (1999). Tripartite synapses: glia, the unacknowledged partner. *Trends Neurosci.,* 22(5), 208-215.

Autry, A. E., Grillo, C. A., Piroli, G. G., Rothstein, J. D., McEwen, B. S., & Reagan, L. P. (2006). Glucocorticoid regulation of GLT-1 glutamate transporter isoform expression in the rat hippocampus. *Neuroendocrinology,* 83(5-6), 371-379.

Banasr, M., Chowdhury, G. M., Terwilliger, R., Newton, S. S., Duman, R. S., Behar, K. L., et al., (2008). Glial pathology in an animal model of depression: reversal of stress-induced cellular, metabolic and behavioral deficits by the glutamate-modulating drug riluzole. *Mol. Psychiatry.*

Banasr, M., Chowdhury, G. M., Terwilliger, R., Newton, S. S., Duman, R. S., Behar, K. L., et al., (2010). Glial pathology in an animal model of depression: reversal of stress-induced cellular, metabolic and behavioral deficits by the glutamate-modulating drug riluzole. *Mol. Psychiatry,* 15(5), 501-511.

Bohn, M. C., Howard, E., Vielkind, U., & Krozowski, Z. (1991). Glial cells express both mineralocorticoid and glucocorticoid receptors. *J. Steroid. Biochem. Mol. Biol.,* 40(1-3), 105-111.

Bridges, N., Slais, K., & Sykova, E. (2008). The effects of chronic corticosterone on hippocampal astrocyte numbers: a comparison of male and female Wistar rats. *Acta Neurobiol. Exp. (Wars),* 68(2), 131-138.

Bruschettini, M., van den Hove, D. L., Gazzolo, D., Bruschettini, P., Blanco, C. E., & Steinbusch, H. W. (2005). A single course of antenatal betamethasone reduces neurotrophic factor S100B concentration in the hippocampus and serum in the neonatal rat. *Brain Res. Dev. Brain Res.,* 159(2), 113-118.

Buckingham, J. C. (2006). Glucocorticoids: exemplars of multi-tasking. *Br. J. Pharmacol.,* 147 Suppl 1, S258-268.

Carrillo-de Sauvage, M. A., Maatouk, L., Arnoux, I., Pasco, M., Sanz Diez, A., Delahaye, M., et al., (2013). Potent and multiple regulatory actions of microglial glucocorticoid receptors during CNS inflammation. *Cell Death Differ.*

Caudle, R. M. (2006). Memory in astrocytes: a hypothesis. *Theor Biol. Med. Model,* 3, 2.

Cutolo, M., Buttgereit, F., & Straub, R. H. (2011). Regulation of glucocorticoids by the central nervous system. *Clin. Exp. Rheumatol.,* 29(5 Suppl 68), S-19-22.

Czeh, B., Muller-Keuker, J. I., Rygula, R., Abumaria, N., Hiemke, C., Domenici, E., et al., (2007). Chronic social stress inhibits cell proliferation in the adult medial prefrontal cortex: hemispheric asymmetry and reversal by fluoxetine treatment. *Neuropsychopharmacology,* 32(7), 1490-1503.

Daneman, R. (2012). The blood-brain barrier in health and disease. *Ann. Neurol.,* 72(5), 648-672.

de Kloet, E. R. (2003). Hormones, brain and stress. *Endocr. Regul.,* 37(2), 51-68.

de Kloet, E. R., Oitzl, M. S., & Joels, M. (1999). Stress and cognition: are corticosteroids good or bad guys? *Trends Neurosci.,* 22(10), 422-426.

De Kloet, E. R., Vreugdenhil, E., Oitzl, M. S., & Joels, M. (1998). Brain corticosteroid receptor balance in health and disease. *Endocr. Rev.,* 19(3), 269-301.

Del Bigio, M. R. (2010). Ependymal cells: biology and pathology. *Acta Neuropathol.,* 119(1), 55-73.

Dimou, L., & Gotz, M. (2012). Shaping barrels: activity moves NG2+ glia. *Nat. Neurosci.,* 15(9), 1176-1178.

Donato, R. (2001). S100: a multigenic family of calcium-modulated proteins of the EF-hand type with intracellular and extracellular functional roles. *Int. J. Biochem. Cell Biol.,* 33(7), 637-668.

Drew, P. D., & Chavis, J. A. (2000). Inhibition of microglial cell activation by cortisol. *Brain Res. Bull.,* 52(5), 391-396.

Edgar, N., & Sibille, E. (2012). A putative functional role for oligodendrocytes in mood regulation. *Transl Psychiatry,* 2, e109.

Ekdahl, C. T. (2012). Microglial activation - tuning and pruning adult neurogenesis. *Front Pharmacol.,* 3, 41.

Elder, G. A., De Gasperi, R., & Gama Sosa, M. A. (2006). Research update: neurogenesis in adult brain and neuropsychiatric disorders. *Mt Sinai J. Med.,* 73(7), 931-940.

Etxeberria, A., Mangin, J. M., Aguirre, A., & Gallo, V. (2010). Adult-born SVZ progenitors receive transient synapses during remyelination in corpus callosum. *Nat. Neurosci.,* 13(3), 287-289.

Fields, R. D., & Stevens-Graham, B. (2002). New insights into neuron-glia communication. *Science,* 298(5593), 556-562.

Fisher, L. A., & Brown, M. R. (1991). Central regulation of stress responses: regulation of the autonomic nervous system and visceral function by corticotrophin releasing factor-41. *Baillieres Clin. Endocrinol. Metab.,* 5(1), 35-50.

Frank, M. G., Baratta, M. V., Sprunger, D. B., Watkins, L. R., & Maier, S. F. (2007). Microglia serve as a neuroimmune substrate for stress-induced potentiation of CNS pro-inflammatory cytokine responses. *Brain Behav. Immun.,* 21(1), 47-59.

Frank, M. G., Watkins, L. R., & Maier, S. F. (2011). Stress- and glucocorticoid-induced priming of neuroinflammatory responses: potential mechanisms of stress-induced vulnerability to drugs of abuse. *Brain Behav. Immun.,* 25 Suppl 1, S21-28.

Frick, L. R., Williams, K., & Pittenger, C. (2013). Microglial dysregulation in psychiatric disease. *Clin. Dev. Immunol.,* 2013, 608654.

Garcia-Segura, L. M., & McCarthy, M. M. (2004). Minireview: Role of glia in neuroendocrine function. *Endocrinology,* 145(3), 1082-1086.

Gianaros, P. J., Jennings, J. R., Sheu, L. K., Greer, P. J., Kuller, L. H., & Matthews, K. A. (2007). Prospective reports of chronic life stress predict decreased grey matter volume in the hippocampus. *Neuroimage,* 35(2), 795-803.

Gonzalez-Perez, O., Chavez-Casillas, O., Jauregui-Huerta, F., Lopez-Virgen, V., Guzman-Muniz, J., Moy-Lopez, N., et al., (2011). Stress by noise produces differential effects on the proliferation rate of radial astrocytes and survival of neuroblasts in the adult subgranular zone. *Neurosci. Res.,* 70(3), 243-250.

Gottschall, P. E., Koves, K., Mizuno, K., Tatsuno, I., & Arimura, A. (1991). Glucocorticoid upregulation of interleukin 1 receptor expression in a glioblastoma cell line. *Am. J. Physiol.,* 261(3 Pt 1), E362-368.

Gould, E., & Tanapat, P. (1999). Stress and hippocampal neurogenesis. *Biol. Psychiatry,* 46(11), 1472-1479.

Hanisch, U. K., & Kettenmann, H. (2007). Microglia: active sensor and versatile effector cells in the normal and pathologic brain. *Nat. Neurosci.,* 10(11), 1387-1394.

Hartmann, C., El-Gindi, J., Lohmann, C., Lischper, M., Zeni, P., & Galla, H. J. (2009). TIMP-3: a novel target for glucocorticoid signaling at the blood-brain barrier. *Biochem. Biophys. Res. Commun.,* 390(2), 182-186.

Huo, Y., Rangarajan, P., Ling, E. A., & Dheen, S. T. (2011). Dexamethasone inhibits the Nox-dependent ROS production via suppression of MKP-1-dependent MAPK pathways in activated microglia. *BMC Neurosci.,* 12, 49.

Iqbal, M., Gibb, W., & Matthews, S. G. (2011). Corticosteroid regulation of P-glycoprotein in the developing blood-brain barrier. *Endocrinology,* 152(3), 1067-1079.

Jauregui-Huerta, F., Garcia-Estrada, J., Ruvalcaba-Delgadillo, Y., Trujillo, X., Huerta, M., Feria-Velasco, A., et al., (2011). Chronic exposure of juvenile rats to environmental noise impairs hippocampal cell proliferation in adulthood. *Noise Health,* 13(53), 286-291.

Jauregui-Huerta, F., Ruvalcaba-Delgadillo, Y., Garcia-Estrada, J., Feria-Velasco, A., Ramos-Zuniga, R., Gonzalez-Perez, O., et al., (2010). Early exposure to noise followed by predator stress in adulthood impairs the rat's re-learning flexibility in Radial Arm Water Maze. *Neuro Endocrinol. Lett.,* 31(4), 538-548.

Jauregui-Huerta, F., Ruvalcaba-Delgadillo, Y., Gonzalez-Castaneda, R., Garcia-Estrada, J., Gonzalez-Perez, O., & Luquin, S. (2010). Responses of glial cells to stress and glucocorticoids. *Curr. Immunol. Rev.,* 6(3), 195-204.

Joels, M., Karst, H., Alfarez, D., Heine, V. M., Qin, Y., van Riel, E., et al., (2004). Effects of chronic stress on structure and cell function in rat hippocampus and hypothalamus. *Stress,* 7(4), 221-231.

Kato, T. A., Hayakawa, K., Monji, A., & Kanba, S. (2013). Missing and Possible Link between Neuroendocrine Factors, Neuropsychiatric Disorders, and Microglia. *Front Integr. Neurosci.,* 7, 53.

Kessler, J. P. (2013). Control of cleft glutamate concentration and glutamate spill-out by perisynaptic glia: uptake and diffusion barriers. *PLoS ONE,* 8(8), e70791.

Kim, H., Lee, J. M., Park, J. S., Jo, S. A., Kim, Y. O., Kim, C. W., et al., (2008). Dexamethasone coordinately regulates angiopoietin-1 and VEGF: a mechanism of glucocorticoid-induced stabilization of blood-brain barrier. *Biochem. Biophys. Res. Commun.,* 372(1), 243-248.

Kim, J. J., & Diamond, D. M. (2002). The stressed hippocampus, synaptic plasticity and lost memories. *Nat. Rev. Neurosci.,* 3(6), 453-462.

Kim, J. K., Kim, S. G., Kim, H. J., & Song, Y. R. (2012). Serum S100B protein is associated with depressive symptoms in patients with end-stage renal disease. *Clin. Biochem.,* 45(18), 1573-1577.

Korte, S. M., Koolhaas, J. M., Wingfield, J. C., & McEwen, B. S. (2005). The Darwinian concept of stress: benefits of allostasis and costs of allostatic load and the trade-offs in health and disease. *Neurosci. Biobehav. Rev.,* 29(1), 3-38.

Kreutzberg, G. W. (1996). Microglia: a sensor for pathological events in the CNS. *Trends Neurosci.,* 19(8), 312-318.

Kroll, S., El-Gindi, J., Thanabalasundaram, G., Panpumthong, P., Schrot, S., Hartmann, C., et al., (2009). Control of the blood-brain barrier by glucocorticoids and the cells of the neurovascular unit. *Ann. NY Acad. Sci.,* 1165, 228-239.

Kumar, S., Cole, R., Chiappelli, F., & de Vellis, J. (1989). Differential regulation of oligodendrocyte markers by glucocorticoids: post-transcriptional regulation of both proteolipid protein and myelin basic protein and transcriptional regulation of glycerol phosphate dehydrogenase. *Proc. Natl. Acad. Sci. USA,* 86(17), 6807-6811.

Lee, Y., Morrison, B. M., Li, Y., Lengacher, S., Farah, M. H., Hoffman, P. N., et al., (2012). Oligodendroglia metabolically support axons and contribute to neurodegeneration. *Nature,* 487(7408), 443-448.

Leventopoulos, M., Ruedi-Bettschen, D., Knuesel, I., Feldon, J., Pryce, C. R., & Opacka-Juffry, J. (2007). Long-term effects of early life deprivation on brain glia in Fischer rats. *Brain Res.,* 1142, 119-126.

Liverani, E., & Paul, C. (2013). Glucocorticoids alter adrenomedullin receptor expression and secretion in endothelial-like cells and astrocytes. *Int. J. Biochem. Cell Biol.*

Lopez, J. F., Akil, H., & Watson, S. J. (1999). Neural circuits mediating stress. *Biol. Psychiatry,* 46(11), 1461-1471.

Lupien, S. J., Fiocco, A., Wan, N., Maheu, F., Lord, C., Schramek, T., et al., (2005). Stress hormones and human memory function across the lifespan. *Psychoneuroendocrinology,* 30(3), 225-242.

Magarinos, A. M., & McEwen, B. S. (1995). Stress-induced atrophy of apical dendrites of hippocampal CA3c neurons: involvement of glucocorticoid secretion and excitatory amino acid receptors. *Neuroscience,* 69(1), 89-98.

Margis, R., Zanatto, V. C., Tramontina, F., Vinade, E., Lhullier, F., Portela, L. V., et al., (2004). Changes in S100B cerebrospinal fluid levels of rats subjected to predator stress. *Brain Res.,* 1028(2), 213-218.

Marin, I., & Kipnis, J. (2013). Learning and memory ... and the immune system. *Learn Mem.,* 20(10), 601-606.

Maschke, C., Rupp, T., & Hecht, K. (2000). The influence of stressors on biochemical reactions--a review of present scientific findings with noise. *Int. J. Hyg. Environ. Health,* 203(1), 45-53.

McEwen, B. S. (2000). Protective and damaging effects of stress mediators: central role of the brain. *Prog. Brain Res.,* 122, 25-34.

McEwen, B. S. (2006). Protective and damaging effects of stress mediators: central role of the brain. *Dialogues Clin. Neurosci.,* 8(4), 367-381.

McLaughlin, K. J., Gomez, J. L., Baran, S. E., & Conrad, C. D. (2007). The effects of chronic stress on hippocampal morphology and function: an evaluation of chronic restraint paradigms. *Brain Res.,* 1161, 56-64.

McLeod, J. D., & Bolton, C. (1995). Dexamethasone induces an increase in intracellular and membrane-associated lipocortin-1 (annexin-1) in rat astrocyte primary cultures. *Cell Mol. Neurobiol.,* 15(2), 193-205.

Minami, M., Kuraishi, Y., Yamaguchi, T., Nakai, S., Hirai, Y., & Satoh, M. (1991). Immobilization stress induces interleukin-1 beta mRNA in the rat hypothalamus. *Neurosci. Lett,* 123(2), 254-256.

Muller, M. B., Lucassen, P. J., Yassouridis, A., Hoogendijk, W. J., Holsboer, F., & Swaab, D. F. (2001). Neither major depression nor glucocorticoid treatment affects the cellular integrity of the human hippocampus. *Eur. J. Neurosci.,* 14(10), 1603-1612.

Munck, A., Guyre, P. M., & Holbrook, N. J. (1984). Physiological functions of glucocorticoids in stress and their relation to pharmacological actions. *Endocr. Rev.,* 5(1), 25-44.

Nair, A., & Bonneau, R. H. (2006). Stress-induced elevation of glucocorticoids increases microglia proliferation through NMDA receptor activation. *J. Neuroimmunol,,* 171(1-2), 72-85.

Napoli, I., & Neumann, H. (2009). Microglial clearance function in health and disease. *Neuroscience,* 158(3), 1030-1038.

Narang, V. S., Fraga, C., Kumar, N., Shen, J., Throm, S., Stewart, C. F., et al., (2008). Dexamethasone increases expression and activity of multidrug resistance transporters at the rat blood-brain barrier. *Am. J. Physiol. Cell Physiol.,* 295(2), C440-450.

Nico, B., & Ribatti, D. (2012). Morphofunctional aspects of the blood-brain barrier. *Curr. Drug Metab.,* 13(1), 50-60.

Nichols, N. R., Agolley, D., Zieba, M., & Bye, N. (2005). Glucocorticoid regulation of glial responses during hippocampal neurodegeneration and regeneration. *Brain Res. Brain Res. Rev.,* 48(2), 287-301.

Niu, H., Hinkle, D. A., & Wise, P. M. (1997). Dexamethasone regulates basic fibroblast growth factor, nerve growth factor and S100beta expression in cultured hippocampal astrocytes. *Brain Res. Mol. Brain Res.,* 51(1-2), 97-105.

O'Callaghan, J. P., Brinton, R. E., & McEwen, B. S. (1991). Glucocorticoids regulate the synthesis of glial fibrillary acidic protein in intact and adrenalectomized rats but do not affect its expression following brain injury. *J. Neurochem.,* 57(3), 860-869.

Ozawa, H. (2005). Steroid Hormones, their receptors and neuroendocrine system. *J. Nippon. Med. Sch.,* 72(6), 316-325.

Pacak, K., & Palkovits, M. (2001). Stressor specificity of central neuroendocrine responses: implications for stress-related disorders. *Endocr. Rev.,* 22(4), 502-548.

Parpura, V., & Verkhratsky, A. (2012). Astrocytes revisited: concise historic outlook on glutamate homeostasis and signaling. *Croat Med. J.*, 53(6), 518-528.

Peferoen, L., Kipp, M., van der Valk, P., van Noort, J. M., & Amor, S. (2013). Review series on immune responses in neurodegenerative diseases: Oligodendrocyte-microglia cross-talk in the CNS. *Immunology*.

Popoli, M., Yan, Z., McEwen, B. S., & Sanacora, G. (2012). The stressed synapse: the impact of stress and glucocorticoids on glutamate transmission. *Nat. Rev. Neurosci.*, 13(1), 22-37.

Pugh, C. R., Nguyen, K. T., Gonyea, J. L., Fleshner, M., Wakins, L. R., Maier, S. F., et al., (1999). Role of interleukin-1 beta in impairment of contextual fear conditioning caused by social isolation. *Behav. Brain Res.*, 106(1-2), 109-118.

Rabat, A., Bouyer, J. J., Aran, J. M., Courtiere, A., Mayo, W., & Le Moal, M. (2004). Deleterious effects of an environmental noise on sleep and contribution of its physical components in a rat model. *Brain Res.*, 1009(1-2), 88-97.

Raff, M. C., Miller, R. H., & Noble, M. (1983). A glial progenitor cell that develops in vitro into an astrocyte or an oligodendrocyte depending on culture medium. *Nature*, 303(5916), 390-396.

Rajkowska, G. (2003). Depression: what we can learn from postmortem studies. *Neuroscientist*, 9(4), 273-284.

Rajkowska, G., & Miguel-Hidalgo, J. J. (2007). Gliogenesis and glial pathology in depression. *CNS Neurol. Disord. Drug Targets*, 6(3), 219-233.

Ramos-Remus, C., Gonzalez-Castaneda, R. E., Gonzalez-Perez, O., Luquin, S., & Garcia-Estrada, J. (2002). Prednisone induces cognitive dysfunction, neuronal degeneration, and reactive gliosis in rats. *J. Investig. Med.*, 50(6), 458-464.

Reagan, L. P., Rosell, D. R., Wood, G. E., Spedding, M., Munoz, C., Rothstein, J., et al., (2004). Chronic restraint stress up-regulates GLT-1 mRNA and protein expression in the rat hippocampus: reversal by tianeptine. *Proc. Natl. Acad. Sci. USA*, 101(7), 2179-2184.

Reichardt, H. M., Gold, R., & Luhder, F. (2006). Glucocorticoids in multiple sclerosis and experimental autoimmune encephalomyelitis. *Expert. Rev. Neurother*, 6(11), 1657-1670.

Rivest, S. (2009). Regulation of innate immune responses in the brain. *Nat. Rev. Immunol.*, 9(6), 429-439.

Robel, S., Berninger, B., & Gotz, M. (2011). The stem cell potential of glia: lessons from reactive gliosis. *Nat. Rev. Neurosci.,* 12(2), 88-104.

Rothermundt, M., Peters, M., Prehn, J. H., & Arolt, V. (2003). S100B in brain damage and neurodegeneration. *Microsc. Res. Tech.,* 60(6), 614-632.

Sabolek, M., Herborg, A., Schwarz, J., & Storch, A. (2006). Dexamethasone blocks astroglial differentiation from neural precursor cells. *Neuroreport,* 17(16), 1719-1723.

Sandi, C., & Pinelo-Nava, M. T. (2007). Stress and memory: behavioral effects and neurobiological mechanisms. *Neural. Plast.,* 2007, 78970.

Sandi, C., Woodson, J. C., Haynes, V. F., Park, C. R., Touyarot, K., Lopez-Fernandez, M. A., et al., (2005). Acute stress-induced impairment of spatial memory is associated with decreased expression of neural cell adhesion molecule in the hippocampus and prefrontal cortex. *Biol. Psychiatry,* 57(8), 856-864.

Sawamoto, K., Wichterle, H., Gonzalez-Perez, O., Cholfin, J. A., Yamada, M., Spassky, N., et al., (2006). New neurons follow the flow of cerebrospinal fluid in the adult brain. *Science,* 311(5761), 629-632.

Scaccianoce, S., Del Bianco, P., Pannitteri, G., & Passarelli, F. (2004). Relationship between stress and circulating levels of S100B protein. *Brain Res.,* 1004(1-2), 208-211.

Schroter, A., Lustenberger, R. M., Obermair, F. J., & Thallmair, M. (2009). High-dose corticosteroids after spinal cord injury reduce neural progenitor cell proliferation. *Neuroscience,* 161(3), 753-763.

Sierra, A., Gottfried-Blackmore, A., Milner, T. A., McEwen, B. S., & Bulloch, K. (2008). Steroid hormone receptor expression and function in microglia. *Glia,* 56(6), 659-674.

Simard, M., Couldwell, W. T., Zhang, W., Song, H., Liu, S., Cotrina, M. L., et al., (1999). Glucocorticoids-potent modulators of astrocytic calcium signaling. *Glia,* 28(1), 1-12.

Sorrells, S. F., & Sapolsky, R. M. (2007). An inflammatory review of glucocorticoid actions in the CNS. *Brain Behav. Immun.,* 21(3), 259-272.

Sugama, S. (2009). Stress-induced microglial activation may facilitate the progression of neurodegenerative disorders. *Med Hypotheses.*

Sugama, S., Fujita, M., Hashimoto, M., & Conti, B. (2007). Stress induced morphological microglial activation in the rodent brain: involvement of interleukin-18. *Neuroscience,* 146(3), 1388-1399.

Tanaka, J., Fujita, H., Matsuda, S., Toku, K., Sakanaka, M., & Maeda, N. (1997). Glucocorticoid- and mineralocorticoid receptors in microglial cells: the two receptors mediate differential effects of corticosteroids. *Glia,* 20(1), 23-37.

Timmermans, W., Xiong, H., Hoogenraad, C. C., & Krugers, H. J. (2013). Stress and excitatory synapses: from health to disease. *Neuroscience,* 248, 626-636.

Tulner, D. M., Smith, O. R., de Jonge, P., van Melle, J. P., Slomp, J., Storm, H., et al., (2009). Circulating cerebral S100B protein is associated with depressive symptoms following myocardial infarction. *Neuropsychobiology,* 59(2), 87-95.

Uher, T., & Bob, P. (2012). Cerebrospinal fluid S100B levels reflect symptoms of depression in patients with non-inflammatory neurological disorders. *Neurosci. Lett.,* 529(2), 139-143.

Vardimon, L., Ben-Dror, I., Avisar, N., Oren, A., & Shiftan, L. (1999). Glucocorticoid control of glial gene expression. *J. Neurobiol.,* 40(4), 513-527.

Vyas, A., Mitra, R., Shankaranarayana Rao, B. S., & Chattarji, S. (2002). Chronic stress induces contrasting patterns of dendritic remodeling in hippocampal and amygdaloid neurons. *J. Neurosci.,* 22(15), 6810-6818.

Woods, A. G., Poulsen, F. R., & Gall, C. M. (1999). Dexamethasone selectively suppresses microglial trophic responses to hippocampal deafferentation. *Neuroscience,* 91(4), 1277-1289.

Zink, M., Vollmayr, B., Gebicke-Haerter, P. J., & Henn, F. A. (2010). Reduced expression of glutamate transporters vGluT1, EAAT2 and EAAT4 in learned helpless rats, an animal model of depression. *Neuropharmacology,* 58(2), 465-473.

Zschocke, J., Bayatti, N., Clement, A. M., Witan, H., Figiel, M., Engele, J., et al., (2005). Differential promotion of glutamate transporter expression and function by glucocorticoids in astrocytes from various brain regions. *J. Biol. Chem.,* 280(41), 34924-34932.

In: Neuro-Immune Interactions ...
Editor: Oscar González-Pérez
ISBN: 978-1-62948-646-8

Chapter 9

IMMUNOMODULATORY ROLE OF ENSHEATHING CELLS IN SPINAL CORD INJURY

Graciela Gudiño-Cabrera, Nidia Carrillo-González, Marcela María J. Rodríguez-Baeza and Gabriela Escobar-Camberos
Laboratorio de Desarrollo y Regeneración Neural,
Departamento de Biología Celular y Molecular, Instituto de Neurobiología,
C.U.C.B.A, Universidad de Guadalajara, Mexico

ABSTRACT

The sense of smell is vital for the survival of organisms. Within the nervous system, the olfactory bulb is the area responsible for receiving and integrating the information from odor particles. However, it is also one of the structures in the central nervous system that is exposed multiple adverse environmental influences, elements that directly affect olfactory receptor neurons. This may explain why these neurons are well protected by the ensheathing glia, which surround and accompany their axons along the trajectory from the nasal cavity to the olfactory bulb, and that regulate their activity. Ensheathing cells, which have significant morphological and functional plasticity, and they are able to respond to several stimuli and protect the nervous system from a large number of pathogens by activating macrophages and by regulating inflammatory reactions. In addition, they are capable of engulfing both bacterial and neuronal debris by phagocytosis, establishing conditions suitable for neurogenesis. Indeed, ensheathing glia participate in neurogenesis by myelinating new axons, secreting growth factors that promote axon growth, and expressing extracellular matrix molecules that correctly guide neurons to the olfactory bulb. These virtues have led the regenerative capacity of ensheathing glia to be assessed in models of spinal cord injury with interesting results, although their possible employment in future human cell therapies is still under study.

Abbreviations

Adap2	Gene encoded Arf-GAP with dual PH domain-containing protein 2
Aif1	Allograft inflammatory factor 1
ATP	Adenosine triphosphate
BDNF	Brain-derived neurotrophic factor
cAMP	Cyclic adenosine monophosphate
CCL2	Chemokine (C-C motif) ligand 2 (CCL2)
CEBPB	CCAAT-enhancer-binding proteins transcription factors
CNS	Central Nervous System
Col5a1	Collagen alpha-1(V) chain
Col5a2	Collagen alpha-2(V) chain
Coro1a	*Gene* encoding Coronin-1A protein
CSPG	Chondroitin sulfate proteoglycan
CX3CL1	C-X3-C motif chemokine 1
CXCL1	C-X-C motif chemokine 1
CXCL12	C-X-C motif chemokine 12
CXCL13	C-X-C motif chemokine 13
CXCR4	C-X-C chemokine receptor type 4
Cyth4	Cytohesin-4
DHA	Docosahexaenoic acid
Dic1	Gene encoding Disrupted-in-schizophrenia 1protein
DNA	Deoxyribonucleic acid
Drp2	Dystrophin Related Protein 2
EC	Ensheathing cell
ECM	Extracellular matrix
EGF	*Epidermal growth factor*
Ephb2	Ephrin type-B receptor 2

Erbb2	V-Erb-B2 Erythroblastic Leukemia Viral Oncogene Homologue 2
FGF-2	Basic fibroblast growth factor
GDNF	Glial cell-derived neurotrophic factor
GFAP	*Glial fibrillary acidic protein*
GM-1	Monosialotetrahexosylganglioside
GM-CSF	*Granulocyte-macrophage colony-stimulating factor*
hCD59	CD59 glycoprotein human also known as MAC-inhibitory protein
HGF	*Hepatocyte growth factor*
IGF-1	*Insulin-like growth factor 1*
IL-1	*Interleukin 1*
IL-10	*Interleukin-10*
IL-1β	*Interleukin-1* beta
IL-3	*Interleukin 3*
IL-6	Interleukin 6
LCG	lactosamine-containing glycans
Lcp2	Gene encoding Lymphocyte cytosolic protein 2
LPS	Lipopolysaccharides
MAG	Myelin-associated *glycoprotein*
MMP-3	Matrix metalloproteinase-3
MMP-9	Matrix metalloproteinase-9
Myo1f	Gene encoding Myosin IF protein
NADP+	*Nicotinamide adenine dinucleotide phosphate*
Ndel1	Gene encodes Nuclear distribution protein nudE-like 1
NF-κB	Nuclear factor kappa-light-chain-enhancer of activated B cells
NG2	Neural/*Glial* Antigen 2
NGF	*Nerve growth factor*
NMDA	N-methyl-D-aspartate
Nogo	Neurite outgrowth inhibitor
NS	Nervous System
NT-3	Neurotrophin-3
NT-4/5	Neurotrophin-4/ neurotrophin-5
NudC	Gene encoding Nuclear Distribution Gene C Homologue protein
OE	Olfactory epithelium
OMgp	Oligodendrocyte-myelin glycoprotein
p75	Low-Affinity Nerve Growth Factor Receptor

PAMPs	Pathogen-associated molecular patterns
PDGF	*Platelet-derived growth factor*
PNS	Peripheral Nervous System
Poly I:C	Polyinosinic-polycytidylic acid
PUFA	*Polyunsaturated fatty acids*
SCI	Spinal cord injury
Sirpa	Gene encoding Signal-Regulatory Protein Alpha
Sparc	Gene encoding Secreted Protein, Acidic, Cysteine-Rich (Osteonectin)
Timp2	Gene encoding TIMP Metallopeptidase Inhibitor 2
TLRs	Toll-like receptors
TNFR1	Tumor necrosis factor receptor1
TNF-α	Tumor necrosis factor

INTRODUCTION

The olfactory bulb is a special structure within the Central Nervous System (CNS) that is responsible for integrating the signals that are received from odor particles. These signals are received by olfactory receptor neurons situated in the olfactory epithelium, neurons that, unlike others, are replaced approximately every 30 days throughout an individual's life. Whenever needed, either during normal cell turnover or following injury, new olfactory receptor neurons are generated from basal progenitor cells in the olfactory epithelium (OE). The new axons produced are bundled together into fascicles, they pass through the cribriform plate of the ethmoid bone [1], and they are targeted to the nerve fiber and glomerular layers where they will make contact and form synapses with olfactory bulb interneurons (Figure 1).

However, the pathway followed by the axons is not random and they travel from the Peripheral Nervous System (PNS) to the CNS in bundles that reach a specific area of the olfactory bulb, maintaining a particular topographical organization [2]. Indeed, each neuron is responsible for detecting a single odor particle at a time. Both their trajectory and their final position is largely determined by olfactory ensheathing cell or ensheathing glia (EC), a particular cell type so-called because of its ability to surrounds axons grouped in bundles and guide them to their correct position within the first two layers of the olfactory bulb: the olfactory nerve fiber and glomerular layers [3]. This ability to surround axons is fundamental to the capacity of the EC to stimulate axon growth by secreting neurotrophic factors and extracellular matrix molecules. In addition to promoting axon growth, the EC also guide, and in some cases inhibit, the growth of axons from olfactory neurons, preventing them from following aberrant pathways. The EC also regulate inflammatory reactions and neuronal death, and they develop an innate immune response that allow them to protect CNS from infections, along with microglia, representing the olfactory system´s first line of defense [4].

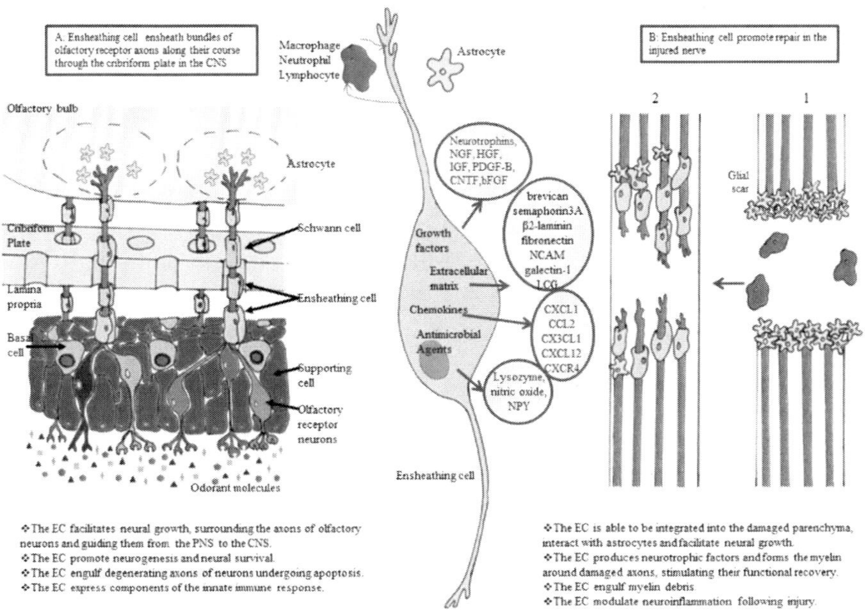

Figure 1. Schematic diagram depicting the adult rat olfactory system. An ensheathing cell is shown at the centre of the diagram, and the names of some of the factors expressed by it are included (this diagram does not include all molecules known to be expressed by the EC). In addition, the interactions between the ECs and astrocytes or cells of the immune system are also depicted. A) In normal conditions, EC within the olfactory bulb. B) Transplanted EC in models of SCI, 1) before and 2) after EC transplantation.

IMMUNOMODULATORY CAPACITY OF ENSHEATHING CELL

Within the CNS, microglial cells are the specialized cells in the immune system that express TLRs and that respond to PAMPs by producing cytokines and nitric oxide. However, in the particular case of primary olfactory nerves, in which uninterrupted neuronal ducts are formed that reach the brain from the nasal cavity, the cells are exposed to a wide variety of particles and pathogens that could potentially reach the CNS, although contamination through this route is not common [4].

There are several mechanisms that prevent infection through this route, such as sneezing, mucus secretion, the presence of antimicrobial molecules on the surface of epithelial cells, the presence of cells of the innate and adaptive immune system, and apoptosis of infected olfactory neurons [5]. Moreover, the EC also offer immune protection in this region, representing an essential component of the innate immune response against bacterial invasion of the CNS via the olfactory nerves, since they can engulf bacteria and disable them by endocytosis when they bind to TLR4 located on the surface of the EC [6]. Indeed, like other immune cells, the ECs are also able to signal in response to bacterial LPS and Poly I:C ligands, inducing nuclear translocation of NF-kB [4].

The EC expresses the antimicrobial peptides lysozyme and NPY, which are components evolutionarily conserved of the innate immune system [7]. NPY has antifungal properties against *Candida albicans* and *E. Coli* [8,9] and lysozyme displays bactericidal activity against both Gram-positive and Gram-negative bacteria given its ability to destroy the bacterial membrane [10]. The EC, like the microglia, can synthesize nitric oxide, which inhibits the production of ATP and DNA, thereby preventing the proliferation of bacteria and fungi [6], making these cells key components of the primary olfactory pathways [5]. EC also express other factors involved in the immune response, such as CEBPB, a transcription factor that regulates the production of nitric oxide, and the chemokines CXCL1 (Gro1), CCL2 (MCP-1), CX3CL1, CXCL12 and CXCR4, which participate in the signalling required for the recruitment of neutrophils and some lymphocytes, respectively [11]. In additions, the EC also fulfill a phagocytotic function *in vivo*, clearing apoptotic and degenerating axons, removing cellular debris and creating space for appropriate neuronal growth [4] that enables new neurons to be generated from progenitors located in the basal epithelium (Figure 1) [12,13].

IMMUNOMODULATORY MOLECULES OF THE ENSHEATHING CELL

The chemokine CX3CL1, also known as fractalkine or neurotactin, participates in cell adhesion and chemotaxis, regulating the branching and migration of monocyte-derived cells in the OE. Although this molecule is present on monocytes, natural killer cells, dendritic cells, macrophages and microglial cells, it is also expressed by olfactory neurons and ensheathing glia, favoring the anti-inflammatory or immunomodulatory activity in the nervous system (NS) [12,14]. The fractalkine receptor (CX3CR1), which in turn is expressed in macrophages and dendritic cells of the OE, plays an important role in the response of macrophages to damage within the primary olfactory pathway. Indeed, in addition to inducing phagocytosis of cellular debris, this receptor helps to maintain a favorable environment by providing an important source of mitogens and differentiation factors to epithelial progenitors that reduce secondary cell death, and that facilitates the replacement of those neurons that are lost by endogenous stem cells [12,14].

The significance of CX3CL1 expression by ECs is enhanced by their neuroprotective activity, given that it inhibits the production of harmful proinflammatory molecules, such as TNF-α, IL-6 and IL-1β, which is especially important given that IL-1β suppresses proliferation of neural precursors [12]. In this sense, a deficiency in CX3CR1 receptors results in the loss of olfactory sensory neurons and reduces the proliferation of progenitor cells. In turn, the lack of signaling through CX3CR1 provokes an excessive increase in the recruitment of macrophages with compromised phagocytotic activity in the OE. These macrophages contain high levels of proinflammatory cytokines (TNF-α, IL-6 and IL-1β), with TNF-α having been shown to induce neuronal apoptosis and IL-1β associated with neurodegeneration. However, The EC is capable of inhibiting the production of some of these cytokines, an activity that depends on the EC expressing the appropriate receptors. Several studies have shown that TNF-α can regulate the migration of different cell types [15] and that when this cytokine is expressed by astrocytes, it acts as a chemoattractant for the EG. Indeed, the EC express TNFR1 (the TNF-α receptor type 1) and their migration is impeded when TNF-α is blocked [16].

REGULATION OF THE NUCLEAR FACTOR KAPPA B BY THE ENSHEATHING CELL

The nuclear factor kappa B (NF-kB) is a key transcriptional regulator of inflammatory genes [17]. Transcription factors of the NF-kB family regulate the inflammation activated by proinflammatory cytokines, reactive oxygen species (ROS), extracellular glutamate, intracellular calcium, and other factors that are intensified after CNS injury [18,19]. NF-kB also regulates astrogliosis, which is associated with an increase in the expression of cytokines, chemokines and adhesion molecules, as well as the synthesis of molecules such as inducible nitric oxide, GM-CSF, GFAP, BDNF and NGF [20,21,22,23], all of which contribute to promote the formation of the glial scar after NS injury.

In conjunction with other growth factors and cytokines induced by regulation of NF-kB, the GM-CSF proinflammatory cytokine induces proliferation and activates the recruitment of leukocytes and microglia, enhancing the secretion of inflammatory cytokines and increasing the levels of nitric oxide and free radicals [22]. It has been shown that moderating inflammation by limiting the activation of NF-kB produces beneficial effects in several models of spinal cord injury [19]. In this context, it has been reported that some soluble factors released by the EC, such as IGF-1, significantly moderate the nuclear translocation of NF-kB in astrocytes, which decreases the transcription of pro-inflammatory cytokines like GM-CSF, as well as diminishing the synthesis of Chondroitin sulfate proteoglycans (CSPGs), proteins that contribute to axonal growth inhibition in the glial scar [17,24]. Notably, when astrocytes are co-cultured with fibroblasts and microglia, enhanced nuclear localization of NF-kB can be observed in the former, while when they are co-cultured with EC, NF-kB remains in its inactive state. Moderate activation of astrocytes represents a mechanism that contributes to neural repair after the transplantation of EC in models of CNS injury [17]. By forming a moderate glial scar and a barrier to axonal growth, reactive astrocytes protect the tissue near the site of injury from cytotoxic conditions, and they facilitate the immune response by isolating the injured tissue from the healthy tissue around it and secreting neurotrophic factors [25].

The Ability of the Ensheathing Cell to Surround Neurons and Promote Axonal Growth

Under normal conditions, myelin contributes to opening up a pathway for some axons during NS development, whereas in adult organisms it surrounds the axons to help them function properly. After injury, damaged neurons may survive if their axons can still extend branches to their original target cells, and if they are remyelinized and make functional synapses having re-established these connections [26,27]. However, after injury the myelin debris from dead cells constitutes an insurmountable barrier to axon regeneration, which can be compensated for by therapeutic transplantation of ECs that are capable of phagocytosing myelin debris, producing neurotrophic factors and remyelinating damaged axons to promote their functional recovery.

Similarly, the EC can synthesize and secrete extracellular matrix (ECM) molecules, such as laminin and fibronectin, which are both components of the cellular parenchyma that promote neurite elongation in *vitro* [28]. In addition, ECs express the lactosamine-containing glycans (LCG), galectin-1, β-2 laminin and semaphorin-3A, and the co-expression of these three latter molecules creates an axon-sorting domain that is capable of promoting and repelling subsets of olfactory axons. In contrast to these, neuropilin-1 expressing axons grow in a complementary pattern, avoiding the ventral nerve layer and projecting medially and laterally [29]. Semaphorin-3A is expressed in the lamina propia surrounding the OE, as well as by the EC in the ventral nerve layer of the olfactory bulb, and it is a molecule that guides axon growth by repelling those of neuropilin-1 expressing neurons [30,31].

LCG expressing axons project to the ventromedial region of the olfactory bulb through a region that is enriched in galectin-1 and laminin [29]. Laminin is a glycoprotein made up of three subunits α, β and γ, and the α2 chain in particular is expressed by tanycytes, the ECs and Schwann cells [32]. In addition, laminin has an EGF-like ligand-binding domain that promotes cell proliferation [33].

Galectins are a family of 15 proteins that are characterized by a well conserved β-galactosidase binding domain, and they are responsible for regulating the survival and proliferation cytotoxic T-cells and effector T helper cells, and the cytokines they synthesize. Galectins are generally known for their pro-adhesive potential and their negative regulation of the proliferation and survival of T-cells [34]. In particular, galectin-1 is a member of the family of β-galactosidase-binding proteins that is expressed by the EC and that mediates the binding of laminin to other neural ligands, stimulating axonal growth and sorting. Indeed, galectin-1 triggers the targeting of discrete subsets of primary olfactory sensory axons to the nerve fiber layer of the olfactory bulb [31,35]. Brevican, is also secreted by ECs and it is a neural proteoglycan involved in the inhibition of axonal growth [36].

In addition, ECs secrete the MMP-3 and MMP-9 metalloproteinases, which makes them capable of degrading many ECM proteins, enabling them to pass through the glial scar formed following injury and to produce a permissive microenvironment for neural regeneration in a site where regeneration is normally inhibited [33]. The glial scar contains diverse ECM molecules, including members of the CSPG family, including neurocan, phosphacan and NG2, among others, each of which is overexpressed following NS injury [37]. This is why it has been postulated that chondroitinase treatment, either alone or in conjunction with a cell therapy like Schwann cell and/or EC transplantation, leads to axonal regeneration [37].

Neural Regeneration-Supporting Growth Factors

The EC respond to several growth factors, a feature that contributes to their ability to facilitate neuronal recovery. Some of these growth factors are secreted by the EC themselves, and others, such as bFGF and heregulins, are secreted by other cells of distinct types. PDGF and IGF-1 stimulate EC proliferation, a process that can be enhanced by forskolin, which increases the intracellular concentrations cAMP [38,39]. The hepatocyte growth factor (HGF) is a potent mitogen for hepatocytes that plays an important role in liver regeneration. However, EC express the HGF receptor, known as c-Met, which contributes to their proliferation *in vitro*, and given that HGF acts as a chemoattractant for migrating cells in a concentration-dependent manner, a similar mechanism is believed to influence the migratory capacity of ECs during development in the olfactory system. In addition, it has been shown that the mitogenic activity of HGF is potentiated by addition of heregulin [38]. In summary, transplantation of EC in spinal cord injury models results in moderate activation of astrocytes, it inhibits the formation of CSPG deposits, it enhances axonal growth within the glial scar, and at the same time, it contributes to the synthesis of neurotrophic factors. Indeed, the possible mechanism by which EC promote axonal regeneration *in vitro* is related to their ability to synthesize and release neurotrophic factors such as GDNF, BDNF, HGF, NGF, and neurotrophins 4 and 5 into the media [40]. In *in vitro* models of cell migration, NGF promotes Schwann cell migration, even through the astrocyte layer, evidence that the NGF released by EC can promote the migration of Schwann cells, even through the astrocytes that may cover them [26].

The low affinity neurotrophin receptor (p75) is expressed by EC, although recent studies have revealed the presence of two distinct EC populations of in the olfactory bulb: one expressing high levels of p75 while the other expresses low levels of this receptor. Microarray studies revealed that populations of ECs expressing high levels of p75 over-express certain genes, such as: Col5a1 and Col5a2, which are involved in the modulation of ECM; SparC that is believed to promote neurite outgrowth; and the Erbb2 and Drp2 genes that are important for axonal fasciculation and defasciculation [41]. Therefore, it is believed that this p75-high expressing population of ECs is involved in the neurogenesis of primary olfactory neurons through processes such as fasciculation, cell separation and the targeting of newly formed olfactory neurons.

Conversely, the ECs that express p75 weakly overexpress genes like, Coro1A and Lcp2, and they secrete the cytokine IL-1 and the chemokine CXCL13, which are involved in activation of immune cells, as well as other genes like Aif1, Sirpa and Timp2 that also regulate the inflammatory response [42]. These cells also express genes involved in axonal guidance, such as the Ndel1, Ephb2 and Cyth4 [43]. Moreover, it has been shown that this population also expresses genes like Dic1, NudC, Myo1f and Adap2, which are involved in the repulsion/adhesion phenomena required during neurogenesis. Thus, both these populations of ECs are involved in neurogenesis in one way or another, although the EC population expressing less p75 is directly involve in controlling the inflammatory response [41]. Given the specific characteristics of the EC, they can be considered to drive the axonal regeneration process that takes place after CNS injury, and particularly, after traumatic injury of the spinal cord [26,33,44].

SPINAL CORD INJURY

The CNS has limited regenerative capacity which explains why neurodegenerative diseases produce a progressive loss of its functions, as does cerebrovascular damage and spinal cord injury. In the case of spinal cord injury (SCI), transplantation of olfactory bulb ECs has been used successfully in experimental models and in clinical studies, and it is currently the best alternative to promote axonal regeneration. Traumatic SCI is a phenomenon that affects both patients and their families, producing severe physical, psychological and social consequences, and an important economic impact on health care services [44,45].

SCI is a complex pathophysiological process characterized by extensive neuronal death and limited axon regeneration [46], which is exacerbated by the neurons inability to undergo self-repair or to self-regenerate, causing permanent paralysis below the level of the lesion [33]. As mentioned above, within the PNS the EC surround the axons of the olfactory receptor neurons generated in the OE, targeting them to the olfactory bulb located in the CNS. The activity of this particular cell type shows some similarities with the neural regeneration-support offered by Schwann cells in the PNS, although unlike these cells, the EC can be integrated into the CNS parenchyma, which has led to the hypothesis that the ECs could promote axonal regeneration following injury [26,33,47].

Traumatic SCI begins with a primary lesion which triggers a series of events that result in the so-called secondary lesion. The primary lesion is the original injury caused by bone and/or ligament displacement and trauma within the medullary cavity. This lesion may generate *flexion*, extension *and* vertebral rotation *distraction* forces, resulting in elongation and/or severing of neural and vascular elements, which will cause the neurological damage [48]. Following the primary injury, the secondary injury involves groups of neurons near the injured area or connected to it, which begin to die, such that the number of neurons lost as a consequence of secondary neuronal death is far greater that the number of neurons lost immediately after the injury. Therefore, secondary injury is probably the main cause responsible for the loss of function in most CNS traumatic injuries [49]. The following events take place during secondary injury and that are responsible for the neuronal loss:

1) Destruction of blood vessels and vascular spasms causing ischemia and its main associated effects: anoxia and hypoglycaemia.
2) Post-traumatic inflammation, which is characterized by the accumulation of macrophages and microglia that contribute to the extent and severity of the injury [50]. This contribution is due to the ability of these cells to cause oxidation or proteolytic damage through the release of various oxidative enzymes, such as myeloperoxidase, *nicotinamide adenine dinucleotide* phosphate ($NADP^+$), and a number

of extracellular matrix metalloproteinase such as MMP9, and the expression of cytokines like IL-1β, TNFα and IL-6 [50,51]. The generation of free radicals and lipid peroxidation can propagate the local destruction of cell membranes, and oxidative stress can fatally disrupt the biochemical and molecular homeostasis of glial cells and neurons.

3) The accumulation of excitatory neurotransmitters, such as glutamate (due to rupture of neuronal and astrocyte cell membranes), which facilitates the influx of Ca^{+2} activating N-methyl-D-aspartate (NMDA) and non-NMDA receptors, ultimately provoking excitotoxicity [49,51]. This cellular hyperexcitation triggers a series of destructive events that promote the release of free radicals, which in turn causes damage to cell membranes and other cellular components resulting in the death of neighboring cells.

Following injury, astrocytes and microglia near the site of injury form a scar to prevent the spread of secondary neuronal death. Astrocytes become hypertrophic and generate robust cytoplasmic extensions full of GFAP. The glial scar seals and isolates the necrotic area from the surrounding intact nerve tissue, while microglia release cytokines that act on astroglia in a paracrine manner to promote their activation and the further production of such trophic factors. Nevertheless, these cells also produce inhibitory molecules that include proteoglycans, tenascins, ephrins, semaphorins, as well as lytic enzymes and free radicals, all of which prevent axonal growth by causing the retraction of growth cones of surviving regenerative neurons [52,53]. Oligodendroglia also hinder axonal regeneration in the NS because once damaged, they release myelin-derived substances, such as the ECM protein Nogo and the MAG glycoprotein [52,54].

The inhibition of regeneration is the final overall effect of all the molecules produced at the site of injury and in its surroundings. This leads to a permanent and irreversible loss of the functions mediated by damaged neurons. The following are some of the experimental treatments that have been designed to promote repair following traumatic SCI [44,46,55]:

1) Blocking of myelin-associated inhibitory molecules, such as using chondroitinase, in order to remove CSPGs from the glial scar, molecules that block Nogo (Nogo A, Nogo 66, MAG) and other myelin components (MAG, OMgp, p75).

2) Addition of neurotrophic factors (NGF, NT-3, FGF-2, GDNF, BDNF, etc), ECM components or biopolymers that promote axonal regeneration.
3) Use of bioactive agents, such as Monosialotetrahexosylganglioside (GM-1), Omega-3 PUFA (polyunsaturated fatty acid omega-3), alpha-linolenic acid and docosahexaenoic acid (DHA), which provide neuroprotection, and thereby reduce the area affected by injury and apoptosis [45]
4) Co-transplantation of ECs and Schwann cells or astrocytes.
5) Stimulation with agents that trigger the activation of neuronal regeneration programs.
6) Ion channel blockers, antioxidants and free radical degrading molecules.

However, it is of crucial importance to be careful when combining such treatments because the administration of some drug combinations may have opposing effects. For example, the administration of methylprednisolone and IL-10 blocks the inflammatory response, which is a process modulated by the EC [55].

Transplants of Ensheathing Cell Promote Regeneration of the Injured Spinal Cord

Transplants of EC in rat models of SCI, performed both during the acute phase (immediately after SCI) and the late phase (one week after the lesion) have been associated with greatly diminished astrocytic gliosis and better functional recovery [55]. ECs have the ability to become integrated into the host parenchyma by infiltrating the site of injury. This phenomenon reduces injury-induced cavity formation, and allows axonal regeneration [56] by reducing the expression of proteoglycans and modulating the reactive astrocytes [57,58]. Following transplantation of ECs after traumatic SCI, reactive astrocytes modulate the migration of the transplanted cells, inducing them to move long distances from where they have been implanted, even passing though the glial scar, to the site of injury where they can be integrated. The EC thereby interact favorably with astrocytes [59]. Furthermore, in co-cultures of astrocytes and EC it has been seen that both cell types intermingle and do not establish boundaries [60]. There is evidence that when astrocytes become reactive that can guide this EC migration and they can secrete and respond to a variety of cytokines including IL-1, IL-6, IL-3 and TNF-α [16].

The EC contribute to preserve the function and morphology of the injured spinal cord by modulating the inflammatory response, and they are also able to mingle with astrocytes and modify the environment of the glial scar. These properties of the EC seem to be due to both the molecular composition of the membrane of these cells, and their ability to secrete neurotrophic factors (Figure 1) [61]. These are features that tell us about the neuroprotective and neuroimmunomodulatory effect of EC, and their ability to interact with the inflammatory cells that are typically present after a lesion. Moreover, the ECs are very plastic, capable of modifying their phenotype (reflecting antigenic differences) depending on their location (e.g., the EC in the lamina propria show a more immature phenotype than in the olfactory bulb) [62], as well as on the age and functional state of a particular individual. Several laboratories are interested in understanding the molecular mechanisms used by this cell type to promote regeneration in order to take advantage of these to enhance neural recovery. Indeed, it is this interest that has prompted researchers to investigate the cellular and molecular characteristics of the EC.

Cell Therapy to Regenerate Injured Tissue

Given the aforementioned virtues of the ECs, these cells are considered excellent candidates for cell therapy to repair SCIs [63]. However, the procedure to obtain these cells from the olfactory bulb of humans involves invasive surgery. Moreover, even if EC could be obtained from the olfactory mucosa, there is also the drawback of cell purity and of the low the number of cells obtained even after their proliferation in the cell culture. In addition, ideally the ECs should be obtained from patient´s own tissue [63,64,65]. An alternative source of ECs for transplantation would be xenotransplantation, although the main hurdle associate with such a process is the problem of tissue rejection via complement activation, which leads to lysis of the transplanted cells. Indeed, although ECs can be obtained from transgenic pigs expressing the complement inhibitory protein (hCD59) [66], the use of transgenic animals is not fully accepted due to the fact that the gene may migrate to other cells with undesirable consequences. Another option is to transplant cells from a EC line, which while retaining all the virtues of the EC, have the disadvantage that their cell immortalization can disrupt their cellular activity [65,67]. Thus, in this context, the transplantation of undifferentiated stem cells or stem cells differentiated into an EC-like phenotype provides a good alternative.

The therapeutic use of undifferentiated stem cells or stem cells that are differentiated *to* the *desired* cellular *phenotype* offers many advantages, particularly as they are cells that can integrate into tissues and promote tissue repair after an injury. These properties of stem cells provide a way to improve the treatments for a wide variety of diseases, including heart disease, diabetes, autoimmune diseases [68], Parkinson's, Alzheimer's, peripheral vascular insufficiency and SCIs [69,70]. The field of regenerative medicine can make use of various sources of stem cells, including mesenchymal stem cells that have many advantages in laboratory studies, such as their integration into a multitude of organs, their specific differentiation into the cell type forming the tissue into which they incorporate, and being located preferentially in damaged regions [68,71]. In addition, mesenchymal stem cells have the advantage of being immunocompatible [72], show immunosuppressive properties and contributing to the dampening of inflammatory processes [68].

The characteristics of mesenchymal stem cells offers large therapeutic advantages, such as the regeneration of damaged tissues, correction of inherited diseases, contribution to reducing chronic inflammation, induction of transplantation tolerance to allogeneic and xenogeneic grafts, transplantation, and serving as vehicle for the delivery of biological agents [73]. Hence, it is clearly important to analyze these cells at the cellular and molecular levels. However, the main limitation in cell therapy *is that stem cells* are *found* in small *numbers* in adult organisms, and thus, the main challenge faced at present is their enrichment, expansion and differentiation into the desired cell phenotypes to improve the outcomes, and to increase the number of conditions that could be potentially treated using this approach [74].

CONCLUSION

Ensheathing cells display unique properties that serve to safeguard the integrity of olfactory neurons. Indeed, in addition to promoting and guiding axonal growth, they guarantee a neuroprotective and immunomodulatory environment by secreting and responding to several cytokines, ECM molecules and growth factors, which allows them to interact with various cell types in both the nervous and the immune system. Thus, EC establish an ideal environment for neurons, both in normal conditions within the olfactory bulb and after transplanting them into lesioned areas, making them an excellent tool to be used in cell therapies to treat conditions such as SCI (Figure 1).

References

[1] Barnett S, Riddell J. Olfactory ensheathing cells (OECs) and the treatment of CNS injury: advantages and possible caveats. *J Anat.* 2004 Jan; 204(1):57-67.

[2] Tenne-Brown J, Puche A, Key B. Expression of galectin-1 in the mouse olfactory system. *Int J Dev Biol.* 1998 Sep; 42(6):791-9.

[3] Doucette JR. The glial cells in the nerve fiber layer of the rat olfactory bulb. *Anat Rec.* 1984 Oct;210(2):385-91.

[4] Vincent AJ, Choi-Lundberg DL, Harris JA, West AK, Chuah MI. Bacteria and PAMPs activate nuclear factor kappaB and Gro production in a subset of olfactory ensheathing cells and astrocytes but not in Schwann cells. *Glia.* 2007 Jul;55(9):905-16.

[5] Leung JY, Chapman JA, Harris JA, Hale D, Chung RS, West AK, Chuah MI. Olfactory ensheathing cells are attracted to, and can endocytose, bacteria. *Cell Mol Life Sci.* 2008 Sep; 65(17):2732-9.

[6] Harris JA, West AK, Chuah MI. Olfactory ensheathing cells: nitric oxide production and innate immunity. *Glia.* 2009 Dec; 57(16):1848-57.

[7] Ubink R, Hökfelt T. Expression of neuropeptide Y in olfactory ensheathing cells during prenatal development. *J Comp Neurol.* 2000 Jul 17;423(1):13-25.

[8] Hansen CJ, Burnell KK, Brodgen KA. Antimicrobial activity of Substance P and Neuropeptide Y against laboratory strains of bacteria and oral microorganisms. *J Neuroimmunol.* 2006 Aug;177(1-2):215-8.

[9] Vouldoukis I, Shai Y, Nicolas P, Mor A. Broad spectrum antibiotic activity of the skin-PYY. *FEBS Lett.* 1996 Feb 19;380(3):237-40.

[10] Ibrahim HR, Yamada M, Matsushita K, Kobayashi K, Kato A. Enhanced bactericidal action of lysozyme to Escherichia coli by inserting a hydrophobic pentapeptide into its C terminus. *J Biol Chem.* 1994 Feb 18;269(7):5059-63.

[11] Chuah MI, Hale DM, West AK. Interaction of olfactory ensheathing cells with other cell types in vitro and after transplantation: glial scars and inflammation. *Exp Neurol.* 2011 May;229(1):46-53.

[12] Ruitenberg MJ, Vukovic J, Blomster L, Hall JM, Jung S, Filgueira L, McMenamin PG, Plant GW. CX3CL1/fractalkine regulates branching

and migration of monocyte-derived cells in the mouse olfactory epithelium. *J Neuroimmunol.* 2008 Dec 15;205(1-2):80-5.

[13] Su Z, Chen J, Qiu, Y, Yuan Y, Zhu F, Zhu Y, Liu X, Pu Y, He C. Olfactory ensheathing cells: the primary innate immunocytes in the olfactory pathway to engulf apoptotic olfactory nerve debris. *Glia.* 2013 Apr;61(4):490-503.

[14] Blomster LV, Vukovic J, Hendrikx DA, Jung S, Harvey AR, Filgueira L, Ruitenberg MJ. CX_3CR1 deficiency exacerbates neuronal loss and impairs early regenerative responses in the target-ablated olfactory epithelium. *Mol Cell Neurosci.* 2011 Nov;48(3):236-45.

[15] Corredor J, Yan F, Shen C, Tong W, John SK, Wilson G, Whitehead R, Polk DB. Tumor necrosis factor regulates intestinal epithelial cell migration by receptor-dependent mechanisms. *Am J Physiol Cell Physiol.* 2003 Apr;284(4):C953-61.

[16] Su Z, Yuan Y, Chen J, Cao L, Zhu Y, Gao L, Qiu Y, He C. Reactive astrocytes in glial scar attract olfactory ensheathing cells migration by secreted TNF-alpha in spinal cord lesion of rat. *PLoS One.* 2009 Dec 3;4(12):e8141.

[17] Hale DM, Ray S, Leung JY, Holloway AF, Chung RS, West AK, Chuah MI. Olfactory ensheathing cells moderate nuclear factor kappaB translocation in astrocytes. *Mol Cell Neurosci.* 2011 Jan;46(1):213-21.

[18] Baeuerle PA, Henkel T. Function and activation of NF-kappa B in the immune system. *Annu Rev Immunol.* 1994;12:141-79.

[19] Bethea JR, Castro M, Keane RW, Lee TT, Dietrich WD, Yezierski RP. Traumatic spinal cord injury induces nuclear factor-kappaB activation. *J Neurosci.* 1998 May 1;18(9):3251-60.

[20] Khrooshi R, Babcock AA, Owens T. NF-kappaB-driven STAT2 and CCL2 expression in astrocytes in response to brain injury. *J Immunol.* 2008 Nov 15;181(10):7284-91.

[21] Bae MK, Kim SR, Lee HJ, Wee HJ, Yoo MA, Ock Oh S, Baek SY, Kim BS, Kim JB, Sik-Yoon, Bae SK. Aspirin-induced blockade of NF-kappaB activity restrains up-regulation of glial fibrillary acidic protein in human astroglial cells. *Biochim Biophys Acta.* 2006 Mar;1763(3):282-9.

[22] Zaheer A, Zaheer S, Sahu SK, Knight S, Khorsravi H, Mathur SN, Lim R. A novel role of glia maturation factor: induction of granulocyte-macrophage colony-stimulating factor and pro-inflammatory cytokines. *J Neurochem.* 2007 Apr;101(2):364-76.

[23] Meeuwsen S, Persoon-Deen C, Bsibsi M, Ravid R, van Noort JM. Cytokine, chemokine and growth factor gene profiling of cultured

human astrocytes after exposure to proinflammatory stimuli. *Glia.* 2003 Sep;43(3):243-53.

[24] Properzi F, Carulli D, Asher RA, Muir E, Camargo LM, van Kuppevelt TH, TEM Dam GB, Furukawa Y, Mikami T, Sugahara K, Toida T, Geller HM, Fawcett JW. Chondroitin 6-sulphate synthesis is up-regulated in injured CNS, induced by injury-related cytokines and enhanced in axon-growth inhibitory glia. *Eur J Neurosci.* 2005 Jan;21(2):378-90.

[25] Sofroniew MV. Reactive astrocytes in neural repair and protection. *Neuroscientist.* 2005 Oct;11(5):400-7.

[26] Cao L, Zhu YL, Su Z, Lv B, Huang Z, Mu L, He C. Olfactory ensheathing cells promote migration of Schwann cells by secreted nerve growth factor. *Glia.* 2007 Jul;55(9):897-904.

[27] Weatherby TM, Davis AD, Hartline DK, Lenz PH. The need for speed. II. Myelin in calanoid copepods. *J Comp Physiol A.* 2000 Apr;186(4):347-57.

[28] Ramón-Cueto A, Avila J. Olfactory ensheathing glia: properties and function. *Brain Res Bull.* 1998 Jun;46(3):175-87.

[29] Crandall JE, Dibble C, Butler D, Pays L, Ahmad N, Kostek C, Püschel AW, Schwarting GA. Patterning of olfactory sensory connections is mediated by extracellular matrix proteins in the nerve layer of the olfactory bulb. *J Neurobiol.* 2000 Dec;45(4):195-206.

[30] Schwarting GA, Kostek C, Ahmad N, Dibble C, Pays L, Püschel AW. Semaphorin 3A is required for guidance of olfactory axons in mice. *J Neurosci.* 2000 Oct 15;20(20):7691-7.

[31] Vincent AJ, West AK, Chuah MI. Morphological and functional plasticity of olfactory ensheathing cells. *J Neurocytol.* 2005 Mar;34(1-2):65-80.

[32] Hagg T, Portera-Cailliau C, Jucker M, Engvall E. Laminins of the adult mammalian CNS; laminin-alpha2 (merosin M-) chain immunoreactivity is associated with neuronal processes. *Brain Res.* 1997 Aug 1;764(1-2):17-27.

[33] Qian LM, Zhang ZJ, Gong AH, Qin RJ, Sun XL, Cao XD, Liu JB, Jiang P, Chen YC. A novel biosynthetic hybrid scaffold seeded with olfactory ensheathing cells for treatment of spinal cord injuries. *Chin Med J* (Engl). 2009 Sep 5;122(17):2032-40.

[34] Cedeno-Laurent F, Dimitroff CJ. Galectins and their ligands: negative regulators of anti-tumor immunity. *Glycoconj J.* 2012 Dec;29(8-9):619-25.

[35] Tenne-Brown J, Puche AC, Key B. Expression of galectin-1 in the mouse olfactory system. *Int J Dev Biol.* 1998 Sep;42(6):791-9.

[36] Yamada H, Fredette B, Shitara K, Hagihara K, Miura R, Ranscht B, Stallcup WB, Yamaguchi Y. The brain chondroitin sulfate proteoglycan brevican associates with astrocytes ensheathing cerebellar glomeruli and inhibits neurite outgrowth from granule neurons. *J Neurosci.* 1997 Oct 15;17(20):7784-95.

[37] Moreno MT, Avila J. The quest to repair the damaged spinal cord. *Recent Pat CNS Drug Discov.* 2006 Jan;1(1):55-63.

[38] Yan H, Nie X, Kocsis JD. Hepatocyte growth factor is a mitogen for olfactory ensheathing cells. *J Neurosci Res.* 2001 Nov 15;66(4):698-704.

[39] Yan H, Rivkees SA. Hepatocyte growth factor stimulates the proliferation and migration of oligodendrocyte precursor cells. J Neurosci Res. 2002 Sep 1;69(5):597-606

[40] Boruch AV, Conners JJ, Pipitone M, Deadwyler G, Storer PD, Devries GH, Jones KJ. Neurotrophic and migratory properties of an olfactory ensheathing cell line. *Glia.* 2001 Mar 1;33(3):225-9.

[41] Honoré A, Le Corre S, Derambure C, Normand R, Duclos C, Boyer O, Marie JP, Guérout N. Isolation, characterization, and genetic profiling of subpopulations of olfactory ensheathing cells from the olfactory bulb. *Glia.* 2012 Mar;60(3):404-13.

[42] Lattin JE, Greenwood KP, Daly NL, Kelly G, Zidar DA, Clark RJ, Thomas WG, Kellie S, Craik DJ, Hume DA, Sweet MJ. Beta-arrestin 2 is required for complement C1q expression in macrophages and constrains factor-independent survival. *Mol Immunol.* 2009 Dec;47(2-3):340-7.

[43] Angot E, Loulier K, Nguyen-Ba-Charvet KT, Gadeau AP, Ruat M, Traiffort E. Chemoattractive activity of sonic hedgehog in the adult subventricular zone modulates the number of neural precursors reaching the olfactory bulb. *Stem Cells.* 2008 Sep;26(9):2311-20.

[44] Moreno-Flores MT, Bradbury EJ, Martín-Bermejo MJ, Agudo M, Lim F, Pastrana E, Avila J, Díaz-Nido J, McMahon SB, Wandosell F. A clonal cell line from immortalized olfactory ensheathing glia promotes functional recovery in the injured spinal cord. *Mol Ther.* 2006 Mar;13(3):598-608.

[45] Lim PA, Tow AM. Recovery and regeneration after spinal cord injury: a review and summary of recent literature. *Ann Acad Med Singapore.* 2007 Jan;36(1):49-57.

[46] Fouad K, Schnell L, Bunge MB, Schwab ME, Liebscher T, Pearse DD. Combining Schwann cell bridges and olfactory-ensheathing glia grafts with chondroitinase promotes locomotor recovery after complete transection of the spinal cord. *J Neurosci.* 2005 Feb 2;25(5):1169-78.

[47] Pastrana E, Moreno-Flores MT, Avila J, Wandosell F, Minichiello L, Diaz-Nido J. BDNF production by olfactory ensheathing cells contributes to axonal regeneration of cultured adult CNS neurons. *Neurochem Int.* 2007 Feb;50(3):491-8.

[48] Harkey HL 3rd, White EA 4th, Tibbs RE Jr, Haines DE. A clinician's view of spinal cord injury. *Anat Rec B New Anat.* 2003 Mar;271(1):41-8.

[49] Verdú E, Nieto-Sampedro M. Lesiones del sistema nervioso; respuesta neuronal y reparación. *En Manual de Neurociencia.* Ed. Sintesis; 1998.

[50] Popa C, Popa F, Grigorean VT, Onose G, Sandu AM, Popescu M, Burnei G, Strambu V, Sinescu C. Vascular dysfunctions following spinal cord injury. *J Med Life.* 2010 Jul-Sep;3(3):275-85.

[51] Stammers AT, Liu J, Kwon BK. Expression of inflammatory cytokines following acute spinal cord injury in a rodent model. *J Neurosci Res.* 2012 Apr;90(4):782-90.

[52] Yamashita T. Molecular mechanism and regulation of axon growth inhibition. *Brain Nerve.* 2007 Dec;59(12):1347-53.

[53] Bovolenta P, Fernaud-Espinosa I, Méndez-Otero R, Nieto-Sampedro M. Neurite outgrowth inhibitor of gliotic brain tissue. Mode of action and cellular localization, studied with specific monoclonal antibodies. *Eur J Neurosci.* 1997 May;9(5):977-89.

[54] Niederöst B, Oertle T, Fritsche J, McKinney RA, Bandtlow CE. Nogo-A and myelin-associated glycoprotein mediate neurite growth inhibition by antagonistic regulation of RhoA and Rac1. *J Neurosci.* 2002 Dec 1;22(23):10368-76.

[55] López-Vales R, Forés J, Verdú E, Navarro X. Acute and delayed transplantation of olfactory ensheathing cells promote partial recovery after complete transection of the spinal cord. *Neurobiol Dis.* 2006 Jan;21(1):57-68. Epub 2005 Jul 26.

[56] Gudiño-Cabrera G, Nieto-Sampedro M. Ensheathing cells: Large scale purification from adult olfactory bulb, freeze-preservation and migration of transplanted cells in adult brain. *Restor Neurol Neurosci.* 1996 Jan 1;10(1):25-34.

[57] O'Toole DA, West AK, Chuah MI. Effect of olfactory ensheathing cells on reactive astrocytes in vitro. *Cell Mol Life Sci.* 2007 May;64(10):1303-9.

[58] García-Alías G, López-Vales R, Forés J, Navarro X, Verdú E. Acute transplantation of olfactory ensheathing cells or Schwann cells promotes recovery after spinal cord injury in the rat. *J Neurosci Res.* 2004 Mar 1;75(5):632-41.

[59] Ramón-Cueto A, Valverde F. Olfactory bulb ensheathing glia: a unique cell type with axonal growth-promoting properties. *Glia.* 1995 Jul;14(3):163-73.

[60] Santos-Silva A, Fairless R, Frame MC, Montague P, Smith GM, Toft A, Riddell JS, Barnett SC. FGF/heparin differentially regulates Schwann cell and olfactory ensheathing cell interactions with astrocytes: a role in astrocytosis. *J Neurosci.* 2007 Jul 4;27(27):7154-67.

[61] Lipson AC, Widenfalk J, Lindqvist E, Ebendal T, Olson L. Neurotrophic properties of olfactory ensheathing glia. *Exp Neurol.* 2003 Apr;180(2):167-71.

[62] Chuah MI, West AK. Cellular and molecular biology of ensheathing cells. *Microsc Res Tech.* 2002 Aug 1;58(3):216-27.

[63] Mackay-Sim A, Féron F, Cochrane J, Bassingthwaighte L, Bayliss C, Davies W, Fronek P, Gray C, Kerr G, Licina P, Nowitzke A, Perry C,Silburn PA, Urquhart S, Geraghty T. Autologous olfactory ensheathing cell transplantation in human paraplegia: a 3-year clinical trial. *Brain.* 2008 Sep;131(Pt 9):2376-86.

[64] Radtke C, Akiyama Y, Brokaw J, Lankford KL, Wewetzer K, Fodor WL, Kocsis JD. Remyelination of the nonhuman primate spinal cord by transplantation of H-transferase transgenic adult pig olfactory ensheathing cells. *FASEB J.* 2004 Feb;18(2):335-7.

[65] DeLucia TA, Conners JJ, Brown TJ, Cronin CM, Khan T, Jones KJ. Use of a cell line to investigate olfactory ensheathing cell-enhanced axonal regeneration. *Anat Rec B New Anat.* 2003 Mar;271(1):61-70.

[66] Imaizumi T, Lankford KL, Burton WV, Fodor WL, Kocsis JD. Xenotransplantation of transgenic pig olfactory ensheathing cells promotes axonal regeneration in rat spinal cord. *Nat Biotechnol.* 2000 Sep;18(9):949-53.

[67] Moreno-Flores MT, Bradbury EJ, Martín-Bermejo MJ, Agudo M, Lim F, Pastrana E, Avila J, Díaz-Nido J, McMahon SB, Wandosell F. A clonal cell line from immortalized olfactory ensheathing glia promotes functional recovery in the injured spinal cord. *Mol Ther.* 2006 Mar;13(3):598-608.

[68] Le Blanc K, Ringdén O. Immunomodulation by mesenchymal stem cells and clinical experience. *J Intern Med.* 2007 Nov;262(5):509-25.

[69] Gögel S, Gubernator M, Minger SL. Progress and prospects: stem cells and neurological diseases. *Gene Ther.* 2011 Jan;18(1):1-6.
[70] Trounson A, Thakar RG, Lomax G, Gibbons D. Clinical trials for stem cell therapies. *BMC Med.* 2011 May 10;9:52.
[71] Hematti P. Role of mesenchymal stromal cells in solid organ transplantation. *Transplant Rev* (Orlando). 2008 Oct;22(4):262-73.
[72] Mizuno H. Adipose-derived stem cells for tissue repair and regeneration: ten years of research and a literature review. *J Nippon Med Sch.* 2009 Apr;76(2):56-66.
[73] Reiser J, Zhang XY, Hemenway CS, Mondal D, Pradhan L, La Russa VF. Potential of mesenchymal stem cells in gene therapy approaches for inherited and acquired diseases. *Expert Opin Biol Ther.* 2005 Dec;5(12):1571-84.
[74] Trounson A, Thakar RG, Lomax G, Gibbons D. Clinical trials for stem cell therapies. *BMC Med.* 2011 May 10;9:52.

EDITOR CONTACT INFORMATON

Dr. Oscar Gonzalez-Perez,
Neuroscience Lab
Facultad de Psicologia, University of Colima
Av. Universidad # 333, Colima,
Col. 28040. Mexico
Tel / Fax (+52) 312-316-1091
osglez@ucol.mx

INDEX

A

B

C

D

E

F

G

H

I

L

M

N

O

P

R

S

T

V